Obesity

Editors

CAROLINE M. APOVIAN
NAWFAL W. ISTFAN

ENDOCRINOLOGY AND METABOLISM CLINICS OF NORTH AMERICA

www.endo.theclinics.com

Consulting Editors
ANAT BEN-SHLOMO
MARIA FLESERIU

September 2016 • Volume 45 • Number 3

ELSEVIER

1600 John F. Kennedy Boulevard • Suite 1800 • Philadelphia, Pennsylvania, 19103-2899

http://www.theclinics.com

ENDOCRINOLOGY AND METABOLISM CLINICS OF NORTH AMERICA Volume 45, Number 3
September 2016 ISSN 0889-8529, ISBN 13: 978-0-323-46255-6

Editor: Jessica McCool
Developmental Editor: Meredith Clinton

Endocrinology and Metabolism Clinics of North America (ISSN 0889-8529) is published quarterly by Elsevier Inc., 360 Park Avenue South, New York, NY 10010-1710. Months of issue are March, June, September, and December. Periodicals postage paid at New York, NY and additional mailing offices. Subscription prices are USD 330.00 per year for US individuals, USD 636.00 per year for US institutions, USD 100.00 per year for US students and residents, USD 415.00 per year for Canadian individuals, USD 787.00 per year for Canadian institutions, USD 480.00 per year for international individuals, USD 787.00 per year for international institutions, and USD 245.00 per year for international and Canadian and foreign students/residents. To receive student/resident rate, orders must be accompanied by name of affiliated institution, date of term, and the signature of program/ residency coordinator on institution letterhead. Orders will be billed at individual rate until proof of status is received. Foreign air speed delivery is included in all *Clinics* subscription prices. All prices are subject to change without notice. **POSTMASTER:** Send address changes to *Endocrinology and Metabolism Clinics of North America*, Elsevier Health Sciences Division, Subscription Customer Service, 3251 Riverport Lane, Maryland Heights, MO 63043. **Customer Service: Telephone: 1-800-654-2452** (U.S. and Canada); **1-314-447-8871** (outside U.S. and Canada). **Fax: 1-314-447-8029. E-mail: journalscustomerservice-usa@elsevier.com (for print support); journalsonlinesupport-usa@elsevier.com (for online support).**

Reprints. For copies of 100 or more, of articles in this publication, please contact the Commercial Rights Department, Elsevier Inc., 360 Park Avenue South, New York, NY 10010-1710; phone: +1-212-633-3874; fax: +1-212-633-3820; E-mail: reprints@elsevier.com.

Endocrinology and Metabolism Clinics of North America is covered in *MEDLINE/PubMed (Index Medicus), EMBASE/Excerpta Medica, Current Contents/Clinical Medicine, Current Contents/Life Sciences, Science Citation Index, ISI/BIOMED, BIOSIS,* and *Chemical Abstracts*.

Contributors

CONSULTING EDITORS

ANAT BEN-SHLOMO, MD
Pituitary Center, Division of Endocrinology, Diabetes, and Metabolism, Cedars Sinai Medical Center, Los Angeles, California

MARIA FLESERIU, MD, FACE
Northwest Pituitary Center, Division of Endocrinology, Diabetes, and Clinical Nutrition, Departments of Medicine and Neurological Surgery, Oregon Health and Science University, Portland, Oregon

EDITORS

CAROLINE M. APOVIAN, MD
Professor of Medicine and Pediatrics, Boston University School of Medicine, Director, Nutrition and Weight Management Center, Section of Endocrinology, Diabetes and Nutrition, Boston Medical Center, Boston, Massachusetts

NAWFAL W. ISTFAN, MD, PhD
Associate Professor of Medicine, Boston University School of Medicine, Section of Endocrinology, Diabetes and Nutrition, Boston Medical Center, Boston, Massachusetts

AUTHORS

NAJI ALAMUDDIN, MD, BCh, MTR
Endocrinology Fellow, Division of Endocrinology, Diabetes, and Metabolism; Center for Weight and Eating Disorders, Perelman School of Medicine, University of Pennsylvania, Philadelphia, Pennsylvania

DAVID B. ALLISON, PhD
Department of Biostatistics, Office of Energetics, Nutrition Obesity Research Center, University of Alabama at Birmingham, Birmingham, Alabama

LOUIS J. ARONNE, MD, FACP, DABOM, FTOS
Sanford I. Weill Professor of Metabolic Research, Comprehensive Weight Control Center, Division of Endocrinology, Diabetes and Metabolism, Weill Cornell Medicine, New York, New York

DAN E. AZAGURY, MD
Assistant Professor of Surgery, Section of Bariatric and Minimally Invasive Surgery, Stanford University School of Medicine, Stanford University, Stanford, California

RACHEL L. BATTERHAM, MBBS, PhD
Department of Medicine, Centre for Obesity Research, Rayne Institute, University College London; University College London Hospitals (UCLH) Bariatric Centre for Weight Loss, Metabolic and Endocrine Surgery; National Institute of Health Research University College London Hospitals Biomedical Research Centre, London, United Kingdom

GEORGE A. BRAY, MD
Boyd Professor Emeritus, Pennington Biomedical Research Center, Louisiana State University, Baton Rouge, Louisiana; Children's Hospital Oakland Research Institute (CHORI), Oakland, California

STACY BRETHAUER, MD
Staff Surgeon, Digestive Diseases Institute, Cleveland Clinic, Cleveland, Ohio

JULIETTA CHANG, MD
Resident Physician, Digestive Diseases Institute, Cleveland Clinic, Cleveland, Ohio

NIRAV K. DESAI, MD
Instructor of Pediatrics, Harvard Medical School; Division of Gastroenterology, Hepatology and Nutrition, Boston Children's Hospital, Boston, Massachusetts

EMILY J. DHURANDHAR, PhD
Department of Kinesiology and Sport Management, Texas Tech University, Lubbock, Texas

GLENN S. GERHARD, MD
Professor and Chair, Department of Medical Genetics and Molecular Biochemistry; Director, Temple Genetics Laboratory and Temple Genetics Clinic; Lewis Katz School of Medicine, Temple University, Philadelphia, Pennsylvania

LEON I. IGEL, MD, FACP, DABOM
Assistant Professor of Clinical Medicine, Comprehensive Weight Control Center, Division of Endocrinology, Diabetes and Metabolism, Weill Cornell Medicine, New York, New York

THOMAS H. INGE, MD, PhD
Professor, Department of Surgery, University of Cincinnati College of Medicine, Cincinnati Children's Hospital Medical Center, Cincinnati, Ohio

SANGEETA R. KASHYAP, MD
Division of Endocrinology, School of Medicine, Department of Endocrinology, Diabetes, and Metabolism, Cleveland Clinic, Cleveland, Ohio

JOHN P. KIRWAN, PhD
Department of Pathobiology, Lerner Research Institute, Cleveland Clinic; Department of Nutrition, School of Medicine, Case Western Reserve University; Metabolic Translational Research Center, Endocrine and Metabolism Institute, Cleveland Clinic, Cleveland, Ohio

REKHA B. KUMAR, MD, MS, DABOM
Assistant Professor of Clinical Medicine, Comprehensive Weight Control Center, Division of Endocrinology, Diabetes and Metabolism, Weill Cornell Medicine, New York, New York

THEODORE K. KYLE, RPh, MBA
ConscienHealth, Pittsburgh, Pennsylvania

JOY A. LEE, MS, RD, LD
Department of Nutrition, Georgia State University, Atlanta, Georgia

JANINE M. MAKARONIDIS, MBChB
Department of Medicine, Centre for Obesity Research, Rayne Institute, University College London; University College London Hospitals (UCLH) Bariatric Centre for Weight Loss, Metabolic and Endocrine Surgery; National Institute of Health Research, University College London Hospitals Biomedical Research Centre, London, United Kingdom

STEVEN K. MALIN, PhD
Assistant Professor, Division of Endocrinology & Metabolism, Department of Kinesiology, Curry School of Education, School of Medicine, University of Virginia, Charlottesville, Virginia

CHRISTOS S. MANTZOROS, MD, DSc, PhD h.c. mult.
Professor of Medicine, Division o f Endocrinology, Diabetes and Metabolism, Department of Internal Medicine, Beth Israel Deaconess Medical Center, Harvard Medical School, Boston, Massachusetts

JOHN MAGAÑA MORTON, MD, MPH, FACS, FASMBS
Chief, Section of Bariatric and Minimally Invasive Surgery, Stanford University School of Medicine, Stanford University, Stanford, California

MEGAN A. McCRORY, PhD, FTOS
Associate Professor, Department of Nutrition, Georgia State University, Atlanta, Georgia

ANNY MULYA, PhD
Department of Pathobiology, Lerner Research Institute, Cleveland Clinic, Cleveland, Ohio

OLIVIER F. NOEL, BS
Lewis Katz School of Medicine, Temple University, Philadelphia, Pennsylvania; Pennsylvania State College of Medicine, Hershey, Pennsylvania; CEO, DNAsimple, Philadelphia, Pennsylvania

STAVROULA A. PASCHOU, MD, PhD
Research Fellow, Division of Endocrinology, Diabetes and Metabolism, Department of Internal Medicine, Beth Israel Deaconess Medical Center, Harvard Medical School, Boston, Massachusetts

HEATHER M. POLONSKY, BS
Project Director, Center for Obesity Research and Education, Temple University College of Public Health, Philadelphia, Pennsylvania

DONNA H. RYAN, MD
Professor Emerita, Pennington Biomedical Research Center, Louisiana State University, Baton Rouge, Louisiana

DAVID B. SARWER, PhD
Associate Dean for Research, Director, Center for Obesity Research and Education, Temple University College of Public Health, Philadelphia, Pennsylvania

KATHERINE H. SAUNDERS, MD
Clinical Fellow in Obesity Medicine, Comprehensive Weight Control Center, Division of Endocrinology, Diabetes and Metabolism, Weill Cornell Medicine, New York, New York

AYLA C. SHAW, MS
Department of Nutrition, Georgia State University, Atlanta, Georgia

ALPANA P. SHUKLA, MD, MRCP (UK)
Assistant Professor of Research in Medicine, Comprehensive Weight Control Center, Division of Endocrinology, Diabetes and Metabolism, Weill Cornell Medicine, New York, New York

PATTY W. SIRI-TARINO, PhD
Associate Staff Scientist, Atherosclerosis Research Program, Children's Hospital Oakland Research Institute (CHORI), Oakland, California

CHRISTOPHER D. STILL, DO
Medical Director, Center for Weight Management; Director, Geisinger Obesity Institute; Associate, Department of Gastroenterology and Nutrition, Geisinger Clinic, Danville, Pennsylvania

GEORGIOS A. TRIANTAFYLLOU, MD
Research Fellow, Division of Endocrinology, Diabetes and Metabolism, Department of Internal Medicine, Beth Israel Deaconess Medical Center, Harvard Medical School, Boston, Massachusetts

THOMAS A. WADDEN, PhD
Albert J. Stunkard Professor of Psychology in Psychiatry, Department of Psychiatry, Director, Center for Weight and Eating Disorders, Perelman School of Medicine, University of Pennsylvania, Philadelphia, Pennsylvania

MARK L. WULKAN, MD
Professor of Surgery and Associate Professor of Pediatrics, Department of Surgery, Emory University School of Medicine, Children's Healthcare of Atlanta, Atlanta, Georgia

Contents

> This article addresses current best practices in obesity management, primarily through the discussion of 5 documents' guidelines: those sponsored by the US National Institutes of Health and the AHA/ACC/TOS, ENDO, ASBP, AACE, and the United Kingdom's NICE. Common to all of these reports is the emphasis on addressing weight management as a pathway to prevention and optimal management of obesity-associated comorbidities (ie, type 2 diabetes and cardiovascular diseases). No one of these documents fits all needs; all have a place. Furthermore, no one of these documents is final. As knowledge advances, all of the documents will require updating.

> In 2013, the American Medical Association recognized obesity as a complex, chronic disease requiring medical attention. Defining obesity as a disease is a very public process, largely driven by expectation of costs and benefits. Although the public has been slow to embrace this definition, evidence is emerging for broader awareness of influencing factors beyond personal choice. This decision seems to be working with other factors to bring more access to care, less blame for people with the condition, and more favorable conditions for research to identify effective strategies for prevention and clinical care to reduce the impact.

> Successful treatment of obesity requires a multidisciplinary approach including diet, exercise and behavioral modification. As lifestyle changes are not sufficient for some patients, pharmacologic therapies should be considered as adjuncts to lifestyle interventions. In this article, we review clinical indications, mechanisms of action, dosing/administration, side effects, drug interactions and contraindications for the six most widely prescribed obesity medications. We also summarize the efficacy data from

phase 3 trials which led to drug approval. As multiple agents are sometimes required for clinically significant weight loss, the future of obesity medicine will likely involve combinations of agents in addition to behavioral counseling.

Bariatric surgery is the only effective treatment for severe obesity. Roux-en-Y gastric bypass (RYGB) and sleeve gastrectomy (SG), the most commonly performed procedures, lead to sustained weight loss, improvements in obesity-related comorbidities and reduced mortality. In humans, the main driver for weight loss following RYGB and SG is reduced energy intake. Reduced appetite, changes in subjective taste and food preference, and altered neural response to food cues are thought to drive altered eating behavior. The biological mediators underlying these changes remain incompletely understood, but changes in gut-derived signals, as a consequence of altered nutrient and/or biliary flow, are key candidates.

Lifestyle modification is the cornerstone treatment of type 2 diabetes in the obese patient, and is highly effective at promoting glucose regulation; however, many individuals struggle over time to maintain optimal glycemic control and/or body weight with lifestyle modification. Therefore, additional therapeutic approaches are needed. Pharmacologic interventions have shown promising results for obesity-related diabetes complications. Not surprisingly though lifestyle modification and pharmacology may become ineffective for treating diabetes over time. Bariatric surgery is considered by some, but not all, to be the most effective and durable treatment for combating obesity. In fact many patients with type 2 diabetes have normalized glucose concentrations within days, postoperation. Taken together, treatment of obesity in the patient with type 2 diabetes requires a multi-faceted approach.

Advisory panels encourage persons with obesity to lose 5% to 10% of body weight, which can be achieved with dietary change, increased physical activity, and behavioral therapy. Patients participate in weekly individual or group treatment sessions delivered in-person or by telephone. Large-scale trials have demonstrated the effectiveness of this approach, with resulting improvement in cardiovascular disease risk factors. Weight regain is common. Several strategies improve weight loss maintenance, including monthly or more frequent follow-up with an interventionist. Digitally-delivered approaches are promising because they have the potential to reach more individuals.

> Diets to treat obesity have been in existence since Hippocrates treated obesity some 2500 years ago. There are currently a wide variety of diets and a common misconception that a single magical diet can cure overweight and obesity. Systematic reviews and meta-analyses indicate that all diets work when adhered to and that initial weight loss can predict the amount of weight lost and maintained for up to 4 years. Individual preferences are thus key in selecting a diet. There are emerging data pinpointing genetic variability in the metabolic responses to variation in macronutrient intake.

> Overweight and obesity are global health problems placing an ever-increasing demand on health care systems. Brown adipose tissue (BAT) is present in significant amounts in adults. BAT has potential as a fuel for oxidation and dissipation as heat production, which makes it an attractive target for obesity therapy. BAT activation results in increased energy expenditure via thermogenesis. The role of BAT/beige adipocyte activation on whole body energy homeostasis, body weight management/regulation, and whole body glucose and lipid homeostasis remains unproven. This paper reviews knowledge on brown/beige adipocytes in energy expenditure and how it may impact obesity therapy and its comorbidities.

> Outcomes after bariatric surgery can vary widely and seem to have a significant genetic component. Only a small number of candidate gene and genome-wide association studies have analyzed bariatric surgery outcomes. The role of bile acids in mediating the beneficial effects of bariatric surgery implicate genes regulated by the farnesoid X receptor transcription factor.

> Leptin, a 167 amino acid adipokine, plays a major role in human energy homeostasis. Its actions are mediated through binding to a leptin receptor and activating the JAK-STAT3 signal transduction pathway. It is expressed mainly in adipocytes, and its circulating levels reflect the body's energy stores in adipose tissue. Recombinant methionyl human leptin has been FDA approved for patients with generalized non-HIV lipodystrophy and for compassionate use in subjects with congenital leptin deficiency. The purpose of this review is to outline the role of leptin in energy homeostasis, as well as its interaction with other hormones.

Over the past 40 years, meal skipping and snacking in adults in the United States has increased, and currently most eating occasions occur later in the day than previously. Whether these changes have played a causal role in the obesity epidemic is poorly understood. Observational studies are largely inconclusive due to methodological limitations. Experimental evidence does not support a causal role for eating frequency, or breakfast skipping in weight control. Emerging evidence suggests that eating irregularity and eating later in the day may be detrimental for weight control, but more studies are needed. This article summarizes studies and highlights areas needing attention.

ENDOCRINOLOGY AND METABOLISM CLINICS OF NORTH AMERICA

ISSUE OF RELATED INTEREST

Primary Care: Clinics in Office Practice, March 2016 (Vol. 43, Issue 1)
Obesity Management in Primary Care
Mark B. Stephens, *Editor*
http://www.primarycare.theclinics.com/

VISIT THE CLINICS ONLINE!
Access your subscription at:
www.theclinics.com

Foreword

Obesity

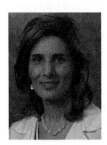 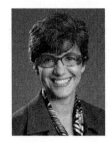

Anat Ben-Shlomo, MD   Maria Fleseriu, MD, FACE
Consulting Editors

Obesity has become a global epidemic. Its incidence is rising in both developed and developing countries, in children and adults of both sexes. Obesity is now considered a chronic disease associated with increased morbidity and mortality and poses a great burden on health systems around the world. This issue on Obesity in *Endocrinology and Metabolism Clinics of North America* summarizes key issues in the field of obesity research and provides important updates on disease pathogenesis and medical management.

Our distinguished guest editors, Caroline Apovian, MD and Nawfal W. Istfan, MD, PhD, from Boston University School of Medicine, both internationally recognized experts in the field, have gathered an outstanding group of clinicians with expertise in various aspects of obesity pathogenesis, comorbidities, treatment guidelines, and management approaches, including lifestyle changes, pharmacotherapy, endoscopic devices, and bariatric surgery.

In the article, "Guidelines for Obesity Management," Dr Ryan presents an overview of several published guidelines for the management of obesity. Guideline emphasis on obesity prevention and associated comorbidities in addition to medical management are discussed and compared.

"Regarding Obesity as a Disease: Evolving Policies and Their Implications," by Drs Kyle, Dhurandhar, and Allison, presents the considerations leading to the 2013 decision of the American Medical Association to recognize obesity as a complex, chronic disease requiring medical attention. The current and future implications on public opinion, public health care, and obesity research are reviewed, as is the debate on merits of this determination.

In "Pharmacotherapy for Obesity," Drs Aronne, Kumar, Igel, Shukla, and Saunders review several FDA-approved pharmacotherapies for obesity that can be used in patients in whom diet, exercise, and behavioral modification approaches are insufficient. Treatment with phentermine, orlistat, phentermine/topiramate ER, lorcaserin, naltrexone SR/bupropion SR, and liraglutide 3.0 mg is discussed in detail, and the

Endocrinol Metab Clin N Am 45 (2016) xiii–xv
http://dx.doi.org/10.1016/j.ecl.2016.06.015
0889-8529/16/$ – see front matter © 2016 Published by Elsevier Inc.

authors present clinical indications, mechanism of action, dosing, adverse events, drug interactions, and contraindications for each agent.

Bariatric surgery is currently considered the most effective treatment for patients with severe obesity. In "Potential Mechanisms Mediating Sustained Weight Loss Following Roux-en-Y Gastric Bypass and Sleeve Gastrectomy," Drs Makaronidis and Batterham discuss mechanisms and possible biological mediators underlying surgery-induced weight reduction following Roux-en-Y gastric bypass and sleeve gastrectomy and review the consequences of reduced energy intake due to altered eating behavior.

In "Type 2 Diabetes Treatment in the Patient with Obesity," Drs Malin and Kashyap discuss the three-tiered medical approach effective in obese patients with type 2 diabetes: lifestyle modification, antidiabetes pharmacotherapy, and antiobesity pharmacotherapy and/or bariatric surgery in selected patients. The authors describe how this combination can be utilized to successfully induce weight loss and improve glycemic control, while recognizing that long-term remission remains a challenge.

Drs Alamuddin and Wadden discuss the significant role of lifestyle modification in the treatment of obese patients in "Behavioral Treatment of the Patient with Obesity." A comprehensive behavioral weight control program treatment approach is overviewed, based on protocols from the LEARN Program for Weight Control, the Diabetes Prevention Program, and Look AHEAD trials. The authors show how such an approach, consisting of tightly monitored caloric restriction, exercise, and behavioral therapy, enables obese patients to shed up to one-tenth of their initial weight in a short period of time.

In the article, "The Role of Macronutrient Content in the Diet for Weight Management," Drs Bray and Siri-Tarino discuss and compare the different established macronutrient-specific diets for weight loss, their benefits, and expected outcomes. The authors emphasize that, despite the fact that all negative energy balance diets based on different macronutrient composition will induce weight loss, individual response varies between patients and is multifactorial.

In "Brown and Beige Adipose Tissue: Therapy for Obesity and Its Comorbidities?" by Drs Mulya and Kirwan, mechanisms underlying the development and activation of brown/beige adipose tissue and its effects on energy expenditure are detailed. The stimulatory effect on this tissue by lifestyle interventions such as dieting, exercise, and gastric bypass surgery is discussed, as is the possibility of targeting brown adipose tissue activation in antiobesity pharmacotherapy.

In the article, "Genetics of Bariatric Surgery Outcomes," Drs Noel, Still, and Gerhard discuss the potential role of genetic predisposition to the pleiotropic effects of bariatric surgery on a number of medical conditions and the observed wide variation in surgical outcomes among patients. The role of a candidate nuclear transcription factor, the farnesoid X receptor, which binds bile acids and retinoid X receptor α, is highlighted.

In "Leptin and Hormones: Energy Homeostasis," Drs Triantafyllou, Paschou, and Mantzoros review leptin central and peripheral signaling and function. They consider its role in energy expenditure and in conditions of hypoleptinemia, such as lipodystrophy, hypothalamic amenorrhea, and congenital leptin deficiency, and also consider the effects of hyperleptinemia accompanying obesity associated with hypothalamic leptin resistance.

Drs Azagury and Morton explain bariatric surgery in their article, "Bariatric Surgery: Overview of Procedures and Outcomes." The authors review the laparoscopic surgical procedures currently available, including Roux-en-Y gastric bypass, sleeve gastrectomy, and adjustable gastric banding. Procedure outcomes are discussed and compared, including postoperative weight loss, resolution of comorbidities, morbidity and mortality, and diabetes control.

In "Medical Devices in the Treatment of Obesity," Drs Chang and Brethauer review the medical devices available for the treatment of selected obese patients, including FDA-approved endoscopically placed intragastric balloon devices and a surgically placed vagal blockade device. Investigational endoscopic devices still in clinical trials are also reviewed. The advantages and disadvantages of each of these devices, and their roles in the treatment of obesity, are discussed.

The utilization of bariatric surgery in obese adolescent patients is discussed by Drs Desai, Wulkan, and Inge in their article, "Update on Adolescent Bariatric Surgery." The authors review eligibility criteria, preoperative preparation, and available surgical procedures for individuals in this age group. Postoperative weight loss and its long-term maintenance, effects on obesity-related comorbidities, and surgical complications are reviewed and compared.

In the article, "The Psychosocial Burden of Obesity," Drs Sarwer and Polonsky consider the psychological aspects of obesity, including its effects on mood, self-esteem, quality of life, and body image, as well as on debilitating medical conditions, such as depression, eating disorders, anxiety, and substance abuse. The authors discuss psychological changes seen after weight loss, including concerning evidence that some patients experience suicide ideation and substance abuse problems despite losing weight after successful bariatric surgery.

In "Energy and Nutrient Timing for Weight Control: Does Timing of Ingestion Matter?" by Drs McCrory, Shaw, and Lee, debate over whether the frequency and timing of meals have a significant effect on obesity is presented, while highlighting the multiple limitations and inconclusive messages of studies done to date. A review of the epidemiology of eating patterns, eating frequency, and the data behind skipping meals is provided.

We hope you will find this issue on *Obesity* in *Endocrinology and Metabolism Clinics of North America* useful in your practice. We thank Caroline Apovian, MD and Nawfal W. Istfan, MD, PhD, for guest-editing this exciting and timely issue, and the Elsevier editorial staff, for their invaluable help.

Anat Ben-Shlomo, MD
Pituitary Center
Division of Endocrinology
Diabetes, & Metabolism
Cedars Sinai Medical Center
8700 Beverly Boulevard
Los Angeles, CA 90048, USA

Maria Fleseriu, MD, FACE
Northwest Pituitary Center
Division of Endocrinology
Diabetes, & Clinical Nutrition
Departments of Medicine
and Neurological Surgery
Oregon Health & Science University
3138 SW Sam Jackson Park Road
Portland, OR 97239, USA

E-mail addresses:
benshlomoa@cshs.org (A. Ben-Shlomo)
fleseriu@ohsu.edu (M. Fleseriu)

Preface

Obesity: Guidelines, Best Practices, New Research

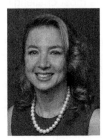 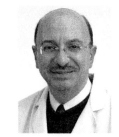

Caroline M. Apovian, MD   Nawfal W. Istfan, MD, PhD
Editors

This issue on obesity includes contributions from the leading clinical experts in obesity clinical treatment, as well as clinical and basic research scientists who have been studying obesity and the control of energy balance. Much has progressed since the discovery of leptin, the hormone that is secreted by adipose tissue, in 1994. This propelled adipose tissue and the connections to energy regulation in the brain to the forefront of obesity research, where it has stayed since then. This, and other discoveries about how the gut, adipose tissue, muscle, and other organs talk to the brain, have translated to the clinical realm and informed the treatment of obesity over the past 20 years. Today, obesity is understood as a chronic disease state, and treatments for this condition have been developed, such as new medications, endoscopic devices, and surgical procedures.

Contributions to this issue include clinical outcomes of the treatments, discussions regarding causes of obesity, psychological aspects, and genetic aspects of the various treatments. New research topics have been added that hold promise of elucidating causes and also informing new treatment ideas. Those practitioners and researchers who are interested in obesity can find in this issue a blueprint of what is known about obesity causes, the latest guidelines on the treatment of obesity, and dietary and behavioral treatment paradigms. Drugs for obesity are discussed, as well as bariatric surgery outcomes and medical devices. Obesity may be treated differently in those with other conditions, such as type 2 diabetes, and different ethnicities have been shown to have variable outcomes for the current treatments. These are discussed in separate articles.

Pediatric obesity has increased at an alarming rate; adolescent bariatric surgery outcomes are discussed.

Finally, obesity as a chronic inflammatory state and the first hormone to be discovered as an adipokine leptin are featured; brown fat as a potential therapy and nutrient-timing discussions are included as well.

Endocrinol Metab Clin N Am 45 (2016) xvii–xviii
http://dx.doi.org/10.1016/j.ecl.2016.06.014
0889-8529/16/$ – see front matter © 2016 Elsevier Inc. All rights reserved.
endo.theclinics.com

We have not included, and could not include, examples of all the research that has burgeoned since the discovery that adipose tissue is an endocrine organ; however, we hope to engender more ideas with this issue for the next generation of obesity medicine specialists and obesity researchers. We hope you see this issue of *Endocrinology and Metabolism Clinics of North America* on obesity as a summary of what has transpired and progressed over the past 10 years in obesity treatment and research into the underlying cause of the obesity epidemic that has become the most challenging nutritional and health case assault of the twenty-first century.

Caroline M. Apovian, MD
Boston Medical Center
Nutrition and Weight Management
88 East Newton Street
Robinson 4400
Boston, MA 02118, USA

Nawfal W. Istfan, MD, PhD
Boston Medical Center
Nutrition and Weight Management
88 East Newton Street
Evans 249
Boston, MA 02118, USA

E-mail addresses:
caroline.apovian@bmc.org (C.M. Apovian)
nawfal.istfan@bmc.org (N.W. Istfan)

Guidelines for Obesity Management

Donna H. Ryan, MD

KEYWORDS

- Obesity guidelines • Obesity clinical practice guidance
- Obesity medication guidelines • Best practices in obesity management
- Medical management of obesity

KEY POINTS

- The current menu of guidance around obesity management is revealing of progress in the field.
- The focus is on health risk assessment, not just body size; and on health improvement, not just reduction in body size.
- Faced with a public health crisis of noncommunicable diseases associated with obesity, governmental entities and professional societies have commissioned guidelines, some backed by systematic evidence reviews, to address how medical practitioners can engage in obesity management.

INTRODUCTION

Countries around the world are challenged by the effects of rising obesity rates on their health care resources. This is particularly urgent in the United States and other developed countries that enjoy high economic status. In response to rising rates of obesity and its health consequences, many countries have developed guidances for obesity management in medical practices. Indeed the author's recent PubMed search revealed obesity guidelines from more than 44 countries. In the past 5 years, US governmental health agencies and professional societies have produced multiple guidelines on medical management of obesity in adults,[1–4] targeting recommendations for both primary care and specialty providers. Those were sponsored by US National Institutes of Health and the American Heart Association, American College of Cardiology, and The Obesity Society (AHA/ACC/TOS),[1] the Endocrine Society (ENDO),[2] the American Society of Bariatric Physicians (ASBP),[3] and the American Association of Clinical Endocrinologists (AACE).[4] In addition, the United Kingdom's National Institute for Health and Care Excellence (NICE) also recently updated with 2 critical questions[5] to their prior obesity guidelines,[6] which were based on systematic evidence review (**Table 1**).

The author has nothing to disclose.
Pennington Biomedical Research Center, 6400 Perkins Road, Baton Rouge, LA 70808, USA
E-mail address: ryandh@pbrc.edu

Endocrinol Metab Clin N Am 45 (2016) 501–510
http://dx.doi.org/10.1016/j.ecl.2016.04.003   **endo.theclinics.com**
0889-8529/16/$ – see front matter © 2016 Elsevier Inc. All rights reserved.

The purpose of this article was to report and compare findings and recommendations across these guidelines, identify areas of controversy and concordance, and suggest how primary care and specialty practices may make use of the most appropriate recommendations for their circumstances. **Table 1** describes, in abbreviated language the methodology, focus, and key recommendations, and whether those recommendations are broad or targeted and areas of controversy for each of the documents.

METHODOLOGY DETERMINES SCOPE

To understand the differences among guidelines, one must understand the methodology used to generate recommendations. There is a movement to make the development process for all guidelines more rigorous.[7,8] Guidelines that use more rigorous methodology can only address a limited range of critical questions because of labor intensity and cost. Those guidelines that rely more on expert opinion can give broader recommendations and respond more quickly to changes in knowledge in an attempt to be more relevant to practitioners. Guidelines that use more rigorous methodology, such as those from AHA/ACC/TOS,[1] ENDO,[2] and NICE,[5] are by necessity more narrow, but are more authoritative; those that rely more on expert opinion of specialists (ASBP[3] and AACE[4]) are not held to the constraints of evidence review methodology and can give broader recommendations and be more timely in an attempt to be more relevant to practitioners. The methodological approach informs the range of recommendation and strength of recommendation possible, as indicated in **Table 1**.

For the purpose of this discussion, we emphasize discrepancies across the guidelines and provide a path to resolve those in application in primary care and specialty offices.

DIAGNOSIS OF OBESITY AND STAGING OF DISEASE: DECIDING APPROPRIATE CANDIDATES FOR MEDICAL INTERVENTION

All guidelines[1-6] use BMI (body mass index, weight in kg/[height in m]^2) as a screening measure. What is new, as compared with guidelines of the past, is that the "BMI centric" approach is fading in influence in all guidelines and BMI is no longer the sole director of treatment choice. In the United States, BMI is a core measure available through the electronic health record at every visit; therefore, the BMI is here to stay. But BMI is only the first step in evaluating risk associated with excess weight. The second step in determining need for medical management is to screen for other risk factors related to excess weight and to make a decision to offer medical treatment based on a combination of body size (BMI) and other risk factor assessment.

If patients meet criteria of overweight (BMI $\geq$25 <30 kg/m^2) and there are risk factors or comorbidities present, then all relevant guidelines[1,3-5] endorse medically directed weight loss intervention as a path to improve health risk. The AHA/ACC/TOS guidelines[1] emphasize the importance of including waist circumference as a risk factor to determine need for weight loss.

Across all guidelines, obesity (BMI $\geq$30 kg/m^2) mandates medical counseling for weight loss, with one exception. A discrepancy arises in guidance for individuals who have BMI of 30 kg/m^2 or higher but have no risk factors. This is sometimes referred to as "metabolically healthy obese" and by AACE[4] as "obesity stage 0." The AACE guidelines[4] are called an "advanced framework" and would *not* recommend medically directed weight loss for this group, whereas other guidelines[1,3] do advise it, based on the rationale that there is likely to be progression over time to development of risk factors and comorbidities. This discrepancy makes sense; patients are not seeking treatment from endocrinologists for a well-patient visit. The AHA/ACC/TOS guidelines[1] were targeted to primary care and routine visits and AACE to specialist care. Where overweight and obesity are present, clinical judgment should rule, after first assessing presence of health risk (eg, blood pressure, laboratory measures, such as glycemia). Certainly specialist care is not appropriate for medically directed weight loss in individuals without any associated health risks, but lifestyle intervention may be appropriately prescribed by primary care providers for individuals with BMI greater than 30 kg/m^2 even without associated health risk, although higher-risk approaches would not be appropriate.

Controversy among guidelines can arise when individuals have comorbidities or risk factors related to excess body fat and have BMI less than 25 kg/m^2. This can be the case in certain racial groups, especially Asian individuals, and all guidelines acknowledge this fact. One advantage of the NICE guidance from 2006[6] and its update in 2013[9] is the discussion of using lower thresholds (23 kg/m^2 to indicate increased risk and 27.5 kg/m^2 to indicate high risk) for BMI to trigger action among Asian (South Asian and Chinese) populations. Although no formal evidence review supports such a recommendation among US immigrants from South Asia and China, the AHA/ACC/TOS guidelines[1] do support such an approach.

CHOICE OF INITIAL TREATMENT APPROACH

The AHA/ACC/TOS guidelines[1] emphasize that comprehensive lifestyle intervention is the cornerstone for treating obesity and adjunctive therapies are reserved for individuals with more health risk who do not succeed with weight loss and maintenance, and this is supported, in general, by all guidelines. However, the AACE Advanced Framework[4] introduces a staging (Obesity 0, Obesity 1, and Obesity 2) that links severity of disease at presentation to amount of weight loss to be achieved. If comorbidities or risk factors are mild, AACE terms this "obesity stage 1." If the associated comorbidities are moderate or severe, the term is "obesity stage 2." This approach promotes the concept is that the intensity of treatment needs to match the severity of disease, rather than the severity of BMI increase, and one should never determine treatment choice based on BMI alone. However, AACE uses the term "obesity" for individuals with weight-related comorbidities and BMI greater than 25 kg/m^2, which is somewhat confusing.

The Obesity Algorithm promoted by ASBP[0] avoids a discussion of criteria for treatment. The emphasis in the ASBP approach is very much on disease management, and BMI is positioned as a predictor for likelihood of health consequences of adiposopathy.[3] The ASBP takes a "holistic approach," with emphasis on concomitant management of obesity-related diseases and weight management, with the obesity specialist positioned as central to a multicomponent approach to chronic weight management.

The specialist approach to intervention is best informed by AACE and ASBP guidelines. Primary care practitioners should take away several important principles from these somewhat different approaches. First, there is more urgency to intervene when patients have health risks or comorbidities associated with excess body weight, and the greater the health risk, the greater the urgency and the more justification for high-intensity approaches. Additionally, the patient's weight management *history* can be used to determine choice of treatment plan. Patients do not need to fail at lifestyle alone under the observation of the health care provider; a history of struggle should be enough justification to add adjuncts, like medications. Finally, because the goal of weight loss is health improvement, the targeted health goal should be the rationale for determining intensity of approach and for judging success of intervention.

Table 1
Comparison of recent clinical treatment guidelines for diagnosis and management of obesity in adults

	2013 AHA/ACC/TOS[1] (Based on Systematic Evidence Review Sponsored by NHLBI)	2015 Endocrine Society Obesity Pharmacotherapy[2]	ASBP (Annual Update)[3]	AACE 2014[4]	2014 NICE[5,6]
	Methodology: stringent; systematic evidence review; graded recommendations	Methodology: stringent; systematic evidence review; graded recommendations	Methodology: consensus of obesity medicine experts; PowerPoint format: downloadable and updated annually	Methodology: consensus of expert endocrinologists; targets treatment recommendations	Methodology: stringent; systematic evidence review; graded recommendations

	Focus: Narrow: 5 critical questions
	• Benefits of weight loss
	• Risks of excess weight
	• Best diet for weight loss
	• Efficacy of lifestyle intervention approaches
	• Efficacy and safety of bariatric surgery
		Focus: Narrow: 2 topical areas
		• Medications approved for weight loss
		• Weight effects of medications used for chronic disease management
			Focus: Broad: many topics. Holistic, comprehensive approach
			• Etiology of obesity and pathophysiology of associated comorbidities
			• Multiple topics in weight management and chronic disease management
				Focus: Conceptual: anthropometric and complications-related evaluation that leads to actionable diagnoses: complications-centric approach to treatment decisions	Focus:
					• 2006: Broad: lifestyle, pharmacotherapy and surgery
					• 2014: Narrow: 2 critical questions
					  ○ VLCD
					  ○ Bariatric surgery for diabetes
					Includes cost-effectiveness considerations

	Recommendations: both broad and narrow; narrow around 5 questions; broad around "Chronic Disease Management Model for Primary Care of Patients With Overweight and Obesity" based on Evidence Statements and Expert Opinion	Recommendations: broad; target an overall approach to medicating the patient with obesity, both to augment weight loss efforts and to minimize weight gain effects of medications for chronic disease prescription	Recommendations: broad; comprehensive and textbook-length with background on etiology, pathogenesis, pathophysiology; broad approach to therapies	Recommendations: broad with focus on staging severity of disease as a guide to treatment planning; more severe disease warrants more aggressive approach	Recommendations: 2006, broad; lifestyle recommendations rely on an earlier review: the 2014 review is an update of 2006 clinical guidelines and is narrowly focused on 2 topical areas (VLCD and bariatric surgery)

Key points:	Key points:	Key points:	Key points:	Key Points:
• BMI is screening tool; waist circumference is a risk factor • It is not necessary to achieve normal weight; health improvements begin with modest weight loss • There is no magic diet • Lifestyle intervention counseling conducted face-to-face in 14 or more sessions in 6 months is the gold standard for weight loss intervention • Bariatric surgery should be discussed with patients who meet criteria and would benefit it and referrals should be made	• Weight-centric prescribing should be done for chronic diseases; in prescribing for chronic diseases avoid medications that promote gain in favor of those that are weight neutral or are associated with weight loss • Medications are useful adjuncts to diet and exercise, when prescribed appropriately • Choosing which medication to use is a shared decision of prescriber and patient	• Obesity specialist is center of multicomponent therapeutic elements that are required for successful weight loss and maintenance • Therapy should be holistic and include management of obesity-related chronic diseases	• Complications of excess body weight should direct intensity of treatment and urgency of treatment • Medications for chronic weight management may be used for patients with more severe disease manifestations as an adjunct to lifestyle (multicomponent) measures as the initial approach	• Do not use VLCD routinely; consider use as part of multicomponent strategy; link use to long-term multicomponent counseling • Offer expedited assessment for bariatric surgery for those who meet criteria; consider bariatric surgery for individuals with type 2 diabetes and BMI $\geq$30 kg/m^2 after surgery monitor annually for nutritional status and offer follow-up for at least 2 y
Areas of controversy:	Areas of controversy:	Areas of controversy:	Areas of controversy:	Areas of controversy:
• Does not include race-specific BMI cut points to assess risk • BMI 30 indicates medical intervention regardless of health status	• Does not indicate stepped approaches to medicating for chronic weight management, for example, all medications given equal consideration for first-line therapy	• No transparency on how evidence drives recommendations	• Specialist focus; no recommendations for screening and early intervention in context of care across the life span • Confusion caused by BMI 25 <30 and risk factors being designated as "obesity"	• Bariatric surgery focus is solely on presence of type 2 diabetes • Amenable to implementation in structured national health care system but difficult to adapt to the United States

Abbreviations: AACE, American Association of Clinical Endocrinologists; AHA/ACC/TOS, American Heart Association, American College of Cardiology, and The Obesity Society; ASBP, American Society of Bariatric Physicians; BMI, body mass index; NHLBI, National Heart, Lung, and Blood Institute; NICE, National Institute for Health and Care Excellence; VLCD, very-low-calorie-diet (less than 800 Kcal/day).

COMPREHENSIVE LIFESTYLE INTERVENTION

It is clear that medical advice to "eat less and exercise more" is not effective for most patients to succeed at weight loss. To succeed at changing behaviors around diet and physical activity, a skill set is required. The term comprehensive refers to simultaneous implementation of 3 elements: dietary change to reduce energy intake, increase in physical activity, and behavioral skill training to affect these changes. The AHA/ACC/TOS guidelines' systematic evidence review[1] of lifestyle intervention was conducted to support inclusion of intensive behavioral therapy for weight management as a part of medical practice. That systematic evidence review demonstrated that when these components are delivered in face-to-face (group or individual) sessions, with at least 14 sessions over 6 months and continued follow-up is provided to 1 year, then average weight loss of 8 kg at 1 year is the result.[1] Although this may seem modest, it translates into clinically significant improvements in blood pressure, triglycerides, high-density lipoprotein cholesterol, measures of glycemic control, and reduction in risk for progression to type 2 diabetes.[1] Based on these and other findings, the US Preventive Services Task Force[10] has recommended that obese individuals with cardiovascular disease risk factors should be referred for lifestyle treatment and the US Centers for Medicare and Medicaid Services promoted policies[11] to reimburse providers for intensive behavioral therapy for obese patients.

Although the best outcomes have been shown with frequent, face-to-face intervention, the practicalities of this in primary care are challenging. Telephonic and Web-based counseling and commercial programs are endorsed as alternatives, although the average weight loss results are less.[1]

DIETS FOR WEIGHT LOSS

The entrenched belief that there is a "magic" diet has stimulated studies that have focused on various macronutrient compositions, including low-fat diets, low-carbohydrate/high-protein diets, low glycemic-index diets, balanced deficit diets, vegetarian, vegan, and various diets based on dietary patterns and eliminating 1 or more major food groups. To address this issue, the AHA/ACC/TOS guidelines performed a systematic evidence review, and of 17 diets evaluated, no one diet was superior.[1] Thus, there are many pathways to successful weight loss. In all those diets that were studied, the best predictor of success was dietary adherence. Providers are advised to prescribe a diet that the patient will adhere to so as to achieve reduced caloric intake and weight loss. This does not mean that diet composition is not important, but merely that without energy deficit, weight loss will not occur. And it does not mean that diet alone should be the focus; a comprehensive approach is required because physical activity is important, too. The goal is health improvement and changes in lifestyle that reduce sedentary behavior and increase physical activity to advance that aim as well as promote weight loss and maintenance. Diet composition is also an important pathway to better health. The provider should consider the patient's health status in recommending diet composition, as well as the patient's personal preferences around food choices. In fact, recent guidelines for Americans from AHA/ACC Lifestyle Guidelines[12] and the Dietary Guidelines for Americans[13] advise consumption of a dietary pattern that emphasizes intake of vegetables, fruits, and whole grains; includes low-fat dairy products, poultry, fish, legumes, nontropical vegetable oils, and nuts; and limits intake of sodium, sweets, sugar-sweetened beverages, and red meats. This can be adapted to a lower carbohydrate or lower glycemic load approach for patients with diabetes mellitus or insulin resistance. Referral to a registered dietitian is endorsed by the AHA/ACC/TOS guidelines[1] when the dietary recommendation has a specific health target.

PHYSICAL ACTIVITY

Increased physical activity is an essential component of a comprehensive lifestyle intervention. The "gold standard programs" reviewed in recent AHA/ACC/TOS guidelines[1] typically prescribe increased aerobic physical activity (such as brisk walking) for more than 150 minutes per week (equal to >30 minutes per day, most days of the week). This echoes the 2001 and 2009 American College of Sports Medicine Position Stand,[14] which also supported 200 to 300 minutes a week for long-term weight loss. That evidence review supports moderate-intensity physical activity between 150 and 250 minutes a week to be effective to prevent weight gain, although that intensity will provide only modest weight loss.[14] This Position Stand found that resistance training does not enhance weight loss but may increase fat-free mass and increased loss of fat mass and is associated with reductions in health risk. Existing evidence indicates that endurance physical activity or resistance training without weight loss improves health risk.[14]

PHARMACOTHERAPY

The best source for authoritative recommendation on use of medications for the patient with obesity comes from the ENDO Guidleines.[2] First is the consideration of the role of medications in weight gain among overweight and obese individuals. As part of evaluation of the patient with obesity, the physician should review the medication list to ensure that the patient is not taking drugs that produce weight gain and to modify where possible, when medications associated with gain are found. Many medications in use for common chronic diseases produce weight gain, and similarly some are associated with weight loss, albeit those medications do not have an obesity indication. Weight-centric medication management of chronic diseases is central to effective obesity management.

All of the guidelines support pharmacotherapy as an adjunct to lifestyle changes to help patients who struggle. Across all guidances,[1–4] the indications for adding pharmacotherapy to a weight loss effort are history of failure to achieve clinically meaningful weight loss and to sustain lost weight, for patients who meet regulatory prescribing guidelines (BMI ≥ 27 kg/m^2 with 1 or more comorbidities or a BMI >30 kg/m^2 with or without metabolic consequences).[1–4]

The ENDO Guidelines on pharmacotherapy for obesity provide recommendations that serve as guiding principles.[2] First, effective lifestyle support for weight loss should be provided during drug use. Medications approved for chronic weight management work to reinforce diets that result in an energy deficit. Second, the patient should be familiar with the drug and its potential side effects. Third, if less than 5% weight loss occurs after 3 months, a new treatment plan should be implemented. No one of the medications approved for chronic weight management is effective in every patient, just as not every patient is appropriate for every medication. And finally, if medications result in improvement in health and weight, they should be continued for the long term.

BARIATRIC SURGERY

The AHA/ACC/TOS guidelines[1] gave the strongest recommendation yet that physicians be proactive in identifying patients who would benefit and referring them to a surgeon. Adult patients with BMI greater than 40 or BMI greater than 35 with obesity-related comorbid conditions are eligible. For individuals at high risk, bariatric surgery can improve many obesity-related comorbidities and reduce risk of mortality. Further, the safety of these procedures has come into acceptable bounds.

The NICE guidelines of 2014[6] had as one critical question the role of bariatric surgery in individuals with recent-onset type 2 diabetes mellitus. Based on a review that considered both clinical and economic evidence, those guidelines recommended, in individuals with recent diagnosis of type 2 diabetes, expedited assessment for bariatric surgery for individuals with BMI of 35 kg/m^2 or higher and *consideration* of bariatric surgery for individuals with BMI of 30 kg/m^2 or higher. Although this is an area of discussion among surgeons in the United States, the AHA/ACC/TOS guidelines[1] supported the strongest recommendation ever that primary care providers advise and refer for bariatric surgery, but at BMI greater than 40 kg/m^2 or greater than 35 kg/m^2 with a comorbidity.

CURRENT CONTROVERSIES AND FUTURE DIRECTION

As this discussion reveals, there is still controversy around risk assessment related to excess body fat as a way to determine treatment intensity. A more sophisticated approach to risk assessment, while not immediately a prospect, would resolve some of the controversy around setting BMI cut points. In the current environment, the best approach to managing patients who do not quite fit BMI cut points is to recognize that sometimes the "rules" need challenging. These guidelines are not laws. They must be challenged when clinical judgment dictates. One active area of controversy is the reexamination of lower BMI cut points for bariatric surgical procedures, especially for patients with type 2 diabetes. We may see the lower BMI for bariatric surgery in type 2 diabetes endorsed in the NICE guidance[5] applied in the United States. Although we have recently made progress in developing new medications for chronic weight management, there are no comparative trials and we have no guidance on stepped or staged approaches to care using these medications. There have also been a number of new devices approved by the Food and Drug Administration for chronic weight management.[15] These include gastric bands, gastric balloons, an electrical stimulating system, and a gastric aspiration device. However, there are no guidelines or best practices that address how to incorporate the use of these tools and how to incorporate their use among other treatment modalities for obesity. Future efforts need to address these issues, and, certainly others.

SUMMARY

The current menu of guidance around obesity management is revealing of progress in the field. The focus is on health risk assessment, not just body size and on health improvement, not just reduction in body size. The various guidances emphasize by their diversity of target audiences the importance of a multilayered approach to addressing the obesity epidemic. There is a need to intervene earlier, in primary care settings, with lifestyle intervention. And further, those interventions will only be effective if they are intensive and comprehensive behavioral therapy approaches. The guidelines emphasize the chronic nature of obesity and the need for long-term care. The guidelines debunk the notion of a magic diet and emphasize the importance of comprehensive approaches to lifestyle change: diet, physical activity, and behavioral changes. Further, the guidelines acknowledge the need for stepping up care when patients struggle and to add adjunctive approaches to lifestyle intervention. We now have the first guidelines based on a systematic evidence review of use of medications in the patient with obesity.[2] The role of bariatric surgical procedures is getting stronger endorsement and there is a clear message that health care providers need to be more proactive in recommending this as a potential pathway to better health for patients with severe obesity. There are guidances for primary care and for specialist care, with specialist care targeting patients with obesity-related complications. The menu illustrates that one size does *not* fit all in terms of where to go for advice. Still, there is remarkable concordance in the overall direction of the guidelines with all making an emphatic statement that it is an obligation for *all* health care providers to participate in obesity management.

REFERENCES

1. Jensen MD, Ryan DH, Donato KA, et al. Guidelines (2013) for managing overweight and obesity in adults. Obesity 2014;22(S2):S1–410.
2. Apovian CM, Aronne LJ, Bessesen DH, et al. Pharmacologic management of obesity: an Endocrine Society clinical practice guideline. J Clin Endocrinol Metab 2015;100(2):342–62.
3. Seger JC, Horn DB, Westman EC, et al. Obesity algorithm, presented by the American Society of Bariatric Physicians, 2014-2015. Available at: www.obesityalgorithm.org. Accessed September 22, 2015.
4. Garvey WT, Garber AJ, Mechanick JI, et al, On behalf of the AACE Obesity Scientific Committee. American Association of Clinical Endocrinologists and American College of Endocrinology position statement on the 2014 advanced framework for a new diagnosis of obesity as a chronic disease. Endocr Pract 2014;20(9):977–89.
5. National Institute for Health and Clinical Excellence. Guidance. Obesity: identification, assessment and management of overweight and obesity in children, young people and adults: partial update of CG43. National Clinical Guideline Centre (UK). London: National Institute for Health and Care Excellence; 2014.
6. National Institute for Health and Clinical Excellence. Obesity Guidance on the prevention of overweight and obesity in adults and children. Issued: December 2006, last modified: 2015. Available at: https://www.nice.org.uk/guidance/cg43/resources/guidance-obesity-pdf. Accessed September 25, 2015.
7. Finding what works in health care standards for systematic reviews. Available at: http://www.iom.edu/Reports/2011/Finding What-Works-in-Health-Care-Standards-for-Systematic-Reviews.aspx. Accessed January 15, 2015.
8. Clinical practice guidelines we can trust. Available at: http://www.iom.edu/Reports/2011/Clinical-Practice-Guidelines-We-Can-Trust.aspx. Accessed January 15, 2015.
9. National Institute for Health and Clinical Excellence: Assessing body mass index and waist circumference thresholds for intervening to prevent ill health and premature death among adults from black, Asian and other minority ethnic groups in the UK. NICE guidelines [PH46]. 2013. Available at: https://www.nice.org.uk/guidance/ph46. Accessed May 10, 2016.
10. LeFevre ML. Behavioral counseling to promote a healthful diet and physical activity for cardiovascular disease prevention in adults with cardiovascular risk factors: U.S. Preventive Services Task Force recommendation statement. Ann Intern Med 2014;161(8):587–93.
11. Decision memo for intensive behavioral therapy for obesity (CAG-00423N). Available at: https://www.cms.gov/medicare-coverage-database/details/nca-decision-memo.aspx?&NcaName=Intensive%20Behavioral%20Therapy%20for%20Obesity&bc=ACAAAAAAIAAA&NCAId=253&. Accessed September 22, 2015.

12. Eckel RH, Jakicic JM, Ard JD, et al, American College of Cardiology/American Heart Association Task Force on Practice Guidelines. 2013 AHA/ACC guideline on lifestyle management to reduce cardiovascular risk: a report of the American College of Cardiology/American Heart Association Task Force on Practice Guidelines. J Am Coll Cardiol 2014;63(25 Pt B):2960–84.
13. The 2015 Dietary Guidelines Advisory Committee (February 2015). Scientific report of the 2015 Dietary Guidelines Advisory Committee. Available at: http://www.health.gov/dietaryguidelines/2015-scientific-report. Accessed September 15, 2015.
14. Donnelly JE, Blair SN, Jakicic JM, et al, American College of Sports Medicine. American College of Sports Medicine Position Stand. Appropriate physical activity intervention strategies for weight loss and prevention of weight regain for adults. Med Sci Sports Exerc 2009;41(2):459–71.
15. FDA approved obesity treatment devices. Available at: http://www.fda.gov/MedicalDevices/ProductsandMedicalProcedures/ObesityDevices/ucm350134.htm. Accessed September 15, 2015.

Regarding Obesity as a Disease

Evolving Policies and Their Implications

Theodore K. Kyle, RPh, MBA[a,*], Emily J. Dhurandhar, PhD[b],
David B. Allison, PhD[c]

KEYWORDS

- Obesity • Health policy • Chronic disease
- Health care economics and organizations • Medicalization • Access to health care
- Social stigma

KEY POINTS

- Defining what is and is not a disease is fundamentally a pragmatic decision; a clear, objective, and widely accepted definition of what is and is not a disease is lacking.
- Obesity is a highly stigmatized condition that has long been generally regarded by the public as a reversible consequence of personal choices.
- As research has documented the genetic, biological, and environmental factors that play important roles in obesity and its resistance to treatment, a growing number of medical and scientific organizations have come to regard obesity as a disease.
- The decision by the American Medical Association (AMA) in 2013 to recognize obesity as a disease state marked a key milestone in progress toward accepting obesity as a disease and advancing evidence-based approaches for its prevention and treatment.
- Some signs of progress are evident following the AMA decision, although diverse stakeholders continue to debate the merits of this determination.

INTRODUCTION

Perhaps because of the close relationship between physical appearance and obesity, intertwined with moral beliefs and class discriminations related to obesity, the social and cultural implications of excess weight have historically received more attention

The authors have nothing to disclose.
[a] ConscienHealth, 2270 Country Club Drive, Pittsburgh, PA 15241, USA; [b] Department of Kinesiology and Sport Management, Texas Tech University, Box 43011, Lubbock, TX 79409-3011, USA; [c] Department of Biostatistics, Office of Energetics, Nutrition Obesity Research Center, University of Alabama at Birmingham, Ryals Building, Room 140J, 1665 University Boulevard, Birmingham, AL 35294, USA
* Corresponding author.
E-mail address: ted.kyle@conscienhealth.org

than its medical implications. Until the mid to late twentieth century in America, undernourishment and hunger were prioritized as more important public health concerns than was obesity. In 1950, the first medical society devoted to clinical management of obesity established itself as the National Obesity Society. The organization subsequently changed its name to the National Glandular Society, the American College of Endocrinology and Nutrition, the American Society of Bariatrics, the American Society of Bariatric Physicians, and now the Obesity Medicine Association.[1] Separately in 1982, the North American Association for the Study of Obesity (NAASO) was founded as a scientific and educational organization. In 2005, NAASO changed its name to become the Obesity Society.

With the recognition that excessive adiposity is responsible for a growing prevalence of chronic diseases, obesity has come to be regarded as "the single greatest threat to public health for this century."[2] Research has provided a deeper understanding of the genetic, metabolic, environmental, and behavioral factors that contribute to obesity. This growing evidence base challenges the dominant public understanding of obesity as a reversible condition resulting primarily from dietary and lifestyle choices that reflect ignorance or limited motivation.

These developments have led obesity to be increasingly described by scientific and medical experts as a complex chronic disease. This article reviews reasons why obesity is regarded as a disease and the implications of this increasingly dominant perspective.

DEFINING WHAT IS A DISEASE

In 2008, the Obesity Society commissioned a panel of experts to consider the question of labeling obesity as a disease and to complete a thorough review of pertinent evidence and arguments.[3] The panel considered 3 distinct approaches to the question.

Scientific

The scientific approach hinges on 2 questions. What are the characteristics that define a disease? And what is the evidence that obesity possesses those characteristics? The panel found that the scientific approach was inadequate for answering this question "because of a lack of a clear, specific, widely accepted, and scientifically applicable definition of 'disease.'"

Forensic

The forensic approach relies on authoritative statements from respected organizations declaring that obesity is or should be considered to be a disease. After an exhaustive search of public statements, the panel found "a clear and strong majority leaning–although not complete consensus–toward obesity being a disease." However, they found that these statements were largely issued as a matter of opinion and lacked arguments or evidence to support a determination of "what is true or what is right."

Utilitarian

The third approach, utilitarian, is a logical analysis of the benefits and harms arising from considering obesity a disease. It formed the basis for the panel's ultimate recommendation.

It follows that the determination of what is a disease is more of a social and policy determination than it is a scientific determination. Policymakers and experts make reasoned judgments about whether or not a condition should be considered a disease based on evidence, as well as explicit and implicit values. Public acceptance (or nonacceptance) of that judgment represents a final step in this process. Randolph Nesse[4] summarized the inherent challenge of defining whether something is a disease:

> *Our social definition of disease will remain contentious, however, because values vary, and because the label "disease" changes judgments about the moral status of people with various conditions, and their rights to medical and social resources.*

MILESTONES IN REGARDING OBESITY AS A DISEASE AND THEIR POLICY IMPLICATIONS

Fig. 1 depicts milestones in regarding obesity as a disease. Each milestone is an example of how labeling a condition as a "disease" or "not a disease" can have significant policy implications. Established in 1977, the Healthcare Financing Administration (predecessor to the Centers for Medicare and Medicaid Services [CMS]) included language in its *Coverage Issues Manual* stating that "obesity is not an illness."[5] This language reflected widely-held beliefs and served as a model for denying coverage of obesity care under both publicly and privately funded health plans.

In 1998, the National Institutes of Health published *Clinical Guidelines on the Identification, Evaluation, and Treatment of Overweight and Obesity in Adults* that stated, "Obesity is a complex multifactorial chronic disease."[6]

In early 2002, the Internal Revenue Service issued a ruling that expenses for obesity treatment would qualify as deductible medical expenses.[7] Later in 2002, the Social Security Administration published an evaluation of obesity stating that "Obesity is a complex, chronic disease characterized by excessive accumulation of body fat."[8] This determination explicitly stated that obesity is a valid medical source of impairment for the purpose of evaluating Social Security disability claims.

A key milestone came in 2004 when the CMS removed language stating that "obesity is not an illness" from its *Coverage Issues Manual.*[5] Although this action did not include a specific determination that obesity is a disease, it removed a significant obstacle to further progress and coverage for obesity-related medical services.

In 2006, CMS issued a National Coverage Determination providing coverage for bariatric surgery under Medicare, a decision that followed as a natural consequence of the agency's 2004 reassessment of obesity.[9]

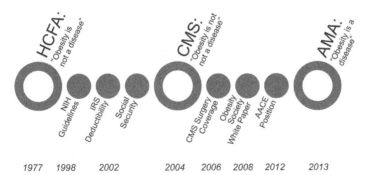

Fig. 1. Milestones toward considering obesity to be a disease. Large open circles represent key milestones; smaller circles represent other noteworthy milestones. AACE, American Association of Clinical Endocrinologists; AMA, American Medical Association; CMS, The Centers for Medicare and Medicaid Services; HCFA, Healthcare Financing Administration; IRS, Internal Revenue Service; NIH, National Institutes of Health.

As previously mentioned, the Obesity Society published a white paper on evidence and arguments for obesity as a disease in 2008, followed in 2012 by a similar position from the American Association of Clinical Endocrinologists.[10]

Finally, in 2013, the American Medical Association (AMA) resolved at its annual House of Delegates meeting to "recognize obesity as a disease state with multiple pathophysiological aspects requiring a range of interventions to advance obesity treatment and prevention."[11] Though this resolution has no legal standing, the AMA has stated that "recognizing obesity as a disease will help change the way the medical community tackles this complex issue." Their leadership in shifting the care model for obesity to a chronic disease model may have a significant impact on the way obesity is addressed.

INITIAL PUBLIC RESPONSE TO THE AMERICAN MEDICAL ASSOCIATION DECISION

The AMA decision to recognize obesity as a disease captured considerable public attention in June of 2013 when it was announced. Though it continued to be discussed and debated among stakeholders in health and obesity policy, interest from the general public quickly faded, as indicated by **Fig. 2**, which depicts Google Trends data for Internet search volume related to obesity and disease.

Much of the public debate about the merits of this decision included 3 distinct viewpoints.

Relief and Agreement

Clinicians, researchers, and individuals with obesity expressed relief that obesity was now being seen as a legitimate health concern, rather than a cosmetic or lifestyle concern. Sarah Bramblette[12] expressed this perspective in *Narrative Inquiry in Bioethics (NIB)*, "I celebrated the American Medical Association's classification of obesity as a disease...I am a real person and deserve the same level of access to health care as other patients."

Concern About Weight Discrimination

Activists in the Fat Acceptance and Health at Every Size movements have consistently expressed opposition to this decision, anticipating that its primary effect would be to promote size and weight discrimination. In another *NIB* essay, Jennifer Hansen expressed this view, "Classifying obesity as a disease provides more ammunition for the 'war on obesity.' From a fat person's perspective, the 'war on obesity' is a war on fat people."[13]

Concern About Personal Responsibility

Michael Tanner captured this perspective in the *National Review*, "At first glance, it's a minor story, hardly worth mentioning, but in reality the AMA's move is a symptom of a

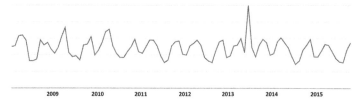

Fig. 2. Interest over time in "obesity disease." The vertical axis is an index of the relative popularity (measured by number of searches) for the search term (obesity disease), compared with all Internet searches completed on Google at a given time. (Google Trends Internet Search Index.)

disease that is seriously troubling our society: the abdication of personal responsibility and an invitation to government meddling."[14]

Research on public perception of obesity following the AMA decision suggests a shift away from the dominant view that obesity is a personal problem of bad choices (**Fig. 3**). However, this research does not suggest that the public is increasingly adopting the view that obesity is a medical problem. Rather, the public is shifting toward a view that obesity is a community problem of bad food and inactivity.[15]

These findings are generally consistent with observations by Puhl and Liu[16] that public awareness of the AMA decision is relatively low. Nonetheless, their study documented more public agreement with statements in support of describing obesity as a disease than with statements opposing it.

POTENTIAL EFFECTS OF REGARDING OBESITY AS A DISEASE

The 2008 white paper commissioned by the Obesity Society concluded:

Considering obesity a disease is likely to have far more positive than negative consequences and to benefit the greater good by soliciting more resources into research, prevention, and treatment of obesity; by encouraging more high-quality caring professionals to view treating the obese patient as a vocation worthy of effort and respect; and by reducing the stigma and discrimination heaped upon many obese persons.

Two years after the decision by the AMA to recognize obesity as a disease, assessing the effects of that decision and comparing those effects to the expected effects is a worthwhile exercise, albeit an exercise that involves a substantial degree of subjective judgments. Certainly, many factors are at work in changes observed since the AMA decision.

Public Understanding of Obesity

Public understanding of obesity has arguably improved as measured by a decline in the dominant view that obesity is simply a personal problem of bad choices. Likewise,

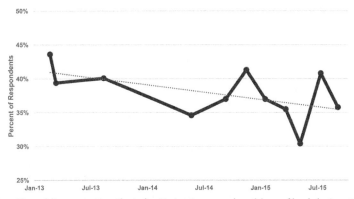

Fig. 3. Trend in public perception that obesity is a "personal problem of bad choices." Between Feb 2013 and Mar 2015, the proportion of the public that viewed obesity primarily as a "personal problem of bad choices" declined modestly ($P = .0004$, binomial regression) from 44% to 36%. (*From* Kyle T, Thomas D, Ivanescu A, et al. Indications of increasing social rejection related to weight bias. Presented at: ObesityWeek. Los Angeles (CA), November 2, 2015. Available at: http://conscienhealth.org/wp-content/uploads/2015/10/Bias-Study-Report.pdf. Accessed November 20, 2015, with permission.)

the research of Puhl and Liu[16] suggests that the public is more supportive of this view of obesity than opposed to it.

Still, public opinion is more focused on risk factors related to the food supply and physical activity than on the medical aspects of obesity.[15] This may be a reflection of the complexity of a disease that remains a challenge to both researchers and health care professionals.

Stigma

Stigma is a prevalent problem for people living with obesity[17] and the evidence for any changes in this phenomenon is mixed. One manifestation of stigma is the idea that "fat shaming," or shaming people with obesity about their weight, will help the individual lose weight. This approach has received considerable attention in popular media and online social networks in the years since the AMA designated obesity as a disease. Fat shaming was hardly recognized before 2012 but interest in the subject has grown dramatically. Assigning the label of "fat shaming" to this idea inherently positions explicit bias against people with obesity as socially unacceptable.

Although explicit shaming of people with obesity may be increasingly rejected, it is not clear that the prevalence of weight bias is changing. In fact, research by the Obesity Action Coalition finds increasing social discomfort toward people who have obesity.[15]

Prevention

Prevention efforts might best be described as experiencing no discernible change in the 2 years since the AMA decision. Writing in *Lancet* (2015), Roberto and colleagues[18] describe "patchy progress" in obesity prevention with only "isolated areas of improvement."

Experimental data published in 2014 suggested that describing obesity as a disease could undermine prevention efforts through a negative effect on self-regulation of dietary behavior.[19]

Treatment

Treatment options for obesity have expanded significantly, with the introduction of 4 new drugs and 3 devices. The Food and Drug Administration has developed a more explicit framework for evaluating benefit-risk tradeoffs for new obesity treatments.[20] Research on new treatment options seems to be growing and multiple national health organizations are working together on guidelines and advocacy for obesity care.[21]

Insurance Reimbursement

Insurance reimbursement remains a significant problem for both patients and providers in obesity care. Nonetheless, some changes have occurred that will influence coverage for obesity care. In 2014, the federal Office of Personnel Management issued guidance to health plans for federal employers that they could no longer exclude obesity care by characterizing obesity as a lifestyle or cosmetic condition. In 2015, the National Conference of Insurance Legislators resolved that state legislatures should provide for "coverage of the full range of obesity treatment."[22]

Medical Education

Medical education has received significant attention from the Bipartisan Policy Center in a report issued in June 2014.[23] In addition, work of the Obesity Society to identify gaps in testing for obesity-related competencies on medical board examinations has resulted in a commitment to address the gaps.[24] Finally, although it has not yet passed, legislation entitled the ENRICH ACT has been introduced to provide grants to medical schools for incorporating obesity education into their curriculum.[25]

Consumer Protection

Consumer protection against fraudulent weight loss products remains a significant problem. Noteworthy actions against dietary supplements by state attorneys general and the US Justice Department have been taken in the last year.[26] The Obesity Society, the Obesity Medicine Association, the Obesity Action Coalition, and the Academy of Nutrition and Dietetics recently issued a joint position calling for more stringent regulation of dietary supplements that make therapeutic claims for obesity.[27]

Discrimination

Discrimination in employment has received increased attention following the AMA decision. Employment law firms have issued opinions that this ruling could create additional risk for employers who discriminate against people with obesity, and the Equal Employment Opportunity Commission has won additional rulings that obesity can be considered a protected disability under the Americans with Disabilities Act.[28]

Credibility

Credibility of obesity research and care is difficult to observe directly. It is worth noting that the numbers of physicians taking the certification examination of the American Board of Obesity Medicine has grown dramatically in the years since the AMA decision. The number applying to take the examination in 2015 grew by 27%, which might be taken as evidence of growing credibility for the emerging specialty of obesity medicine.[29] In addition, the Commission on Dietetic Registration is preparing to offer a certification examination in obesity and weight management for allied health professionals.[30]

IMPLICATIONS FOR OBESITY RESEARCH

The National Institutes of Health has recognized that obesity is a chronic disease since 1998, and this is reflected in the *Strategic Plan for NIH Obesity Research* released by the NIH Obesity Task Force in 2011.[31] The main highlights of the research agenda outlined include a need for more probative research to better understand the fundamental causes of obesity, to develop new and more effective treatments for obesity, to empirically test strategies for obesity prevention in the real-world settings for which they are intended, and to improve technology to overcome many challenges in obesity research. This agenda demonstrates acknowledgement of a chronic and relatively unaddressed disease that is still in great need of further probative research to improve outcomes.

However, whether or not progress is being made on this probative research agenda, and if the AMA decision to recognize obesity as a disease has influenced the research agenda and resources for obesity research thus far, is unclear. Ultimately, this research agenda demonstrates insightful leadership and is well informed but will not influence which research is conducted until individuals participating in the grant review process view obesity as a disease.

If strides in the medicalization of obesity treatment through improved education in medical schools and insurance coverage of treatments following the decision continue to progress, this may eventually lead to more demand for, and better coordination of, data collection on evidence-based care models. Similarly, if the disease decision continues to lessen the view that obesity is an issue of personal responsibility, this may eventually be reflected in the treatment and prevention approaches that are being pursued through research.

SUMMARY

Defining what is and is not a disease is necessarily a pragmatic decision. A clear, objective, and widely accepted definition of what is and is not a disease, which adequately captures things conventionally accepted as diseases and excludes things that are not, is lacking. Obesity is a highly stigmatized condition that has long been generally regarded by the public as a reversible consequence of personal choices. As research has documented the genetic, biological, and environmental factors that play important roles in obesity and its resistance to treatment, a growing number of medical and scientific organizations have come to regard obesity as a disease. The decision by the AMA in 2013 to recognize obesity as a disease state marked a key milestone in progress toward accepting obesity as a disease and advancing evidence-based approaches for its prevention and treatment. Some signs of progress are evident following the AMA decision, although diverse stakeholders continue to debate the merits of this determination.

REFERENCES

1. Eknoyan G. A history of obesity, or how what was good became ugly and then bad. Adv Chronic Kidney Dis 2006;13(4):421–7.
2. U.S. Department of Health and Human Services. Dietary guidelines for Americans, 2010. 7th edition. Washington, DC: U.S. Government Printing Office; 2010.
3. Allison DB, Downey M, Atkinson RL, et al. Obesity as a disease: a white paper on evidence and arguments commissioned by the Council of the Obesity Society. Obesity (Silver Spring) 2008;16(6):1161–77.
4. Nesse RM. On the difficulty of defining disease: a Darwinian perspective. Med Health Care Philos 2001;4(1):37–46.
5. Tillman K. National coverage analysis (NCA) tracking sheet for obesity as an illness (CAG-00108N). Baltimore (MD): CMS.gov; 2004. Available at: https://www.cms.gov/medicare-coverage-database/details/nca-details.aspx? NCAId=57&TAId=23&IsPopup=y&. Accessed November 20, 2015.
6. National Heart, Lung, and Blood Institute. Clinical guidelines on the identification, evaluation, and treatment of overweight and obesity in adults–The evidence report. National Institutes of Health. Obes Res 1998;6(Suppl 2):51S–209S. Publication no. 98-4083. Available at: http://www.nhlbi.nih.gov/guidelines/obesity/ob_gdlns.pdf.
7. Anderson C. Obesity is tax deductible. New York (NY): CBSnews.com; 2002. Available at: http://www.cbsnews.com/news/obesity-is-tax-deductible/. Accessed November 20, 2015.
8. SSA.gov. Social Security Administration Program Operations Manual (POMS) - DI 24570.001 Evaluation of Obesity. 2002. Available at: https://secure.ssa.gov/poms.nsf/lnx/0424570001. Accessed November 20, 2015.
9. Phurrough S, Salive M. Decision memo for bariatric surgery for the treatment of morbid obesity (CAG-00250R). Baltimore (MD): CMS.gov; 2006. Available at: www.cms.gov/medicare-coverage-database/details/nca-decision-memo.aspx? NCAId=160&ver=32&NcaName=Bariatric+Surgery+for+the+Treatment+of+Morbid+Obesity+(1st+Recon)&bc=BEAAAAAAEAgA. Accessed November 20, 2015.

10. Mechanick JI, Garber AJ, Handelsman Y, et al. American Association of Clinical Endocrinologists' position statement on obesity and obesity medicine. Endocr Pract 2012;18(5):642–8.

11. Pollack A. AMA recognizes obesity as a disease. NYTimescom 2013. Available at: http://nyti.ms/1Guko03. Accessed November 20, 2015.

12. Bramblette S. I am not obese. I am just fat. Narrat Inq Bioeth 2014;4(2):85–8.

13. Hansen J. Explode and die! A fat woman's perspective on prenatal care and the fat panic epidemic. Narrat Inq Bioeth 2014;4(2):99–101.

14. Tanner M. Obesity is not a disease. National Review Online 2013. Available at: http://www.nationalreview.com/article/352626/obesity-not-disease-michael-tanner. Accessed November 20, 2015.

15. Kyle T, Thomas D, Ivanescu A, et al. Indications of Increasing Social Rejection Related to Weight Bias. Presented at: ObesityWeek. Los Angeles (CA), November 2, 2015. Available at: http://conscienhealth.org/wp-content/uploads/2015/10/Bias-Study-Report.pdf. Accessed November 20, 2015.

16. Puhl RM, Liu S. A national survey of public views about the classification of obesity as a disease. Obesity (Silver Spring) 2015;23(6):1288–95.

17. Puhl R, Kyle T. Pervasive bias: an obstacle to obesity solutions. Washington, DC: National Academy of Medicine; 2014. Available at: http://nam.edu/perspectives-2015-pervasive-bias-an-obstacle-to-obesity-solutions/. Accessed November 20, 2015.

18. Roberto CA, Swinburn B, Hawkes C, et al. Patchy progress on obesity prevention: emerging examples, entrenched barriers, and new thinking. Lancet. 2015; 385(9985):2400–9.

19. Hoyt CL, Burnette JL, Auster-gussman L. "Obesity is a disease": examining the self-regulatory impact of this public-health message. Psychol Sci 2014;25(4): 997–1002.

20. Ho MP, Gonzalez JM, Lerner HP, et al. Incorporating patient-preference evidence into regulatory decision making. Surg Endosc 2015;29(10):2984–93.

21. Smith S. AMA joins call for coverage of obesity treatments and medications - TOS connect. Obes Soc 2014. Available at: http://tosconnect.obesity.org/news/press-releases/new-item2. Accessed November 21, 2015.

22. National Conference of Insurance Legislators. NCOIL Legislators Adopt Resolution Encouraging Coverage For Obesity Treatment. 2015. Available at: http://www.ncoil.org/HomePage/2015/07292015ObesityResolutionPR.pdf. Accessed November 20, 2015.

23. Glickman D, Shalala D. Teaching nutrition and physical activity. In: Tatsutani M, editor. Medical school: training doctors for prevention-oriented care. Washington, DC: Bipartisan Policy Center; 2014. Available at: http://bipartisanpolicy.org/wp-content/uploads/sites/default/files/Med_Ed_Report.PDF. Accessed November 20, 2015.

24. Kushner R, Butsch S, Aronne L, et al. Review of Obesity-Related Items on the United States Medical Licensing Examination (USMLE) Examinations for Medical Students: What is Being Tested? Presented at: ObesityWeek. Los Angeles (CA), November 2, 2015. Available at: https://guidebook.com/guide/48144/poi/4317961/?pcat=185403. Accessed November 20, 2015.

25. Glickman D, Shalala D. The ENRICH Act will provide better tools to fight obesity epidemic. TheHill 2015. Available at: http://thehill.com/blogs/congress-blog/healthcare/236479-the-enrich-act-will-provide-better-tools-to-fight-obesity. Accessed November 20, 2015.

26. Lorenzetti L. Justice department charges dietary supplements maker. Fortune 2015. Available at: http://fortune.com/2015/11/17/doj-dietary-supplements/. Accessed November 20, 2015.

27. The Obesity Society. Dietary Supplements Sold as Medicinal or Curative for Obesity. 2015. Available at: http://www.obesity.org/publications/position-and-policies/medicinal-or-curative. Accessed November 20, 2015.

28. Katz D. Another judge finds that obesity may be a "disability" under the ADA (Americans with Disabilities Act). Natl L Rev 2015. Available at: http://www.natlawreview.com/article/another-judge-finds-obesity-may-be-disability-under-ada-americans-disabilities-act. Accessed November 20, 2015.

29. Burke J. Record number of physicians to sit for 2015 ABOM exam. Denver (CO): American Board of Obesity Medicine; 2015. Available at: http://abom.org/record-number-of-physicians-to-sit-for-2015-abom-exam/. Accessed November 20, 2015.

30. Commission on Dietetic Registration. CDR's New Interdisciplinary Certification in Obesity and Weight Management. 2015. Available at: https://www.cdrnet.org/interdisciplinary. Accessed November 20, 2015.

31. NIH Obesity Research. Strategic Plan for NIH Obesity Research. 2011. Available at: http://obesityresearch.nih.gov/about/strategic-plan.aspx. Accessed November 20, 2015.

Pharmacotherapy for Obesity

Katherine H. Saunders, MD*, Alpana P. Shukla, MD, MRCP (UK), Leon I. Igel, MD, DABOM, Rekha B. Kumar, MD, MS, DABOM, Louis J. Aronne, MD, DABOM, FTOS

KEYWORDS

- Obesity • Weight management • Pharmacotherapy • Orlistat
- Phentermine/topiramate ER • Lorcaserin • Naltrexone SR/bupropion SR
- Liraglutide

KEY POINTS

- Obesity treatment requires a multidisciplinary approach, which can include pharmacotherapy.
- There are several obesity medications approved by the Food and Drug Administration and the newer agents have been approved for long-term therapy.
- Successful pharmacotherapy depends on tailoring treatment to a patient's behaviors and comorbidities.

INTRODUCTION

Successful treatment of obesity requires a multidisciplinary approach, including diet, exercise, and behavioral modification. Even with significant lifestyle changes, weight loss is a challenge for many patients, as reduced calorie consumption and increased energy expenditure are counteracted by adaptive physiologic responses.[1–3] Reduction in body mass causes an increase in appetite and a decrease in energy expenditure, which is out of proportion to the weight loss. These changes are associated with alterations in a range of hormones.[4,5]

According to the 2013 American Heart Association, American College of Cardiology, and The Obesity Society Guideline for the Management of Overweight and Obesity in Adults, pharmacotherapy for the treatment of obesity can be considered if a patient has

Disclosure Statement: Katherine H. Saunders, Alpana P. Shukla and Leon I. Igel declare that they have no conflict of interest. Rekha B. Kumar is a speaker for Jansen Pharmaceuticals and a shareholder in Zafgen and Myos Corporation. Louis J. Aronne declares consultant/advisory board work with Jamieson Labs, Pfizer Inc, Novo Nordisk A/S, Eisai, VIVUS, GI Dynamics, JOVIA Health, and Gelesis. He is a shareholder of Zafgen, Gelesis, Myos Corporation, and Jamieson Labs, and he is on the Board of Directors of MYOS Corporation and Jamieson Labs. He has received research funding from Aspire Bariatrics and Eisai.
Comprehensive Weight Control Center, Division of Endocrinology, Diabetes and Metabolism, Weill Cornell Medicine, 1165 York Avenue, New York, NY 10065, USA
* Corresponding author.
E-mail address: kph2001@med.cornell.edu

Endocrinol Metab Clin N Am 45 (2016) 521–538
http://dx.doi.org/10.1016/j.ecl.2016.04.005
0889-8529/16/$ – see front matter
endo.theclinics.com

- A body mass index (BMI) $\geq$30 kg/m^2
- A BMI $\geq$27 kg/m^2 with weight-related comorbidities, such as hypertension, type 2 diabetes, dyslipidemia, and obstructive sleep apnea.[6]

In 2015, the Endocrine Society published clinical practice guidelines on pharmacologic management of obesity.[7] These evidence-based guidelines include recommendations for individualized weight management and ongoing evaluation of medication efficacy.

The development and approval of new antiobesity medications is challenging. As many weight loss drugs have been withdrawn over the years due to side effects and adverse events, the Food and Drug Administration (FDA) has strict criteria for medication approval.[8,9] A new agent must induce at least 5% statistically significant placebo-adjusted weight loss at 1 year or 35% or more of patients must achieve at least 5% weight loss (which must be at least twice that induced by placebo). The FDA also requires evidence that a medication improves metabolic biomarkers including blood pressure, lipids, and glycemia.

The following are the 6 most widely prescribed obesity medications approved by the FDA:

- Phentermine
- Orlistat
- Phentermine/topiramate extended release (ER)
- Lorcaserin
- Naltrexone sustained release (SR)/bupropion SR
- Liraglutide 3.0 mg (**Table 1**)

Most of the antiobesity medications affect appetite mechanisms, signaling through serotonergic, dopaminergic, or noradrenergic pathways. They primarily target the arcuate nucleus of the hypothalamus to stimulate anorexigenic pro-opiomelanocortin (POMC) neurons, which promote satiety. Orlistat is the only medication that is not significantly absorbed systemically; it blocks absorption of fat calories.

In the past, medications for obesity were used as short-term treatment. However, newer agents have been approved for long-term therapy, as obesity is now considered to be a chronic disease.[10] Phentermine/topiramate ER, lorcaserin, naltrexone SR/bupropion SR, and liraglutide 3.0 mg are indicated for chronic weight management, as an adjunct to a reduced-calorie diet and increased physical activity.[11–14] Phentermine is the only medication approved as a short-term adjunct,[15] and orlistat has the added indication to reduce risk for weight regain after prior weight loss.[16]

The aim of this article was to review current pharmacotherapy for obesity. Medications approved for weight management should be viewed as useful additions to diet and exercise for patients who have been unsuccessful with lifestyle changes alone.

PHENTERMINE

Phentermine was approved by the FDA in 1959 and has been the most commonly prescribed antiobesity medication in the United States. It was approved only for short-term use (3 months) as there are no long-term safety trials of phentermine monotherapy; however, many practitioners prescribe phentermine for longer durations as off-label therapy for continued weight management. In addition, phentermine was approved in combination with topiramate ER for chronic weight management in 2012. Other antiobesity medications, such as diethylpropion and phendimetrazine are also available in the United States, but use and data are minimal.

Phentermine is an adrenergic agonist that promotes weight loss by activation of the sympathetic nervous system. Norepinephrine release causes increased resting energy expenditure and appetite suppression.[17] In the 1990s, it was prescribed in combination with the serotonin-releasing medication, fenfluramine; however, fenfluramine was withdrawn in 1997 because of cardiac valvulopathy.[18]

Studies evaluating monotherapy with phentermine published in the 1960s and 1970s overestimated efficacy, as they presented only completer analyses despite high dropout rates.[19] In a 28-week, randomized controlled trial comparing the combination of phentermine and topiramate ER with its components as monotherapies in adults with obesity, phentermine (15 mg daily) alone was associated with a 6.0 kg weight loss at 28 weeks[20]; 46% of subjects in this group achieved 5% or more weight loss and 21.8% achieved 10% or more weight loss.

The efficacy of continuous versus intermittent phentermine treatment was evaluated in a 36-week, double-blind, placebo-controlled study of 108 women who were overweight or obese.[21] One group received phentermine continuously, a second group alternated phentermine and placebo every 4 weeks, and a third group received placebo continuously. Compared with a 4.8 kg weight loss in the placebo group, the mean weight loss was 12.2 kg and 13.0 kg in patients who received phentermine continuously and intermittently, respectively (**Fig. 1**). Similar to other studies around the same time, attrition was 41% and data were presented for completers only. Nevertheless, the study illustrated that there is no advantage of continuous compared with intermittent phentermine treatment.

Dosing/Administration

The recommended dosage of phentermine is 15.0 to 37.5 mg orally once daily before breakfast or 1 to 2 hours after breakfast. The standard adult dosage is 1 tablet (37.5 mg) daily; however, dosage should be individualized to achieve adequate response with the lowest effective dose. For some patients, a quarter tablet (9.375 mg) or a half tablet (18.75 mg) may be adequate. A split dose of a half tablet 2 times daily is also an option, but administration of the second dose in the late evening should be avoided to prevent insomnia.

Phentermine is a Schedule IV controlled substance and is not recommended for use in pediatric patients 16 years or younger.

Side Effects

The most common treatment-emergent adverse events (TEAEs) with phentermine include the following:

- Dizziness
- Dry mouth
- Difficulty sleeping
- Irritability
- Nausea/vomiting
- Diarrhea
- Constipation

Drug-Drug Interactions

- Monoamine oxidase inhibitors (MAOIs) (during or within 14 days following administration)
- Other sympathomimetic amines

Table 1
Overview of antiobesity medications approved by the Food and Drug Administration

Medication	Phentermine	Orlistat (Xenical)	Phentermine/ Topirimate ER (Qsymia)	Lorcaserin (Belviq)	Naltrexone SR/ Bupropion SR (Contrave)	Liraglutide 3.0 mg (Saxenda)
Mechanism	Adrenergic agonist	Lipase inhibitor	Adrenergic agonist/ neurostabilizer	5-HT$_{2c}$ receptor agonist	Opioid receptor antagonist/ dopamine and NE reuptake inhibitor	GLP-1 analog
Estimated % weight loss (medication compared with placebo, ITT data)	5.1% at 28 wk[20] 15 mg daily	3.1% at 1 y[19] 120 mg TID	6.6% at 1 y[30] 7.5/46 mg daily	3.6% at 1 y[34] 10 mg BID	4.8% at 56 wk[38] 16/180 mg BID	5.4% at 56 wk[44] 3 mg daily
Dosage/ administration	15 mg or 37.5 mg daily (can also use $^1\!/_4$ or ½ pill)	120 mg TID with meals	3.75/23 mg daily with gradual dose escalation (7.5/46 mg daily, then 11.25/69 mg daily, then 15/92 mg daily)	10 mg BID	8/90 mg daily (in the morning) with dose escalation (8/90 mg BID then 16/180 mg in the morning, 8/90 mg in the evening then 16/180 mg BID)	0.6 mg daily with gradual dose escalation (1.2 mg daily then 1.8 mg daily then 2.4 mg daily then 3.0 mg daily)
Available formulations	Capsule, tablet, powder	Capsule	Capsule	Tablet	Tablet	Prefilled pen for SC injection
Approved for long-term use	No	Yes	Yes	Yes	Yes	Yes
Schedule IV controlled substance	Yes	No	Yes	Yes	No	No

Side effects	Dizziness, dry mouth, difficulty sleeping, constipation, irritability	Bloating, diarrhea	Paresthesia, dizziness, dysgeusia, insomnia, constipation, dry mouth	Headache, dizziness, fatigue, nausea, dry mouth, constipation, hypoglycemia, back pain, cough, fatigue	Nausea, constipation, headache, vomiting, dizziness, insomnia, dry mouth, diarrhea	Nausea, hypoglycemia, diarrhea, constipation, vomiting, headache, dyspepsia, fatigue, dizziness, abdominal pain, increased lipase
Contraindications	Pregnancy, nursing, CVD, during or within 14 d of MAOIs, hyperthyroidism, glaucoma, agitated states, history of drug abuse	Pregnancy, chronic malabsorption syndrome, cholestasis	Pregnancy, glaucoma, hyperthyroidism, during or within 14 d of MAOIs	Pregnancy	Pregnancy, uncontrolled HTN, history of seizures or at risk of seizure, bulimia or anorexia, use of opioid agonists or partial agonists, during or within 14 d of MAOIs	Pregnancy, personal or family history of medullary thyroid carcinoma or multiple endocrine neoplasia syndrome type 2

Abbreviations: 5-HT$_{2C}$, serotonin; BID, twice daily; CVD, cardiovascular disease; ER, extended release; GLP-1, glucagon-like peptide-1; HTN, hypertension; ITT, intention-to-treat; MAOI, monoamine oxidase inhibitor; NE, norepinephrine; SC, subcutaneous; SR, sustained release; TID, 3 times daily.

Adapted from Apovian CM, Aronne L, Powell AG. Clinical management of obesity. West Islip (NY): Professional Communications, Inc; 2015. p. 186–92; with permission.

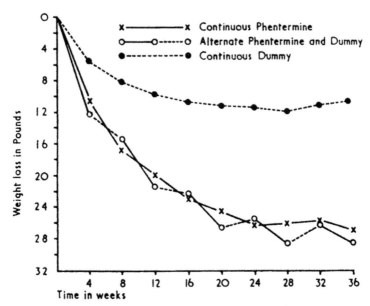

Fig. 1. Weight loss with continuous versus intermittent treatment with phentermine. (*From* Munro JF, MacCuish AC, Wilson EM, et al. Comparison of continuous and intermittent anorectic therapy in obesity. Br Med J 1968;1(5588):354; with permission.)

Contraindications

- Pregnancy/nursing
- History of cardiovascular disease (eg, coronary artery disease, stroke, arrhythmias, congestive heart failure, uncontrolled hypertension)
- Hyperthyroidism
- Glaucoma
- Agitated states
- History of drug abuse
- Concomitant alcohol use
- Known hypersensitivity or idiosyncrasy to sympathomimetic amines

ORLISTAT (XENICAL)

Orlistat was approved by the FDA in 1999 for chronic weight management and remained the only FDA-approved weight loss medication for chronic use until 2012. It is also available as an over-the-counter medication called Alli at half the prescription dose.[22] Unlike the other weight loss agents that enhance energy expenditure and/or reduce appetite, orlistat has a unique mechanism of action. It reduces fat absorption from the gastrointestinal tract by inhibiting pancreatic and gastric lipases. At the recommended dose, orlistat blocks absorption of about 30% of ingested fat.[23]

The efficacy of orlistat was demonstrated in the XENDOS trial, a 4-year, double-blind, prospective study in which 3305 patients were randomized to lifestyle changes with either orlistat 120 mg or placebo 3 times daily.[24] Patients had a BMI of 30 or more; 21% had prediabetes and 79% had normal glucose tolerance. Mean weight loss after 4 years was significantly greater with orlistat (5.8 kg vs 3.0 kg with placebo; *P*<.001) and similar in those with and without prediabetes.

Orlistat not only promotes weight loss, but it also improves insulin sensitivity and lowers serum glucose levels. In the XENDOS trial, the cumulative incidence of diabetes was 6.2% with orlistat and 9.0% with placebo, corresponding to a risk reduction of 37.3% (*P*<.0032). In addition to improving glycemic control and reducing the incidence of diabetes, orlistat was found to improve concentrations of total cholesterol, low density lipoprotein cholesterol, and blood pressure in a Cochrane systematic review.[25]

Although the gastrointestinal side effects associated with steatorrhea can limit patient tolerability and long-term use, orlistat can be an attractive medication for patients with constipation. The medication can be started once daily and titrated up if tolerated. Alternatively, the addition of a psyllium fiber supplement can reduce side effects.

Dosing/Administration

The recommended dosage of orlistat is one 120-mg capsule (Xenical) or one 60-mg capsule (Alli) 3 times a day with each main meal containing fat. It can be taken during or up to 1 hour after the meal. Patients should be advised to follow a nutritionally balanced, reduced-calorie diet with approximately 30% of calories from fat. Additionally, the daily intake of fat, carbohydrate, and protein should be distributed over 3 meals. As orlistat decreases the absorption of fat-soluble vitamins (A, D, E, and K), patients should take a multivitamin (separately from the medication) to ensure adequate nutrition.

Side Effects

The most common TEAEs with orlistat include the following:

- Oily spotting
- Flatus with discharge
- Fecal urgency
- Fatty/oily stool
- Oily evacuation
- Increased defecation
- Fecal incontinence

Drug-Drug Interactions

- Cyclosporine (should be taken 2 hours before or after orlistat dose)
- Levothyroxine
- Warfarin
- Antiepileptic drugs

Contraindications

- Pregnancy
- Chronic malabsorption syndrome
- Cholestasis
- Known hypersensitivity to orlistat or to any component of the product

PHENTERMINE/TOPIRAMATE EXTENDED RELEASE (QSYMIA)

The fixed-dose combination of phentermine and topiramate ER was approved by the FDA in 2012 as the first combination medication for chronic weight management. As obesity is a complex disorder that involves multiple signaling pathways, targeting different sites simultaneously can have an additive effect on weight loss. In addition, the smaller doses of each medication reduce the side-effect profile.

Topiramate, which was approved for epilepsy in 1996 and migraine prophylaxis in 2004, has been found to decrease caloric intake. Randomized controlled trials illustrate that topiramate monotherapy produces weight loss among subjects with obesity of 6 to 8 kg at 24 weeks and improves glycemic control, lipids, and blood pressure.[26,27] The mechanism responsible for weight loss is uncertain, but thought to be mediated through its modulation of gamma-aminobutyric acid receptors, inhibition of carbonic anhydrase, and antagonism of glutamate to reduce food intake.[28]

The efficacy of phentermine/topiramate ER on weight loss was assessed in two 1-year randomized, double-blind, placebo-controlled studies, EQUIP and CONQUER,[29,30] as well as a 2-year extension trial, SEQUEL.[31] The CONQUER trial randomized 2487 patients who were overweight or obese to treatment with placebo, 7.5/46 mg of phentermine/topiramate ER or 15/92 mg phentermine/topiramate ER. Compared with placebo, both dosages resulted in significantly greater weight loss throughout the 56-week course of treatment (9.8 kg with 15/92 mg, 7.8 kg with 7.5/46 mg and 1.2 kg with placebo, P<.0001). Forty-eight percent of patients in the highest dose group lost 10% or more of their baseline weight compared with 37% in the lower-dose group and 7% in the placebo group.

The SEQUEL trial demonstrated ongoing weight loss with phentermine/topiramate ER 2 years after completion of the CONQUER study. The mean percentage changes from baseline body weight were significantly greater in the 2 treatment groups compared with placebo (10.5%, 9.3%, and 1.8% with 15/92 mg, 7.5/46 mg, and placebo, respectively, P<.0001) (**Fig. 2**).

In the CONQUER study, phentermine/topiramate ER 15/92 mg compared with placebo resulted in significant changes in waist circumference, systolic and diastolic blood pressure, lipids, fasting glucose, and fasting insulin. Improvements in risk factors were most pronounced in patients with preexisting comorbidities. In patients without diabetes at baseline, the SEQUEL trial demonstrated a 54% reduction in the progression to type 2 diabetes.

Dosing/Administration

Phentermine/topiramate ER is available in 4 doses, which are considerably lower than the maximum recommended doses of the individual medications for other indications. Phentermine/topiramate ER should be taken once daily in the morning with or without food. Evening administration should be avoided to prevent insomnia associated with phentermine.

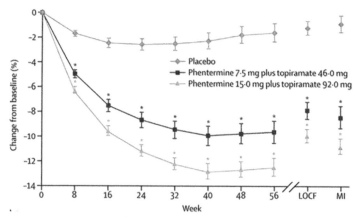

Fig. 2. Weight loss with phentermine 7.5 mg/topiramate 46 mg and phentermine 15 mg/topiramate 92 mg compared with placebo. (*From* Gadde KM, Allison DB, Ryan DH, et al. Effects of low-dose, controlled-release, phentermine plus topiramate combination on weight and associated comorbidities in overweight and obese adults (CONQUER): a randomised, placebo-controlled, phase 3 trial. Lancet 2011;377(9774):1345; with permission.)

Gradual dose escalation, which helps minimize risks and adverse events, should be done as follows:

- 3.75/23 mg daily for 14 days then 7.5/46 mg daily
- At 12 weeks: option to increase to 11.25/69 mg daily then 15/96 mg daily

The medication should be discontinued or the dose should be escalated if 3% weight loss is not achieved after 12 weeks at 7.5/46 mg daily. In addition, if 5% weight loss is not achieved after 12 weeks on the maximum dose (15/92 mg), the medication should be discontinued. Gradual discontinuation is recommended to prevent seizure from rapid withdrawal of topiramate.

All formulations of phentermine/topiramate ER are listed in Schedule IV of the Controlled Substances Act because phentermine is a Schedule IV drug.

The medication is pregnancy category X, and the FDA requires a Risk Evaluation and Mitigation Strategy (REMS) to inform prescribers and women of reproductive potential about the following:

- Increased risk of congenital malformation, specifically orofacial clefts, in infants exposed to phentermine/topiramate ER during the first trimester of pregnancy
- Importance of pregnancy prevention for women of reproductive potential receiving phentermine/topiramate ER
- Need to discontinue phentermine/topiramate ER immediately if pregnancy occurs[32]

Side Effects

The most common TEAEs with phentermine/topiramate ER include the following:

- Paresthesia
- Dizziness
- Dysgeusia
- Insomnia
- Constipation
- Dry mouth

Drug-Drug Interactions

- MAOIs
- Sympathomimetic amines

Contraindications

- Pregnancy (recommend pregnancy test before starting followed by monthly tests in appropriate patients)
- Glaucoma
- Hyperthyroidism
- Use during or within 14 days of taking MAOIs

LORCASERIN (BELVIQ)

Lorcaserin was also approved by the FDA in 2012 for chronic weight management. It is a serotonin receptor agonist thought to reduce food intake and increase satiety by selectively activating receptors on anorexigenic POMC neurons in the hypothalamus. At the recommended dose, lorcaserin selectively binds to 5-HT_{2C} receptors instead of 5-HT_{2A} and 5-HT_{2B} receptors, which are associated with hallucinations and cardiac valve insufficiency, respectively.[33]

Three randomized, double-blind, placebo-controlled trials of 1-year or 2-years duration, evaluated the effects of lorcaserin on weight as well as secondary cardiovascular outcomes. The BLOOM and BLOSSOM trials enrolled patients who were overweight and obese,[34,35] and BLOOM-DM enrolled patients with type 2 diabetes (baseline hemoglobin A1c of 7%–10%).[36]

The BLOOM trial randomized 3182 patients with a mean BMI of 36.2 kg/m^2 to receive lorcaserin 10 mg twice daily or placebo along with diet and exercise counseling for 52 weeks. At week 52, patients in the placebo group continued to receive placebo, but patients in the lorcaserin group were randomly reassigned to receive either lorcaserin or placebo for an additional 52 weeks. After 1 year, mean weight loss in the lorcaserin group was significantly greater than in the placebo group (5.8 kg compared with 2.2 kg, respectively; $P<.001$) (**Fig. 3**). Among patients in the lorcaserin group who achieved 5% or more weight loss at 1 year (47.5% vs 20.3% with lorcaserin and placebo, respectively), more patients were able to maintain their weight loss at the end of 2 years compared with those who were switched to placebo (67.9% vs 50.3%, $P<.001$).

The BLOOM study also demonstrated significant changes in cholesterol, blood pressure, heart rate, fasting glucose, fasting insulin, hemoglobin A1c, and waist circumference. In the BLOOM-DM study, there was a mean reduction of hemoglobin A1c of 0.9% in the treatment group compared with 0.4% reduction in the placebo group. Interestingly, this A1c reduction is also observed with 10 mg daily, which is half of the recommended dose.

To evaluate for theoretic risk of valvulopathy, patients in the trials were monitored by serial echocardiograms. In both the BLOOM and BLOOM-DM studies, FDA-defined valvulopathy developed in 2.3% in the placebo group compared with 2.7% in the lorcaserin group after 1 year ($P = .70$).

Dosing/Administration

The recommended dosage of lorcaserin is 10 mg twice daily with or without food. The medication should be discontinued if 5% or more weight loss is not

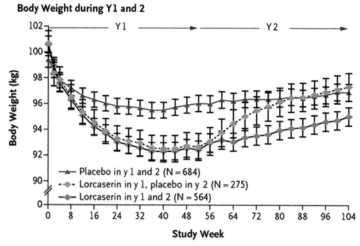

Fig. 3. Weight loss with lorcaserin, lorcaserin/placebo, and placebo. (*From* Smith SR, Weissman NJ, Anderson CM, et al. Multicenter, placebo-controlled trial of lorcaserin for weight management. N Engl J Med 2010;363(3):250; with permission.)

achieved after 12 weeks. Lorcaserin is listed in Schedule IV of the Controlled Substances Act.

Side Effects

The most common TEAEs with lorcaserin in nondiabetic patients include the following:

- Headache
- Dizziness
- Fatigue
- Nausea
- Dry mouth
- Constipation

The most common TEAEs with lorcaserin in patients with diabetes include the following:

- Hypoglycemia
- Headache
- Back pain
- Cough
- Fatigue

Drug-Drug Interactions

- Serotonergic drugs (coadministration may lead to the development of potentially life-threatening serotonin syndrome or neuroleptic malignant syndromelike reactions, although none were reported in phase 3 studies)

Contraindications

- Pregnancy
- Valvular heart disease (but no significant risk of valvulopathy was found during phase 3 studies)

BUPROPION SUSTAINED RELEASE/NALTREXONE SUSTAINED RELEASE (CONTRAVE)

Bupropion SR/naltrexone SR was approved by the FDA in 2014. Bupropion is a dopamine/norepinephrine reuptake inhibitor that was approved on its own for depression in the 1980s and smoking cessation in 1997. Naltrexone is an opioid receptor agonist approved for opiate dependency in 1984 and alcohol addiction in 1994. Naltrexone antagonizes an inhibitory feedback loop that limits bupropion's anorectic properties so the 2 medications have a synergistic effect.[37] The combination works synergistically to activate POMC neurons in the arcuate nucleus. This causes release of alpha-melanocyte–stimulating hormone (a potent anorectic neuropeptide), which projects to other hypothalamic areas involved in feeding and body weight control.

Four 56-week phase 3 multicenter, double-blind, placebo-controlled trials were conducted to evaluate the effect of bupropion SR/naltrexone SR in subjects who were obese or overweight with at least 1 weight-related comorbidity:

- Contrave Obesity Research I (COR-I)[38]
- Contrave Obesity Research II (COR-II)[39]
- Contrave Obesity Research Behavioral Modification (COR-BMOD)[40]
- Contrave Obesity Research Diabetes (COR-Diabetes).[41]

In the COR-I trial, mean change in body weight was 6.1% in the naltrexone 32 mg plus bupropion group compared with 1.3% in the placebo group (*P*<.0001) **(Fig. 4)**.

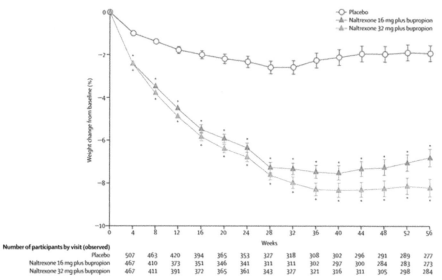

Number of participants by visit (observed)														
	0	4	8	12	16	20	24	28	32	36	40	44	48	52	56
Placebo	507	463	420	394	365	353	327	318	308	302	296	291	289	277
Naltrexone 16 mg plus bupropion	467	410	373	351	346	341	311	311	302	297	300	284	283	273
Naltrexone 32 mg plus bupropion	467	411	391	372	365	361	343	327	321	316	311	305	298	284

Fig. 4. Weight loss with naltrexone/bupropion 16/360 mg and naltrexone/bupropion 32/360 mg compared with placebo. (*From* Greenway FL, Fujioka K, Plodkowski RA, et al. Effect of naltrexone plus bupropion on weight loss in overweight and obese adults (COR-I): a multicentre, randomised, double-blind, placebo-controlled, phase 3 trial. Lancet 2010;376(9741):599; with permission.)

Forty-eight percent of the subjects in the naltrexone 32 mg plus bupropion group had a decrease in body weight of 5% or more compared with 16% assigned to placebo (*P*<.0001).

The COR-Diabetes study illustrated similar weight loss results: bupropion SR/naltrexone SR resulted in significantly greater weight reduction (5.0% vs 1.8%; *P*<.001) and greater proportion of patients achieving 5% or more weight loss (44.5% vs 18.9%, *P*<.001) compared with placebo. In addition, bupropion SR/naltrexone SR resulted in significantly greater HbA1c reduction (0.6%) compared with placebo (0.1%, *P*<.001).

In the COR-BMOD trial, participants who received an intensive group behavioral modification program (BMOD) with placebo lost an average of 5.1% of initial weight in 56 weeks of treatment. The addition of bupropion SR/naltrexone SR to BMOD significantly increased weight loss to 9.3% and resulted in 66.4% of participants losing 5% or more of initial weight, as compared with 42.5% of those who received placebo with BMOD.

All of the trials illustrated significant improvements in high-density lipoprotein and triglycerides and all trials besides COR-Diabetes found significant improvements in fasting insulin, insulin resistance index (HOMA-IR), and waist circumference.

Dosing/Administration

Naltrexone SR/bupropion SR tablets contain 8 mg naltrexone and 90 mg bupropion. Initial prescription should be for 1 tablet daily with instructions to increase by 1 tablet a week to a maximum dosage of 2 tablets in the morning, 2 tablets in the evening (32/360 mg):

- Week 1: 1 tablet in the morning
- Week 2: 1 tablet twice daily

- Week 3: 2 tablets in the morning, 1 table in the evening
- Week 4: 2 tablets twice daily

The medication should be discontinued if a patient has not achieved 5% weight loss at 12 weeks.

Side Effects

The most common TEAEs with naltrexone SR/bupropion SR include the following:

- Nausea/vomiting
- Constipation
- Headache
- Dizziness
- Insomnia
- Dry mouth
- Diarrhea

Drug-Drug Interactions

- MAOIs (use during or within 14 days of administration)
- Opioids, opioid agonists, opioid partial agonists (effect might be antagonized by naltrexone SR/bupropion SR; medication might provide inadequate pain relief)
- Abrupt discontinuation of alcohol, benzodiazepines, barbiturates, and antiepileptic drugs

Contraindications

- Pregnancy
- Uncontrolled hypertension
- Seizure disorder or history of seizures
- Use of other bupropion-containing products
- Bulimia or anorexia nervosa
- Known allergy to bupropion, naltrexone, or any other component of the drug
- History of suicidal behavior (black box warning for bupropion when used for smoking cessation and depression, but no evidence of suicidality was found in phase 3 studies)

LIRAGLUTIDE (SAXENDA)

Liraglutide is a glucagon-like peptide-1 (GLP-1) analog with 97% homology to human GLP-1, a gut-derived incretin hormone. Native GLP-1 has a half-life of only 1 to 2 minutes; however, liraglutide has a half-life of approximately 13 hours. Liraglutide was approved in 2010 for the treatment of type 2 diabetes under the brand name Victoza at dosages up to 1.8 mg daily. It improves hemoglobin A1c, blood pressure, and lipids. Because many patients on the liraglutide lost weight in a dose-dependent manner, it appeared to be a desirable treatment option for obesity.[42] In 2014, the FDA approved liraglutide as Saxenda at 3.0 mg for chronic weight management in patients with obesity. Weight loss is mediated by reduced appetite and energy intake rather than increased energy expenditure.[43]

SCALE Obesity and Prediabetes and SCALE Diabetes evaluated the effect of liraglutide 3.0 mg on subjects who were overweight or obese with prediabetes and diabetes, respectively.[44,45] Both 56-week, randomized, placebo-controlled, double-blind clinical trials illustrated significantly greater mean weight loss than placebo (8.0% vs 2.6% in SCALE Obesity and Prediabetes and 5.9% vs 2.0% in SCALE Diabetes, $P<.0001$).

The efficacy of liraglutide in maintaining weight loss was examined in the SCALE Maintain study.[46] A total of 422 subjects who were overweight or obese and lost 5% or more of their initial body weight on a low-calorie diet were randomly assigned to liraglutide 3.0 mg daily or placebo for 56 weeks. Mean weight loss on the initial diet was 6.0%. By the end of the study, participants in the liraglutide group lost an additional 6.2% compared with 0.2% with placebo (*P*<.0001) (**Fig. 5**).

Gastrointestinal symptoms, such as nausea, vomiting, and abdominal pain, were the most common reason subjects withdrew from the trials. None of the patients in SCALE Diabetes or SCALE Maintain developed pancreatitis; however, 11 subjects in SCALE Obesity and Prediabetes developed pancreatitis: 10 (0.4%) of 2841 in the liraglutide group compared with 1 (<0.1%) of 1242 in the placebo group. Increased rates of cholecystitis and cholelithiasis were also observed in phase 3 studies, but it is unclear whether the cases were related to the medication or to weight loss. Although liraglutide is associated with improvements in blood pressure and lipids, it was found to increase heart rate by 2.0/min in SCALE Diabetes.

Dosing/Administration

Liraglutide is administered as a subcutaneous injection once daily into the abdomen, thigh, or upper arm irrespective of meals. It is initiated at 0.6 mg daily for 1 week with instructions to increase by 0.6 mg weekly until 3.0 mg is reached. Slower dose titration is effective in managing gastrointestinal side effects.

The medication should be discontinued if a patient has not achieved 4% weight loss at 16 weeks.

Side Effects

The most common TEAEs with liraglutide 3.0 mg include the following:

- Nausea/vomiting
- Hypoglycemia

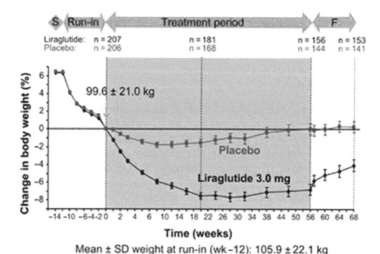

Fig. 5. Weight loss with liraglutide 3.0 mg compared with placebo after initial diet-induced weight loss. (*From* Wadden TA, Hollander P, Klein S, et al. Weight maintenance and additional weight loss with liraglutide after low-calorie-diet-induced weight loss: the SCALE Maintenance randomized study. Int J Obes (Lond) 2013;37(11):1447; with permission.)

- Diarrhea
- Constipation
- Headache
- Decreased appetite
- Dyspepsia
- Fatigue
- Dizziness
- Abdominal pain
- Increased lipase

Drug-Drug Interactions

- Insulin (risk of hypoglycemia, although studies evaluating coadministration are ongoing)

Contraindications

- Pregnancy
- Personal or family history of medullary thyroid carcinoma or multiple endocrine neoplasia syndrome type 2 (black box warning because C-cell tumors were found in rodents given liraglutide, but there is no evidence in humans)
- Prior serious hypersensitivity reaction to liraglutide or to any of the product components

FUTURE CONSIDERATIONS/SUMMARY

As multiple agents are sometimes required for clinically significant weight loss, the future of obesity medicine will likely involve combinations of agents in addition to behavioral counseling. In a recent pilot study, the addition of phentermine to lorcaserin resulted in twice as much weight loss compared with lorcaserin alone.[47] Other combined treatments are also expected.

Another medication in the pipeline is beloranib, an injectable agent that inhibits methionyl aminopeptidase 2 (MetAP2). Beloranib promotes intracellular reduction in fat biosynthesis and increased fat oxidation and lipolysis.[48] In a phase 2, double-blind, randomized controlled trial, beloranib resulted in dose-dependent progressive weight loss of 5.5, 6.9, and 10.9 kg for 0.6, 1.2, and 2.4 mg beloranib, respectively, compared with 0.4 kg with placebo (all $P < .0001$ vs placebo).[49] The study also illustrated reductions in waist circumference and body fat mass, as well as improvements in lipids, high-sensitivity C-reactive protein, and blood pressure. While generally well tolerated, there has been an association with venous thromboembolic events, which is currently being investigated.

Successful pharmacotherapy for obesity depends on tailoring treatment to a patient's behaviors and comorbidities. When choosing a medication, it is also essential to consider medication interactions, contraindications, and risk of potential adverse effects. The challenges of weight maintenance justify a long-term approach with chronic treatment and follow-up to prevent relapses.

REFERENCES

1. Hinkle W, Cordell M, Leibel R, et al. Effects of reduced weight maintenance and leptin repletion on functional connectivity of the hypothalamus in obese humans. PLoS One 2013;8(3):e59114.

2. Rosenbaum M, Hirsch J, Gallagher DA, et al. Long-term persistence of adaptive thermogenesis in subjects who have maintained a reduced body weight. Am J Clin Nutr 2008;88(4):906–12.

3. Rosenbaum M, Goldsmith R, Bloomfield D. Low-dose leptin reverses skeletal muscle, autonomic, and neuroendocrine adaptations to maintenance of reduced weight. J Clin Invest 2005;115(12):3579–86.

4. Sumithran P, Prendergast LA, Delbridge E, et al. Long-term persistence of hormonal adaptations to weight loss. N Engl J Med 2011;365(17):1597–604.

5. Goldsmith R, Joanisse DR, Gallagher D. Effects of experimental weight perturbation on skeletal muscle work efficiency, fuel utilization, and biochemistry in human subjects. Am J Physiol Regul Integr Comp Physiol 2010;298(1):R79–88.

6. Jensen MD, Ryan DH, Apovian CM, et al. 2013 AHA/ACC/TOS guideline for the management of overweight and obesity in adults: a report of the American College of Cardiology/American Heart Association Task Force on Practice Guidelines and The Obesity Society. J Am Coll Cardiol 2014;63(25 Pt B):2985–3023.

7. Apovian CM, Aronne LJ, Bessesen DH, et al. Pharmacological management of obesity: an Endocrine Society clinical practice guideline. J Clin Endocrinol Metab 2015;100(2):342–62.

8. Golden J. FDA 2007 Draft Guidance for Industry. Developing products for weight management. Silver Spring (MD): U.S. Department of Health and Human Services, Food and Drug Administration; 2007. Available at: http://www.fda.gov/downloads/AdvisoryCommittees/CommitteesMeetingMaterials/Drugs/EndocrinologicandMetabolicDrugsAdvisoryCommittee/UCM299133.pdf. Accessed September 22, 2015.

9. Heal DJ, Gosden J, Smith SL. Regulatory challenges for new drugs to treat obesity and comorbid metabolic disorders. Br J Clin Pharmacol 2009;68(6):861–74.

10. American Medical Association. Policy H-440.842. Recognition of Obesity as a Disease; 2013. Available at: https://www.ama-assn.org/ssl3/ecomm/PolicyFinderForm.pl?site=www.ama-assn.org&uri=/resources/html/PolicyFinder/policyfiles/HnE/H-440.842.HTM.

11. Qsymia [package insert]. Mountain View, CA: VIVUS, Inc; 2012.

12. Belviq [package insert]. Zofingen, Switzerland: Arena Pharmaceuticals; 2012.

13. Contrave [package insert]. Deerfield, IL: Takeda Pharmaceuticals America, Inc; 2014.

14. Saxenda [package insert]. Plainsboro, NJ: Novo Nordisk; 2014.

15. Suprenza [package insert]. Cranford, NJ: Akrimax Pharmaceuticals, LLC; 2013.

16. Xenical [package insert]. South San Francisco, CA: Genentech USA, Inc; 2015.

17. Rothman RB, Baumann MH, Dersch CM, et al. Amphetamine-type central nervous system stimulants release norepinephrine more potently than they release dopamine and serotonin. Synapse 2001;39(1):32–41.

18. Bachorik L. FDA announces withdrawal fenfluramine and dexfenfluramine (Fen-Phen). Silver Spring (MD): U.S Food and Drug Administration; 1997. Available at: http://www.fda.gov/Drugs/DrugSafety/PostmarketDrugSafetyInformationforPatientsandProviders/ucm179871.htm. Accessed September 22, 2015.

19. Yanovski SZ, Yanovski JA. Long-term drug treatment for obesity: a systematic and clinical review. JAMA 2014;311(1):74–86.

20. Aronne LJ, Wadden TA, Peterson C, et al. Evaluation of phentermine and topiramate versus phentermine/topiramate extended-release in obese adults. Obesity (Silver Spring) 2013;21(11):2163–71.

21. Munro JF, MacCuish AC, Wilson EM, et al. Comparison of continuous and intermittent anorectic therapy in obesity. Br Med J 1968;1(5588):352–4.
22. Alli [package insert]. Moon Township, PA: GlaxoSmithKline Consumer Healthcare, LP; 2015.
23. Zhi J, Melia AT, Guerciolini R, et al. Retrospective population-based analysis of the dose-response (fecal fat excretion) relationship of orlistat in normal and obese volunteers. Clin Pharmacol Ther 1994;56(1):82–5.
24. Torgerson JS, Hauptman J, Boldrin MN, et al. XENical in the prevention of diabetes in obese subjects (XENDOS) study: a randomized study of orlistat as an adjunct to lifestyle changes for the prevention of type 2 diabetes in obese patients. Diabetes Care 2004;27(1):155–61.
25. Rucker D, Padwal R, Li SK, et al. Long term pharmacotherapy for obesity and overweight: updated meta-analysis. BMJ 2007;335(7631):1194–9.
26. Wilding J, Van Gaal L, Rissanen A, et al, OBES-002 Study Group. A randomized double-blind placebo-controlled study of the long-term efficacy and safety of topiramate in the treatment of obese subjects. Int J Obes Relat Metab Disord 2004; 28:1399–410.
27. Bray GA, Hollander P, Klein S, et al. A 6-month randomized, placebo controlled, dose-ranging trial of topiramate for weight loss in obesity. Obes Res 2003;11: 722–33.
28. Kushner RF. Weight loss strategies for treatment of obesity. Prog Cardiovasc Dis 2014;56(4):465–72.
29. Allison DB, Gadde KM, Garvey WT, et al. Controlled-release phentermine/topiramate in severely obese adults: a randomized controlled trial (EQUIP). Obesity (Silver Spring) 2012;20(2):330–42.
30. Gadde KM, Allison DB, Ryan DH, et al. Effects of low-dose, controlled-release, phentermine plus topiramate combination on weight and associated comorbidities in overweight and obese adults (CONQUER): a randomised, placebo-controlled, phase 3 trial. Lancet 2011;377(9774):1341–52.
31. Garvey WT, Ryan DH, Look M, et al. Two-year sustained weight loss and metabolic benefits with controlled-release phentermine/topiramate in obese and overweight adults (SEQUEL): a randomized, placebo-controlled, phase 3 extension study. Am J Clin Nutr 2012;95(2):297–308.
32. Qsymia Risk Evaluation and Mitigation Strategy (REMS). VIVUS, Inc. Available at: http://www.qsymiarems.com/. Accessed October 12, 2015.
33. Connolly HM, Crary JL, McGoon MD, et al. Valvular heart disease associated with fenfluramine-phentermine. N Engl J Med 1997;337(9):581–8.
34. Smith SR, Weissman NJ, Anderson CM, et al. Multicenter, placebo-controlled trial of lorcaserin for weight management. N Engl J Med 2010;363(3):245–56.
35. Fidler MC, Sanchez M, Raether B, et al. A one-year randomized trial of lorcaserin for weight loss in obese and overweight adults: the BLOSSOM trial. J Clin Endocrinol Metab 2011;96(10):3067–77.
36. O'Neil PM, Smith SR, Weissman NJ, et al. Randomized placebo-controlled clinical trial of lorcaserin for weight loss in type 2 diabetes mellitus: the BLOOM-DM study. Obesity (Silver Spring) 2012;20(7):1426–36.
37. Greenway FL, Whitehouse MJ, Guttadauria M, et al. Rational design of a combination medication for the treatment of obesity. Obesity (Silver Spring) 2009;17(1): 30–9.
38. Greenway FL, Fujioka K, Plodkowski RA, et al. Effect of naltrexone plus bupropion on weight loss in overweight and obese adults (COR-I): a multicentre,

randomised, double-blind, placebo-controlled, phase 3 trial. Lancet 2010; 376(9741):595–605.

39. Apovian CM, Aronne L, Rubino D, et al. A randomized, phase 3 trial of naltrexone SR/bupropion SR on weight and obesity-related risk factors (COR-II). Obesity (Silver Spring) 2013;21(5):935–43.

40. Wadden TA, Foreyt JP, Foster GD, et al. Weight loss with naltrexone SR/bupropion SR combination therapy as an adjunct to behavior modification: the COR-BMOD trial. Obesity (Silver Spring) 2011;19(1):110–20.

41. Hollander P, Gupta AK, Plodkowski R, et al. Effects of naltrexone sustained-release/bupropion sustained-release combination therapy on body weight and glycemic parameters in overweight and obese patients with type 2 diabetes. Diabetes Care 2013;36(12):4022–9.

42. Nauck M, Frid A, Hermansen K, et al. Efficacy and safety comparison of liraglutide, glimepiride, and placebo, all in combination with metformin, in type 2 diabetes: the LEAD (liraglutide effect and action in diabetes)-2 study. Diabetes Care 2009;32(1):84–90.

43. van Can J, Sloth B, Jensen CB, et al. Effects of the once-daily GLP-1 analog liraglutide on gastric emptying, glycemic parameters, appetite and energy metabolism in obese, non-diabetic adults. Int J Obes (Lond) 2014;38(6):784–93.

44. Pi-Sunyer X, Astrup A, Fujioka K, et al. A randomized, controlled trial of 3.0 mg of liraglutide in weight management. N Engl J Med 2015;373(1):11–22.

45. Davies MJ, Bergenstal R, Bode B, et al. Efficacy of liraglutide for weight loss among patients with type 2 diabetes: the SCALE Diabetes randomized clinical trial. JAMA 2015;314(7):687–99.

46. Wadden TA, Hollander P, Klein S, et al. Weight maintenance and additional weight loss with liraglutide after low-calorie-diet-induced weight loss: the SCALE Maintenance randomized study. Int J Obes (Lond) 2013;37(11):1443–51.

47. Smith SR, Garvey WT, Greenway F, et al. Combination weight management (WM) pharmacotherapy with lorcaserin (LOR) and immediate release (IR) Phentermine (phen) [abstract]. Poster presented at Obesity Week. Boston, MA, November 2–7, 2014.

48. Hughes TE, Kim DD, Marjason J, et al. Ascending dose-controlled trial of beloranib, a novel obesity treatment for safety, tolerability, and weight loss in obese women. Obesity (Silver Spring) 2013;21(9):1782–8.

49. Kim DD, Krishnarajah J, Lillioja S, et al. Efficacy and safety of beloranib for weight loss in obese adults: a randomized controlled trial. Diabetes Obes Metab 2015; 17(6):566–72.

Potential Mechanisms Mediating Sustained Weight Loss Following Roux-en-Y Gastric Bypass and Sleeve Gastrectomy

CrossMark

Janine M. Makaronidis, MBChB[a,b,c], Rachel L. Batterham, MBBS, PhD[a,b,c],*

KEYWORDS

- Obesity • Bariatric surgery • Sleeve gastrectomy • Roux-en-Y gastric bypass
- Gut hormones • Bile acids • Eating behavior • Microbiome

KEY POINTS

- Reduced energy intake, as a result of altered eating behavior, is the main driver for weight loss in humans following Roux-en-Y gastric bypass and sleeve gastrectomy.
- The biological mediators underlying altered eating behavior after surgery remain incompletely understood, but changed gut-derived signals as a consequence of altered nutrient and/or biliary flow are key candidates.
- Understanding the interplay between gut hormones, bile acids, and the microbiome and their relative roles will enable the development of nonsurgical treatment options for obesity.

INTRODUCTION

Bariatric surgery is currently the only effective treatment for severe obesity, which is defined by a body mass index (BMI) equal to or greater than 40 kg/m^2, or greater than 35 kg/m^2 in the presence of obesity-related complications.[1] Bariatric surgery involves surgical manipulation of the gastrointestinal (GI) tract, which alters nutrient

The authors have nothing to disclose.
[a] Department of Medicine, Centre for Obesity Research, Rayne Institute, University College London, Rayne Building, 5 University Street, London WC1E 6JF, UK; [b] University College London Hospitals (UCLH) Bariatric Centre for Weight Loss, Metabolic and Endocrine Surgery, UCLH, Ground Floor West Wing, 250 Euston Road, London NW1 2PG, UK; [c] National Institute of Health Research University College London Hospitals Biomedical Research Centre, 149 Tottenham Court Road, Kings Cross, London W1T 7DN, UK
* Corresponding author. Centre for Obesity Research, University College London, Rayne Building, 5 University Street, London WC1E 6JF, UK.
E-mail address: r.batterham@ucl.ac.uk

Endocrinol Metab Clin N Am 45 (2016) 539–552
http://dx.doi.org/10.1016/j.ecl.2016.04.006
0889-8529/16/$ – see front matter © 2016 Elsevier Inc. All rights reserved.

flow and affects GI biology. These changes engender beneficial effects on energy and glucose homeostasis.[2–4]

Gaining an understanding of the mechanisms underlying the sustained weight loss and metabolic benefits produced by bariatric surgery may hold the key to developing novel nonsurgical treatments for obesity and type 2 diabetes (T2D). In particular, it is now clear that altered eating behavior plays a key role in mediating the weight loss following sleeve gastrectomy (SG) and Roux-en-Y gastric bypass (RYGB) in humans.[5,6] This has led to intense research efforts focused on delineating how SG and RYGB affect the drive to eat.

HISTORICAL PERSPECTIVES

The concept of bariatric surgery emerged in the 1950s from the observation that small intestine resection resulted in weight loss.[7] The first procedure aimed specifically at inducing weight loss, a jejunoileal bypass (JIB), in which most of the small intestine was bypassed, was performed in 1953.[8] The theoretic basis driving the development of the JIB was that weight loss would be achieved through malabsorption. This indeed was the case; however, weight loss was coupled with electrolyte imbalances, nutritional deficiencies, diarrhea, and liver failure, necessitating the development of less malabsorptive surgical procedures.[8] In addition, patients with peptic ulcer disease who underwent gastric resection and/or bypass were also observed to lose weight. In these patients, reduced stomach capacity (restriction) and decreased digestion were suggested to drive weight loss.[8] This led Mason and colleagues[9] to perform the first gastric bypass procedure for weight loss in 1967.[8] These 2 different approaches formed the basis for subsequent "malabsorptive" and "restrictive" procedures or "hybrid" procedures, combining these 2 mechanisms; for example, the RYGB, which has evolved over the ensuing 60 years.[7,8] However, it is now recognized that most bariatric procedures engender weight loss and metabolic improvements by mechanisms other than restriction and/or malabsorption.

Over the past decade, the beneficial effects of bariatric surgery on weight and obesity-associated comorbidities have resulted in a marked increase in the number of bariatric procedures undertaken, with approximately 460,000 operations performed in 2013.[10] The choice of surgical procedure has, and still is, evolving, guided by technical advances, the beneficial clinical outcomes achieved, short-term and long-term complication rates, and by the evidence regarding the physiology underpinning their success. Currently, the most common procedures undertaken globally are RYGB, SG, adjustable gastric banding (AGB), and biliopancreatic duodenal switch.[10] Purely restrictive procedures, such as AGB and vertical banded gastroplasty, are now less commonly performed. RYGB and SG represent the vast majority of procedures undertaken and form the focus of this review (**Fig. 1**).

ROUX-EN-Y GASTRIC BYPASS

In RYGB, a small gastric pouch of approximately 20 mL is created through dividing the stomach. This is anastomosed with the mid-jejunum, creating the Roux limb, allowing ingested nutrients to bypass most of the stomach, duodenum, and proximal jejunum.[11] Anastomosis of the biliopancreatic limb with the jejunum allows drainage of bile acids and pancreatic secretions, which mix with the ingested nutrients in the jejunum.[11] RYGB is established as an efficient treatment for severe obesity, with the long-term (>20 years) outcome data demonstrating sustained weight loss and favorable metabolic outcomes, particularly relating to T2D.[12,13]

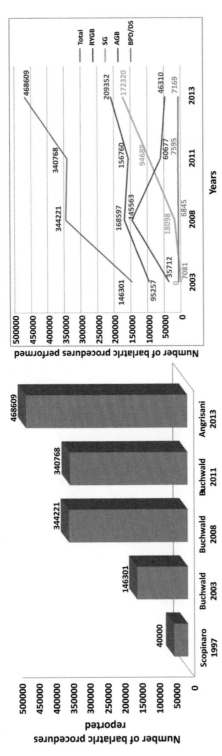

Fig. 1. Left: Number of bariatric procedures performed by published surveys. Right: Numbers of procedures performed worldwide. (*From* Angrisani L, Santonicola A, Iovino P, et al. Bariatric surgery worldwide 2013. Obes Surg 2015;25(10):1824 and 1829; with permission.)

SLEEVE GASTRECTOMY

SG, intended as a purely restrictive procedure, was initially performed as a first-stage procedure to reduce weight in patients with BMI greater than 50 kg/m². Following weight loss, this was then transformed into a hybrid procedure, such as RYGB. However, SG alone resulted in significant sustained weight loss and metabolic benefits, leading to the adoption of SG as a standalone procedure.[10,14,15] SG involves transection along the greater curvature of the stomach and removing 80% to 90% of the total stomach volume, including the fundus and body, without intervention to the small intestine.[16] Gastric contents pass rapidly into the duodenum.

SG is technically easier than RYGB, associated with fewer complications and perioperative and nutritional complications and produces similar short-term weight-loss and clinical outcomes compared with RYGB.[14,17,18] Consequently, the proportion of SG has increased from 0% to 37% from 2003 to 2013 and is anticipated to become the most common bariatric procedure undertaken.[10] Randomized control trials are currently under way, comparing outcomes post-RYBG against SG in severely obese individuals and comparing the efficacy of the 2 procedures with regard to resolution of T2D[19,20] (**Fig. 2, Table 1**).

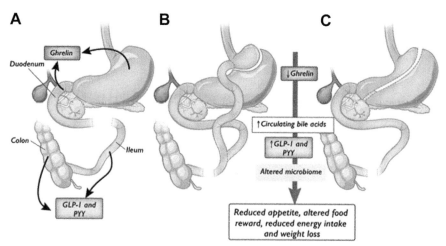

Fig. 2. Illustrations of (*A*) normal GI tract, (*B*) RYGB, and (*C*) SG. (*A*) Multiple hormones are secreted from the GI tract. Ghrelin is secreted from the P/D1 cells of the gastric fundus, whereas GLP-1 and PYY are secreted from L-cells located predominantly in the ileum and colon. (*B*) RYGB; nutrients bypass most of the stomach and flow directly into the mid-jejunum. Anastomosis of the biliopancreatic limb with the jejunum allows drainage of bile acids into the common limb, where ingested nutrients and bile acids mix. (*C*) SG; nutrients pass rapidly from the gastric sleeve into the duodenum with unaltered flow of bile acids. Following RYGB and SG, circulating ghrelin levels are reduced, meal-stimulated PYY and GLP-1 are increased. Bile acid secretion is enhanced and the microbiome is altered. These changes in gut-derived factors are thought to drive reduced appetite and altered food reward value, leading to a decreased energy intake and weight loss.

Table 1
Weight loss, type 2 diabetes remission, and complications following Roux-en-Y gastric bypass (RYGB) and sleeve gastrectomy (SG)

Outcome	RYGB, %	SG, %
Weight loss (%WL)		
STAMPEDE (3 y)[17]	24.5 ± 9.1	21.1 ± 8.9
BOLD data 6 mo[14]	26.8	24
BOLD data 12 mo[14]	34.2	29.5
Type 2 diabetes remission at 3 y		
STAMPEDE[17]	38	24
Complications (BOLD data)[14]		
All complications	10	6.3 (P<.001)
Serious complications	2.5	2.4 (P = .736)

The Surgical TreAtment and Medications Potentially Eradicate Diabetes Efficiently[17] (STAMPEDE) trial, investigated 3-year weight loss and remission of type 2 diabetes in patients with type 2 diabetes, randomised to medical therapy or medical therapy plus either RYGB or SG.[17] The Bariatric Outcomes Longitudinal Database (BOLD) compared weight loss and complications following SG and RYGB.[14]
    Data from Refs.[14,17,72]

BODY WEIGHT REGULATION AND THE IMPACT OF OBESITY

The mechanisms regulating body weight are complex and involve neural circuits controlling energy homeostasis as well as reward-related pathways. Regulatory brain centers continually integrate peripheral signals relating to energy stores and nutrient availability to determine feeding behavior.[4] Leptin, insulin, and gut-derived factors are established as key regulators of energy homeostasis.[21] Peripheral long-term signals, providing information regarding availability of energy stores via insulin and leptin secretion in response to adiposity, and short-term signals regarding nutrient and meal-derived energy availability modulate hunger and satiety perception.[22]

Gut hormones are secreted from the GI enteroendocrine cells in response to nutrient ingestion and act as autocrine, paracrine, and endocrine regulators of energy and glucose homeostasis.[4,23] The anorectic hormone peptide YY3-36 (PYY) and glucagonlike peptide-1 (GLP-1), an incretin hormone, are both secreted in response to nutrient ingestion from enteroendocrine L-cells present throughout the GI tract.[5,23] PYY has potent anorectic effects, with exogenous administration shown to reduce food intake.[24] Evidence from experimental imaging and translational studies indicate that PYY mediates its anorectic effects predominantly by acting on central appetite-regulating circuits and brain regions involved in food reward.[25] There is also evidence that circulating GLP-1 has appetite-suppressing effects by modulating neural activity within homeostatic and reward brain centers, in a manner additive to PYY.[26] The orexigenic hormone ghrelin, produced by P/D1 cells in oxyntic glands in the gastric fundus, also acts on homeostatic and reward centers involved in appetite regulation to control energy intake.[27] Circulating ghrelin levels increase in the fasted state and decrease postprandially.[23,27] Elevations in ghrelin levels have been shown to enhance the hedonic responses to eating.[28]

Bile acids, in addition to their role in lipid metabolism, influence glucose and energy homeostasis, through signaling and nutrient sensing in the hepatoportal circulation.[29] Furthermore, bile acids directly affect the intestinal microbiome through local effects on the intestinal milieu.[30] The microbiome, which has recently been implicated in the pathophysiology of several disease processes, also contributes toward energy homeostasis.[29,31] A dysbiotic relationship between host and micriobiome could contribute to the development of obesity through increasing intestinal permeability and energy absorption.[29]

Taste and olfactory signals influence food selection and, consequently, energy intake.[32] Interestingly, there is emerging evidence for an interplay between signals of energy homeostasis and taste and smell. Insulin leptin, GLP-1, PYY and ghrelin have been found in saliva and their cognate receptors identified on taste buds and olfactory neurons.[32] It is now also clear that rewarding food-related sensory stimuli can override satiety signals leading to excess energy intake. Chronic excess energy intake leads to deregulation of the homeostatic mechanisms that normally control body weight. Thus, an obese individual is predisposed to gain more weight.[28] Physiologic changes in obesity include resistance to the effects of both leptin and insulin, blunted circulating gut hormone responses to nutrient ingestion, with reduced plasma PYY and GLP-1 levels, dysregulation of circulating ghrelin, reduced circulating bile acids levels, altered gut microbiome, and decreased vagal signal transmission.[33]

Obese individuals perceive foods high in sugar and fat content more pleasurable compared with lean individuals.[34] Furthermore, brain-imaging studies have shown increased stimulation of central reward pathways in response to eating or food cues in obese compared with normal-weight individuals.[34–36] Consequently, eating behavior in obesity becomes dissociated form perceptions of satiety and hunger.[37]

Why Is Weight Loss Maintenance Through Nonsurgical Means So Difficult?

Weight loss through intentional caloric restriction results in compensatory changes that aim to defend the higher body weight.[36] These include decreased energy expenditure, due to reduced lean muscle mass and reduced sympathetic activity,[38] reduced circulating leptin, GLP-1 and PYY levels with increased ghrelin levels,[36] and altered brain neural response to food cues. Moreover, these changes are sustained in the long term.[36] **Table 2** compares physiologic responses to weight loss though dieting with bariatric surgery.

Sustained Weight Loss Following Bariatric Surgery

In contrast to weight loss though calorie-restricted dieting, bariatric surgery poses an effective treatment for severe obesity with significant weight loss, sustained in the long-term. The 20-year outcome data from the Swedish Obese Subjects (SOS) study showed that patients who received bariatric surgery achieved a significantly greater mean body weight reduction of 18% ($\pm$11%) compared with 1% ($\pm$3%) in patients who received standard medical treatment through their local health centers.[12] However, it is important to note that the weight loss achieved after surgery follows a wide and normal distribution, and studying the extreme responders may provide key insights into the mechanisms involved (**Fig. 3**).[39]

Mechanisms Other Than Restriction and Malabsorption Are at Play

The multifactorial mechanisms promoting weight loss and improvements in obesity-related comorbidities following RYGB/SG are incompletely understood. However, it is now clear that the beneficial effects of bariatric surgery are not achieved through restriction and malabsorption alone.[40,41] Reduced energy intake, as a result of altered eating behavior, is the main driver for weight loss in humans.[5,23,42] Here we review the key eating behavior changes that occur following RYGB and SG together with the potential mechanisms by which RYGB and SG impact on central appetite-regulating circuits.

Table 2
Comparison of the effects of weight loss due to "dieting" or following bariatric surgery on signals of energy balance and appetite

Measure	Weight Loss Through Dieting	Weight Loss Through Bariatric Surgery
Ghrelin	Levels increase with dieting[36,55]	Reduction with SG, possible reduction with RYGB in the immediate postoperative period[54]
PYY	Reduced levels[29,36]	Increased levels[18,54,73]
GLP-1	Reduced levels[29,36]	Increased levels[18,23,54]
Leptin	Reduced levels[72]	Reduced levels[72] Suggestion that leptin sensitivity may improve[21]
Bile acids	Unclear. Blunted bile acid response in obesity with no significant difference following AGB[74]	Increased secretion
Intestinal microbiome	Improvement with weight loss[75]	Altered ("leaner") microbiome[30,75]
Perceived hunger	Increased hunger[36]	Reduced hunger[44]
Perceived satiety	Lower satiety[36]	Increased satiety[6]
Food aversions	—	Altered food preference[48]
Long-term sustainability	Average 80% weight regain in 5 y[76]	Average weight loss of 25% at 10% and 18% at 20 y post-RYGB[3,12]
Body weight regulation	Homeostatic mechanisms defend higher body weight[36,76]	Resets body weight "set point" to lower weight[5]

Abbreviations: AGB, adjustable gastric banding; RYGB, Roux-en-Y gastric bypass; SG, sleeve gastrectomy.

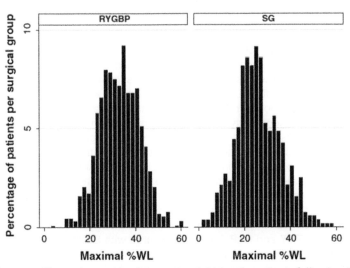

Fig. 3. Histogram illustrating maximal percent weight loss in patients following RYGB and SG. WL, weight loss. (*From* Manning S, Pucci A, Carter NC, et al. Early postoperative weight loss predicts maximal weight loss after sleeve gastrectomy and Roux-en-Y gastric bypass. Surg Endosc 2015;29(6):1487; with permission.)

EATING BEHAVIOR CHANGES FOLLOWING ROUX-EN-Y GASTRIC BYPASS AND SLEEVE GASTRECTOMY

Changes in eating behavior following bariatric surgery were first suggested by Bray and colleagues[43] in 1980, who observed a reduction in food intake following intestinal bypass. They proposed that "oral" (taste or smell), "gastrointestinal" (mechanical distension or nutrient composition) and "postingestional" (nutrient or hormonal satiety mediators) factors as possible mediators.[43] Following RYGB and SG, patients report appetite changes with reduced hunger and increased satiety.[44–46] After surgery, altered subjective taste and smell, together with the food aversions, are common and are thought to drive a change in food preferences away from sweet and high-fat foods.[6,47,48] Moreover, the reward value of food-related stimuli is decreased after surgery.[6,49] A study using progressive ratio tasks to assess reward values of food before and after RYGB, revealed a significant reduction in the reward value of sweet and high-fat foods after surgery, compared with a control group.[50] Studies using functional MRI scanning have shown lower brain-hedonic responses to food following RYGB compared with AGB, associated with lower palatability of high-fat and energy-dense foods.[49,51,52] Consequently, a change in the way food is perceived is considered a key contributor toward the altered food preference leading to a lower energy intake after surgery.

POTENTIAL MECHANISMS UNDERLYING EATING BEHAVIOR CHANGES AFTER SURGERY IN HUMANS

Altered eating behavior after RYGB and SG results in a lower energy intake, which is the main driver for weight loss in humans.[23,53] The biological mediators underlying these changes remain incompletely understood, but gut-derived signals as a consequence of altered nutrient and/or biliary flow are key candidates. Interestingly, although RYGB and SG differentially alter GI anatomy, they lead to comparable outcomes in terms of weight loss and metabolic benefits.[18,54]

Gut Hormones

A landmark publication by Cummings and colleagues[55] in 2002, showed that circulating ghrelin levels rose with calorie-restricted diets but reduced markedly post-RYGB. These findings acted as the catalyst for investigating the role of gut hormones as mediators of the beneficial effects of surgery. Subsequently, there has been some controversy regarding post-RYGB circulating ghrelin levels. However, these differences reflect methodological variability in terms of duration after surgery and sample processing techniques, as the active from of ghrelin, acyl-ghrelin, is highly labile and requires specific processing to accurately measure circulating levels.[56,57] SG, which involves removing most ghrelin-producing cells, leads to sustained and greater reduction in circulating acyl-ghrelin levels than RYGB.[54] Both RYGB and SG are associated with marked increase in nutrient-stimulated circulating levels of PYY and GLP-1.[54,58] These changes occur before and are independent of weight loss, pointing toward a procedure-related mechanism. Comparative studies suggest that RYGB leads to greater post-meal PYY and GLP-1 levels compared with SG.[54]

Cross-sectional studies have shown that patients with poor weight loss exhibit higher subjective hunger, lower subjective satiety, higher ghrelin, and lower PYY and GLP-1 compared with patients with good weight loss.[59,60] Furthermore, inhibition of PYY and GLP-1 with somatostatin analogue, octreotide, leads to return of appetite and increased energy intake and weight gain.[61]

Gut hormone receptors for PYY, GLP-1, and ghrelin are expressed on taste buds and there is emerging evidence that these hormones modulate taste.[62,63] Given that the postoperative changes in eating behavior and taste perception overlap with the known effects of changes in gut hormones, it is biologically plausible that these changes can be attributed to increased gut hormone secretion and signaling through gut hormone receptors. Favorable gut hormone responses after surgery, with increased meal-stimulated PYY and GLP-1 levels, combined with lower ghrelin levels, are clearly associated with higher weight loss.[54] However, the causative factor of this effect is not yet established.

RYGB and SG have been undertaken in transgenic rodents so as to provide mechanistic insights into the role of altered gut hormones. Somewhat surprisingly, global GLP-1 receptor knockout mice exhibit similar weight loss and glycemic improvement following SG and RYGB to their wild-type littermates.[64,65] Similarly, global ghrelin knockout mice respond in a similar manner following SG to their wild-type control mice.[66] However, PYY knockout mice exhibit reduced early postoperative weight loss and glycemic improvement compared with wild-type mice.[4,66] These observations suggest that weight loss and metabolic improvements are at least partially mediated by postoperative modulation of PYY.

Other gut hormones with effects on feeding behavior have also been studied. Oxyntomodulin, a pro-glucagon–derived peptide with parallel actions to GLP-1 and anorectic effects, has been shown to increase post-RYGB.[23] The anorexigenic hormone cholecystokinin has been suggested to act synergistically with leptin, and amylin, a pancreatic hormone cosecreted with insulin, may also exhibit anorectic effects.[21] However, the extent of their role in mediating the effects of post-bariatric surgery has not been established.

Bile Acids and Microbiome

Both RYGB and SG induce changes in the interaction between ingested nutrients and bile acids. Despite their anatomic differences, they exert similar effects on bile acids, altering both their composition and secretion.[30] RYGB and SG both lead to increased bile acid secretion, which has been linked to improved lipid and glucose metabolism.[29]

The metabolic effects of bile acids are mediated through signaling via 2 receptors; the cell surface G protein-coupled receptor 5 (TGR5) and farnesoid X receptor (FXR).[30] TGR5 is expressed on L-cells and activation of the receptor leads to GLP-1 release. Increased TGR5 activation is a proposed mechanism contributing to higher GLP-1 levels following bariatric surgery.[29] The FXR pathways have several functions, including regulating bile acid synthesis, secretion, conjugation, and regulation of the intestinal microbiome.[29,30,67,68] The latter influences energy absorption, through altering intestinal mucosal permeability, and energy expenditure by intracellular thyroid hormone activation via FXR signaling.[29,69] Following RYGB and SG, the intestinal microbiome is altered. Moreover, the finding that transplant of feces from RYGB-treated to germ-free mice resulted in significantly greater weight loss compared with mice receiving feces from sham-surgery treated mice suggests that the altered microbiome per se contributes to weight loss.[70] However, significant differences exist between the rodent and the human microbiome, as well as in the physiologic processes driving weight loss. Thus, the relationship between postoperative weight loss and bile acids, FXR signaling, and intestinal bacteria in humans remains to be clarified.

Enteroplasticity

Enteroplasticity refers to the postsurgical adaptations, including remodeling of the intestinal mucosa, morphologic changes, and alterations in innervation.[30] Increased postoperative nutrient exposure of intestinal L-cells as a consequence of rapid gastric emptying and/or anatomic GI tract rearrangements lead to enhanced secretion of PYY, GLP-1 and oxyntomodulin.[29,30] In addition, there is evidence that L-cells proliferate following RYGB and SG and that L-cells exhibit increased nutrient sensitivity, releasing more PYY and GLP-1 for a given nutrient stimulant.[71] Neurophysiological studies suggest that vagus nerve signaling also increases post-RYGB.[33] These intestinal adaptations may contribute to the sustained metabolic effects of bariatric surgery.

THE FUTURE: KNIFELESS SURGERY?

Bariatric surgery is a safe and highly effective treatment for obesity and T2D. Nevertheless, it requires long-term follow-up and monitoring for complications, nutritional deficiencies, and development or relapse of T2D. Despite the increasing numbers of procedures performed, there is high geographic variability in accessibility to surgery. In addition, although bariatric surgery is highly effective, at the individual level, clinical response is highly variable. Therefore, developing novel therapies that mimic the post–bariatric surgery internal milieu poses an appealing therapeutic aim. Understanding the interplay among gut hormones, bile acids, and the microbiome will be key to fully elucidate the success of bariatric surgery and the reasons behind the variability in response. Such findings would enable the development of nonsurgical treatment options for obesity, leading to sustainable weight loss and reduction in obesity-related morbidity and mortality.

REFERENCES

1. Gloy VL, Briel M, Bhatt DL, et al. Bariatric surgery versus non-surgical treatment for obesity: a systematic review and meta-analysis of randomised controlled trials. BMJ 2013;347:f5934.
2. Buchwald H, Avidor Y, Braunwald E, et al. Bariatric surgery: a systematic review and meta-analysis. JAMA 2004;292(14):1724–37.
3. Buchwald H, Estok R, Fahrbach K, et al. Weight and type 2 diabetes after bariatric surgery: systematic review and meta-analysis. Am J Med 2009;122(3): 248–56.e5.
4. Miras AD, le Roux CW. Mechanisms underlying weight loss after bariatric surgery. Nat Rev Gastroenterol Hepatol 2013;10(10):575–84.
5. Manning S, Pucci A, Batterham RL. Roux-en-Y gastric bypass: effects on feeding behavior and underlying mechanisms. J Clin Invest 2015;125(3):939–48.
6. le Roux CW, Bueter M. The physiology of altered eating behaviour after Roux-en-Y gastric bypass. Exp Physiol 2014;99(9):1128–32.
7. Saber AA, Elgamal MH, McLeod MK. Bariatric surgery: the past, present, and future. Obes Surg 2008;18(1):121–8.
8. Buchwald H. The evolution of metabolic/bariatric surgery. Obes Surg 2014;24(8): 1126–35.
9. Mason EE, Ito C. Gastric bypass in obesity. Surg Clin North Am 1967;47(6): 1345–51.
10. Angrisani L, Santonicola A, Iovino P, et al. Bariatric surgery worldwide 2013. Obes Surg 2015;25(10):1822–32.
11. Olbers T, Lonroth H, Fagevik-Olsen M, et al. Laparoscopic gastric bypass: development of technique, respiratory function, and long-term outcome. Obes Surg 2003;13(3):364–70.

12. Sjostrom L. Review of the key results from the Swedish Obese Subjects (SOS) trial—a prospective controlled intervention study of bariatric surgery. J Intern Med 2013;273(3):219–34.
13. Sjostrom L, Peltonen M, Jacobson P, et al. Association of bariatric surgery with long-term remission of type 2 diabetes and with microvascular and macrovascular complications. JAMA 2014;311(22):2297–304.
14. Sczepaniak JP, Owens ML, Shukla H, et al. Comparability of weight loss reporting after gastric bypass and sleeve gastrectomy using BOLD data 2008-2011. Obes Surg 2015;25(5):788 95.
15. Carlin AM, Zeni TM, English WJ, et al. The comparative effectiveness of sleeve gastrectomy, gastric bypass, and adjustable gastric banding procedures for the treatment of morbid obesity. Ann Surg 2013;257(5):791–7.
16. Abu-Jaish W, Rosenthal RJ. Sleeve gastrectomy: a new surgical approach for morbid obesity. Expert Rev Gastroenterol Hepatol 2010;4(1):101–19.
17. Schauer PR, Bhatt DL, Kirwan JP, et al. Bariatric surgery versus intensive medical therapy for diabetes-3-year outcomes. N Engl J Med 2014;370(21):2002–13.
18. Peterli R, Steinert RE, Woelnerhanssen B, et al. Metabolic and hormonal changes after laparoscopic Roux-en-Y gastric bypass and sleeve gastrectomy: a randomized, prospective trial. Obes Surg 2012;22(5):740–8.
19. Göteborg University. Sleeve gastrectomy and Roux-en-Y gastric bypass in the treatment of type 2 diabetes mellitus ClinicalTrials.gov [Internet]. Bethesda (MD): National Library of Medicine (US); 2015. Available at: https://clinicaltrials.gov/ct2/show/NCT01984762?term=Sleeve+Gastrectomy+and+Roux-en-Y+Gastric+Bypass+in+the+Treatment+of+Type+2+Diabetes+Mellitus&rank=1.
20. Strasbourg IHU. Laparoscopic sleeve gastrectomy versus Roux-en-Y gastric bypass ClinicalTrials.gov. Bethesda (MD): National Library of Medicine (US); 2015. Available at. https://clinicaltrials.gov/ct2/show/record/NCT02475590?term=obesity+sleeve+gastrectomy+roux-en-y&rank=3.
21. Suzuki K, Jayasena CN, Bloom SR. Obesity and appetite control. Exp Diabetes Res 2012;2012:824305.
22. Morton GJ, Meek TH, Schwartz MW. Neurobiology of food intake in health and disease. Nat Rev Neurosci 2014;15(6):367–78.
23. Scott WR, Batterham RL. Roux-en-Y gastric bypass and laparoscopic sleeve gastrectomy: understanding weight loss and improvements in type 2 diabetes after bariatric surgery. Am J Physiol Regul Integr Comp Physiol 2011;301(1):R15–27.
24. Batterham RL, Cowley MA, Small CJ, et al. Gut hormone PYY(3-36) physiologically inhibits food intake. Nature 2002;418(6898):650–4.
25. Batterham RL, ffytche DH, Rosenthal JM, et al. PYY modulation of cortical and hypothalamic brain areas predicts feeding behaviour in humans. Nature 2007; 450(7166):106–9.
26. Manning S, Pucci A, Batterham RL. GLP-1: a mediator of the beneficial metabolic effects of bariatric surgery? Physiology (Bethesda) 2015;30(1):50–62.
27. Muller TD, Nogueiras R, Andermann ML, et al. Ghrelin. Mol Metab 2015;4(6):437–60.
28. Berthoud HR. Metabolic and hedonic drives in the neural control of appetite: who is the boss? Curr Opin Neurobiol 2011;21(6):888–96.
29. Dixon JB, Lambert EA, Lambert GW. Neuroendocrine adaptations to bariatric surgery. Mol Cell Endocrinol 2015;418(Pt 2):143–52.
30. Seeley RJ, Chambers AP, Sandoval DA. The role of gut adaptation in the potent effects of multiple bariatric surgeries on obesity and diabetes. Cell Metab 2015; 21(3):369–78.

31. Aron-Wisnewsky J, Clement K. The effects of gastrointestinal surgery on gut microbiota: potential contribution to improved insulin sensitivity. Curr Atheroscler Rep 2014;16(11):454.

32. Cummings DE. Taste and the regulation of food intake: it's not just about flavor. Am J Clin Nutr 2015;102(4):717–8.

33. Browning KN, Fortna SR, Hajnal A. Roux-en-Y gastric bypass reverses the effects of diet-induced obesity to inhibit the responsiveness of central vagal motoneurones. J Physiol 2013;591(Pt 9):2357–72.

34. Rissanen A, Hakala P, Lissner L, et al. Acquired preference especially for dietary fat and obesity: a study of weight-discordant monozygotic twin pairs. Int J Obes Relat Metab Disord 2002;26(7):973–7.

35. Shin AC, Townsend RL, Patterson LM, et al. "Liking" and "wanting" of sweet and oily food stimuli as affected by high-fat diet-induced obesity, weight loss, leptin, and genetic predisposition. Am J Physiol Regul Integr Comp Physiol 2011;301(5): R1267–80.

36. Sumithran P, Prendergast LA, Delbridge E, et al. Long-term persistence of hormonal adaptations to weight loss. N Engl J Med 2011;365(17):1597–604.

37. Barkeling B, King NA, Naslund E, et al. Characterization of obese individuals who claim to detect no relationship between their eating pattern and sensations of hunger or fullness. Int J Obes (Lond) 2007;31(3):435–9.

38. Leibel RL, Hirsch J. Diminished energy requirements in reduced-obese patients. Metabolism 1984;33(2):164–70.

39. Manning S, Pucci A, Carter NC, et al. Early postoperative weight loss predicts maximal weight loss after sleeve gastrectomy and Roux-en-Y gastric bypass. Surg Endosc 2015;29(6):1484–91.

40. Dirksen C, Damgaard M, Bojsen-Moller KN, et al. Fast pouch emptying, delayed small intestinal transit, and exaggerated gut hormone responses after Roux-en-Y gastric bypass. Neurogastroenterol Motil 2013;25(4). 346–e255.

41. Odstrcil EA, Martinez JG, Santa Ana CA, et al. The contribution of malabsorption to the reduction in net energy absorption after long-limb Roux-en-Y gastric bypass. Am J Clin Nutr 2010;92(4):704–13.

42. Lutz TA, Bueter M. The physiology underlying Roux-en-Y gastric bypass: a status report. Am J Physiol Regul Integr Comp Physiol 2014;307(11):R1275–91.

43. Bray GA, Dahms WT, Atkinson RL, et al. Factors controlling food intake: a comparison of dieting and intestinal bypass. Am J Clin Nutr 1980;33(2 Suppl):376–82.

44. Warde-Kamar J, Rogers M, Flancbaum L, et al. Calorie intake and meal patterns up to 4 years after Roux-en-Y gastric bypass surgery. Obes Surg 2004;14(8): 1070–9.

45. Mathes CM, Spector AC. Food selection and taste changes in humans after Roux-en-Y gastric bypass surgery: a direct-measures approach. Physiol Behav 2012;107(4):476–83.

46. Laurenius A, Larsson I, Bueter M, et al. Changes in eating behaviour and meal pattern following Roux-en-Y gastric bypass. Int J Obes (Lond) 2012;36(3): 348–55.

47. Thomas JR, Marcus E. High and low fat food selection with reported frequency intolerance following Roux-en-Y gastric bypass. Obes Surg 2008;18(3):282–7.

48. Holinski F, Menenakos C, Haber G, et al. Olfactory and gustatory function after bariatric surgery. Obes Surg 2015;25(12):2314–20.

49. Scholtz S, Miras AD, Chhina N, et al. Obese patients after gastric bypass surgery have lower brain-hedonic responses to food than after gastric banding. Gut 2014; 63(6):891–902.

50. Miras AD, Jackson RN, Jackson SN, et al. Gastric bypass surgery for obesity decreases the reward value of a sweet-fat stimulus as assessed in a progressive ratio task. Am J Clin Nutr 2012;96(3):467–73.

51. Ochner CN, Kwok Y, Conceicao E, et al. Selective reduction in neural responses to high calorie foods following gastric bypass surgery. Ann Surg 2011;253(3):502–7.

52. Ochner CN, Stice E, Hutchins E, et al. Relation between changes in neural responsivity and reductions in desire to eat high-calorie foods following gastric bypass surgery. Neuroscience 2012;209:128–35.

53. Shin AC, Berthoud HR. Obesity surgery: happy with less or eternally hungry? Trends Endocrinol Metab 2013;24(2):101–8.

54. Yousseif A, Emmanuel J, Karra E, et al. Differential effects of laparoscopic sleeve gastrectomy and laparoscopic gastric bypass on appetite, circulating acyl-ghrelin, peptide YY3-36 and active GLP-1 levels in non-diabetic humans. Obes Surg 2014;24(2):241–52.

55. Cummings DE, Weigle DS, Frayo RS, et al. Plasma ghrelin levels after diet-induced weight loss or gastric bypass surgery. N Engl J Med 2002;346(21):1623–30.

56. Chandarana K, Drew ME, Emmanuel J, et al. Subject standardization, acclimatization, and sample processing affect gut hormone levels and appetite in humans. Gastroenterology 2009;136(7):2115–26.

57. Hosoda H, Kangawa K. Standard sample collections for blood ghrelin measurements. Meth Enzymol 2012;514:113–26.

58. Ramon JM, Salvans S, Crous X, et al. Effect of Roux-en-Y gastric bypass vs sleeve gastrectomy on glucose and gut hormones: a prospective randomised trial. J Gastrointest Surg 2012;16(6):1116–22.

59. Dirksen C, Jorgensen NB, Bojsen-Moller KN, et al. Gut hormones, early dumping and resting energy expenditure in patients with good and poor weight loss response after Roux-en-Y gastric bypass. Int J Obes (Lond) 2013;37(11):1452–9.

60. le Roux CW, Welbourn R, Werling M, et al. Gut hormones as mediators of appetite and weight loss after Roux-en-Y gastric bypass. Ann Surg 2007;246(5):780–5.

61. Pucci A, Wui Hang C, Jenny J, et al. A case of severe anorexia, excessive weight loss and high peptide YY levels after sleeve gastrectomy. Endocrinol Diabetes Metab Case Rep 2015;2015:150020.

62. Mathes CM, Bueter M, Smith KR, et al. Roux-en-Y gastric bypass in rats increases sucrose taste-related motivated behavior independent of pharmacological GLP-1-receptor modulation. Am J Physiol Regul Integr Comp Physiol 2012;302(6):R751–67.

63. Miras AD, le Roux CW. Bariatric surgery and taste: novel mechanisms of weight loss. Curr Opin Gastroenterol 2010;26(2):140–5.

64. Mokadem M, Zechner JF, Margolskee RF, et al. Effects of Roux-en-Y gastric bypass on energy and glucose homeostasis are preserved in two mouse models of functional glucagon-like peptide-1 deficiency. Mol Metab 2014;3(2):191–201.

65. Ye J, Hao Z, Mumphrey MB, et al. GLP-1 receptor signaling is not required for reduced body weight after RYGB in rodents. Am J Physiol Regul Integr Comp Physiol 2014;306(5):R352–62.

66. Chandarana K, Gelegen C, Karra E, et al. Diet and gastrointestinal bypass-induced weight loss: the roles of ghrelin and peptide YY. Diabetes 2011;60(3):810–8.

67. Dutia R, Embrey M, O'Brien S, et al. Temporal changes in bile acid levels and 12alpha-hydroxylation after Roux-en-Y gastric bypass surgery in type 2 diabetes. Int J Obes (Lond) 2015;39(5):806–13.

68. Kuipers F, Groen AK. FXR: the key to benefits in bariatric surgery? Nat Med 2014; 20(4):337–8.

69. Watanabe M, Houten SM, Mataki C, et al. Bile acids induce energy expenditure by promoting intracellular thyroid hormone activation. Nature 2006;439(7075): 484–9.

70. Tremaroli V, Karlsson F, Werling M, et al. Roux-en-Y gastric bypass and vertical banded gastroplasty induce long-term changes on the human gut microbiome contributing to fat mass regulation. Cell Metab 2015;22(2):228–38.

71. Cavin JB, Couvelard A, Lebtahi R, et al. Differences in alimentary glucose absorption and intestinal disposal of blood glucose after Roux-en-Y gastric bypass vs sleeve gastrectomy. Gastroenterology 2016;150(2):454–64.e9.

72. Sweeney TE, Morton JM. Metabolic surgery: action via hormonal milieu changes, changes in bile acids or gut microbiota? A summary of the literature. Best Pract Res Clin Gastroenterol 2014;28(4):727–40.

73. le Roux CW, Aylwin SJ, Batterham RL, et al. Gut hormone profiles following bariatric surgery favor an anorectic state, facilitate weight loss, and improve metabolic parameters. Ann Surg 2006;243(1):108–14.

74. Pournaras DJ, Glicksman C, Vincent RP, et al. The role of bile after Roux-en-Y gastric bypass in promoting weight loss and improving glycaemic control. Endocrinology 2012;153(8):3613–9.

75. Rosenbaum M, Knight R, Leibel RL. The gut microbiota in human energy homeostasis and obesity. Trends Endocrinol Metab 2015;26(9):493–501.

76. Leibel RL, Seeley RJ, Darsow T, et al. Biologic responses to weight loss and weight regain: report from an American Diabetes Association research symposium. Diabetes 2015;64(7):2299–309.

Type 2 Diabetes Treatment in the Patient with Obesity

Steven K. Malin, PhD[a], Sangeeta R. Kashyap, MD[b],*

KEYWORDS

- Insulin resistance • β- cell function • Glycemic control • Exercise • Diet
- Pharmacology • Bariatric surgery

KEY POINTS

- Lifestyle modification is effective at promoting weight loss and glycemic control in patients with type 2 diabetes, although long-term adherence remains challenging.
- Many pharmacologic interventions (eg, metformin, SLGT2 inhibitors, lorcaserin, liraglutide 3.0 mg) have promising results for obesity and related diabetes complications.
- Bariatric surgery is the most effective and durable treatment for individuals with obesity and type 2 diabetes; however, long-term remission of diabetes remains questionable.

INTRODUCTION

An estimated 347 million adults live with type 2 diabetes (T2D) worldwide, about half of whom are undiagnosed.[1] Although the cause for T2D is multifactorial, nearly 80% of all people with T2D are obese. This strongly suggests that obesity may play a central role in the progression from normal glucose tolerance to frank T2D. The mechanism by which obesity promotes T2D is an area of intense research but inadequate compensation of the β cells in response to an increasingly insulin-resistant skeletal muscle and liver characterize T2D. It is now recognized that individuals with impaired glucose tolerance (prediabetes) have lost upward of 80% of their β-cell function and have comparable degrees of insulin resistance to clinical T2D.[2] In addition, adipose tissue is considered a chief culprit in the development of multiorgan insulin resistance and β-cell dysfunction through increased circulatory factors (free fatty acids, leptin, and so forth) that promote hyperglycemia.[3] Newer understandings of T2D pathophysiology acknowledge that the gastrointestinal tract (eg, small intestine), kidney, and

The authors have nothing to disclose.

[a] Division of Endocrinology & Metabolism, Department of Kinesiology, Curry School of Education, School of Medicine, University of Virginia, 203 Memorial Gymnasium, Charlottesville, VA 22904, USA; [b] Division of Endocrinology, School of Medicine, Department of Endocrinology, Diabetes, and Metabolism, Cleveland Clinic, 9500 Euclid Avenue, NE40, Cleveland, OH 44195, USA
* Corresponding author.
E-mail address: kashyas@ccf.org

Endocrinol Metab Clin N Am 45 (2016) 553–564
http://dx.doi.org/10.1016/j.ecl.2016.04.007
0889-8529/16/$ – see front matter
endo.theclinics.com

brain in addition to the aforementioned organs collectively play an important role in the progression to T2D. Thus, identification of end-organ targets that promote hyperglycemia is critical to the advancement of successful treatment strategies. As a result, efforts are needed to make clinical decisions based on the underlying pathophysiologic abnormality.

Recently obesity has been considered a "disease" by major health organizations, although others consider obesity to be simply a side effect of energy imbalance.[4] In either case, it is reasonable that current focus be placed on intensifying efforts to improve weight management and glycemic control to combat the increased incidence of cardiovascular disease (CVD) in people with T2D. Here, we discuss studies relevant to addressing antiobesity therapeutic options for the individual with T2D and dual actions to improve glycemic control. We present evidence suggesting that lifestyle modification directly and successfully induces meaningful weight loss by inducing a negative energy balance. Also highlighted are recent advances in the understanding of pharmacologic interventions that drive weight loss and improve insulin sensitivity and β-cell function with or without lifestyle modification. Lastly, we discuss the inclusion of bariatric surgery into the algorithm for diabetes therapy, and close with a discussion of the clinical importance of combining exercise and diet with pharmacology or bariatric surgery as needed disease modification.

MANAGEMENT OF TYPE 2 DIABETES FOLLOWING LIFESTYLE MODIFICATION

A central goal of diabetes care is to aid individuals in making better lifestyle decisions that lead to healthier body weights because obesity is the basic risk factor for T2D. Indeed, sedentary behavior and increased caloric intake are two key factors known to trigger insulin resistance and force the β-cell to secrete more insulin. In contrast, lifestyle intervention consisting of increased physical activity and low-fat diet reducing weight by approximately 5 kg for 2 years or beyond lowers diabetes risk by 30% to 60%.[5] Weight loss of 2% to 5% over 1 to 4 years decreases hemoglobin (Hb) A_{1c} by 0.2% to 0.3%. Moreover, losses of 5% to 10% at 1 year are associated with reductions in HbA$_{1c}$ of 0.6% to 1.0%.[5] The Finnish Diabetes Prevention Study provided advice for subjects to lose greater than 5% weight loss by decreasing total fat less than 30% of total calorie intake (with <10% coming from saturated fat), increasing fiber consumption (ie, 15 g per 1000 kcal), and increasing physical activity (30 min/d).[6] This lifestyle prescription lowered the cumulative incidence of diabetes by 58% in people with prediabetes compared with control subjects.[6] In another landmark trial, the US Diabetes Prevention Program (DPP) Study, which recommended people with prediabetes exercise 150 min/wk and loss of 7% of weight showed that new diabetes cases were lowered by 58%.[7] However, subjects who lost the most weight and met physical activity/diet targets had greater than 90% risk reductions of diabetes.[8] These reports are consistent with recent work showing that the combination of a well-balanced diet (eg, low-fat and high-fiber diet) promoting approximately 5% to 8% weight loss with increased physical activity is a well-established strategy for managing T2D because higher doses of physical activity generally increase insulin sensitivity[9,10] and β-cell function.[11] Although caloric restriction is arguably the most important factor driving weight loss, it remains possible that low carbohydrate intake per se may yield greater reductions in circulating blood glucose and body weight, particularly during the first few months of a lifestyle program.[12,13] Nevertheless, increased physical activity is a primary determinant of maintaining the lost weight. As such, structured exercise interventions in particular have been shown to significantly improve HbA$_{1c}$ levels,[14,15] although some work suggests that not all people with hyperglycemia respond favorably to standard lifestyle interventions.[16,17] This latter point is an important consideration because weight loss may be the most important contributor to T2D prevention.[18,19] Further work is required to understand why some people with hyperglycemia do not respond to traditional lifestyle modification and to determine the optimal exercise prescription for diabetes prevention and treatment.

MANAGEMENT OF TYPE 2 DIABETES USING PHARMACOLOGY

Despite randomized clinical trials showing the clear efficacy of lifestyle modification on weight loss, long-term adherence to diet and exercise remains difficult.[20] Less than 50% of people with T2D achieve adequate glucose control (HbA$_{1c}$ <7.0%) through this regimen,[21] and many people regain weight over time.[22] Alarmingly, this traditional approach does not decrease the incidence of cardiovascular events in obese adults with T2D,[23] and may not be adequate for maintaining improved insulin sensitivity or β-cell function. Thus, pharmacologic agents that target insulin resistance, β-cell dysfunction, and obesity are usually needed for T2D management.

Insulin Sensitizers

Metformin is the most widely prescribed drug to treat hyperglycemia in children and adults with T2D.[24] In fact, metformin is the first-line oral antidiabetic medication recommended by the American Diabetes Association, and individuals with prediabetes and at least one CVD risk factor (eg, hypertension, dyslipidemia, and so forth) are also encouraged to be treated with metformin.[25] Current evidence suggests that the biguanidine increases insulin sensitivity through the suppression of hepatic gluconeogenesis and opposition of glucagon action and stimulation of peripheral glucose uptake through activation of AMPK.[24] In the setting of T2D and obesity, metformin is an attractive therapeutic choice because of its ability to promote weight loss.[26] To date, the longest and best study of metformin on body weight comes from the Diabetes Prevention Program. Within the first 3 years of this double-blind randomized trial, the metformin group lost approximately 2.9 kg versus 0.42 kg in the control group.[7] Impressively, this weight loss effect persisted up to 15 years.[27] Thus, metformin is a useful first-line pharmacotherapy for T2D to manage blood glucose and reduce body weight, although it is worth noting that interactions of metformin pharmacotherapy with lifestyle changes is an area of needed research because studies report that metformin enhances, blunts, or has no effect on exercise-induced improvements in insulin sensitivity and glucose homeostasis.[24] Whether there is an optimal combination of metformin with exercise and/or diet remains to be determined.

Thiazolidinediones

Thiazolidinediones (TZDs; ie, pioglitazone) act on peroxisome proliferator–activated receptor γ, and are effective at improving insulin sensitivity (eg, adipose, liver, and muscle) and improving/restoring pancreatic β-cell function.[2] Despite these glycemic benefits, many health care providers have reservations about prescribing TZDs because they promote substantial weight gain. However, this storage of excess fat is in part the mechanism by which TZDs increase insulin sensitivity and β-cell function. TZDs are known to lower circulating lipids (eg, free fatty acids) thereby reducing ectopic lipids (eg, intramuscular fat) and visceral fat while distributing circulating free fatty acids to subcutaneous fat in people with hyperglycemia.[28] In line with this redistribution of body fat, TZDs also have potent antiatherogenic effects that lower overall risk for CVD and even slow down the progression from prediabetes to T2D.[29] Thus, given the moderate weight gain with this agent, low-dose TZDs should be considered only as a second-line therapy for individuals who do not achieve glycemic control with metformin plus lifestyle modification.

Insulin Secretagogues and β-Cell Function Agonists

Sulfonylureas

Sulfonylureas (SFUs) enhance insulin secretion through binding receptors associated with potassium channels on β cells.[30] Use of SFUs along with metformin in patients with T2D may be prudent to prevent further β-cell failure. However, it was shown in the UK Prospective Diabetes Study that SFUs had no protective effects on the pancreatic β-cell in newly diagnosed patients with T2D. HbA_{1c} levels showed a continuous rise regardless of SFU treatment when compared with control. This decline in glycemic control was paralleled by a deterioration in β-cell function (via HOMA-β) such that approximately 50% of people required additional therapeutic agents to maintain HbA_{1c} less than 7.0% at 3 years later.[31] Given that SFU usage carries a risk of inducing hypoglycemia, does not preserve pancreatic function, and promotes weight regain compared with usage of oral insulin-sensitizing agents,[30,32] SFUs should be used with caution particularly in the setting of obesity.

Incretin analogues

Glucagon-like polypeptide (GLP)-1 and glucose-dependent insulinotropic peptide are incretin hormones that account for approximately 60% of the meal-stimulated insulin secretion, and are important for delaying gastric emptying and reducing postprandial glucose levels by stimulating pancreatic function.[33] GLP-1 is considered the key incretin hormone and receptor agonists (eg, exenatide and liraglutide) are currently approved pharmacologic agents that simulate the action of GLP-1 or share 97% homology to native GLP-1 thereby extending the circulating half-life of GLP-1 from 1 to 2 minutes to 13 hours.[34] Given the capacity of GLP-1 to promote pancreatic β-cell insulin secretion and promote significant weight loss, research effort to understand the mechanism of improvement in glycemic control and weight loss observed has intensified.[35–37] In addition, a recent meta-analysis demonstrated that GLP-1 receptor agonists provided the greatest benefit to glycemic control when compared with various antidiabetic drugs added to existing metformin regimens.[38] Although GLP-1-centered therapies are encouraging, they are potentially associated with an increased risk of pancreatitis and pancreatic cancer.[39] Thus, given that hypoglycemia is mediated by combination therapies designed to increase insulin sensitivity and incretin hormones, caution regarding potential hypoglycemia must be taken before initiating therapy with incretin analogues.

Dipeptidyl-pepidase-IV inhibitors

Dipeptidyl-pepidase-IV (DPP-IV) is an enzyme that cleaves GLP-1, thereby limiting the glucoregulatory benefits of this incretin hormone action. Inhibitors of DPP-IV also increase GLP-1 concentrations.[40,41] This is physiologically relevant because DPP-IV is thought to not only impair β-cell function but also worsen insulin resistance in adults with metabolic syndrome and prediabetes/T2D.[42] However, the action of DPP-IV inhibitors depends on endogenous secretion of GLP-1. Thus, DPP-IV-inhibitor-induced rises in GLP-1 are usually lower than GLP-1 analogue-related rises (see above). Although there are limited data on the long-term utility of DPP-IV inhibitors, several studies show that this class of pharmacologic agents improve postprandial glucose metabolism. The effectiveness of DPP-IV inhibitors on glycemic control is consistent with recent work demonstrating that lifestyle modifications in part lower CVD risk by reducing DPP-IV concentrations.[42] Nevertheless, DPP-IV inhibitors have no effect on weight loss, so this treatment regimen seems unique to glycemia per se and may not be appropriate for combating the obesity often associated with T2D.

Insulin

Patients with less than adequate responses to insulin sensitizers or secretagogues should be considered for treatment with basal insulin and prandial insulin as necessary. Like SFUs, insulin use carries risk of hyperinsulinemic-induced hypoglycemia and weight gain.[43] However, evidence suggests that personalizing insulin titration in conjunction with oral hypoglycemic agents promotes better glycemic benefit in patients who do not respond to other oral agents. For instance, obese patients with insulin-requiring T2D after gastric bypass surgery showed higher rates of complete remission at 1 year postsurgery with personalized insulin titration schedules and metformin compared with patients whose postsurgical medical care did not involve protocol-driven pharmacologic treatment.[44] Although additional work is required to understand the optimal combination of pharmacologic and lifestyle therapy to improve glucose homeostasis, the collective literature does indicate that combinations of existing T2D therapeutics can provide adequate glycemic control despite the tendency of insulin use to cause weight gain of 2 kg to 9 kg within 6 to 12 months of treatment.[2]

Novel Glycemic Medication: Sodium-Glucose Cotransporter 2 Inhibitors

The kidney plays an important role in filtering approximately 160 g of glucose each day, and nearly 90% of all glucose is reabsorbed in the body by sodium-glucose cotransporter (SGLT)-2 transporters located in the promixmal tubule.[2] The result is less glucose excretion in urine. New work shows that SGLT2 inhibitors, or gliflozins, are novel antidiabetes agents that block glucose reabsorption in the renal tubules and promote loss of glucose in the urine. A meta-analysis of 25 randomized trials concluded that use of SGLT2 inhibitors for T2D is associated with significant improvement in glycemic control and blood pressure and reduction in body weight.[45] This is consistent with other work in patients with poorly controlled T2D showing that SGLT2 treatment as an add-on therapy to metformin improves many CVD risk factors.[46] However, use of these drugs increases the risk of genital mycotic infections and lower urinary tract infections.[47] Nevertheless, given the favorable effects of SGLT2 inhibitors on glycemic control, weight loss, and blood pressure, SGLT2 inhibitors constitute an attractive treatment modality in patients with T2D and obesity.

Weight Loss Agents that Provide Glycemic Benefit

Phentermine-topiramate

Phentermine is a sympathomimetic drug that reduces appetite by stimulating norepinephrine action in the hypothalamus. Topiramate is a carbonic anhydrase inhibitor and a monosaccharide that lowers food cravings, decreases lipogenesis, and increases energy expenditure.[48] In the SEQUEL trial, which is an extension of the CONQUER trial, phentermine-topiramate induced greater weight loss and HbA$_{1c}$ improvements in patients with T2D compared with patients treated with placebo alone.[49] In fact, study participants with prediabetes, metabolic syndrome, or both who underwent treatment with phentermine-topirimate also had significant weight loss and reduced risk of T2D progression.[50] Therefore, because phentermine-topiramate seems to induce beneficial effects on weight loss and glycemic control, it warrants consideration as a potential obesity-related therapy for T2D.

Orlistat

Orlistat is a gastric and pancreatic lipase inhibitor that blocks dietary fat absorption from the gastrointestinal system by approximately 30%. Randomized trials and meta-analyses have demonstrated that orlistat treatment can produce weight loss and reduce the incidence of T2D in people with impaired glucose tolerance.[51] A recent randomized controlled trial over 1 year reported greater weight loss and improvements in insulin sensitivity in patients treated with orlistat as compared with those treated with placebo.[52] Several mechanisms have been proposed to account for the antidiabetic effect of orlistat, such as improved insulin sensitivity, incomplete dietary fat digestion, partial stimulation of GLP-1 release, and decreases in visceral adiposity.[53] However, orlistat use predisposes patients to fecal urgency, mild steatorrhea, and flatus with discharge, and the drug may interfere with absorption of fat-soluble vitamins.[43] As such, orlistat should be used with caution to ensure healthy nutrient intake for the patient.

Lorcaserin

Lorcaserin is a selective agonist of the serotonin 2C receptor. It activates central serotonin 2C receptors with a functional selectivity of approximately 15 and 100 times over that for serotonin receptors 2A and 2B, respectively. It reduces appetite and food intake thereby reducing body weight in men and women.[54] Currently, this treatment is recommended for obese (body mass index ≥ 30 kg/m^2) individuals or overweight (body mass index ≥ 27 kg/m^2) people who suffer from at least one weight-related complication, such as hypertension, T2D, or dyslipidemia.[55] In a randomized trial called BLOOM-DM, 604 patients with T2D were randomly assigned to lorcaserin (10 mg once daily or twice daily) or placebo, and most patients were treated with metformin, an SFU, or both. After 1 year, more patients lost greater than or equal to 5% of their body weight with lorcaserin compared with placebo (44.7%, 37.5%, and 16.1%, respectively). There was also a significant reduction in HbA$_{1c}$ (-1.0%, -0.9%, and -0.4% points, respectively) and fasting blood glucose (-28.4, -27.4, and -11.9 mg/dL) in the lorcaserin compared with placebo group.[56] Because lorcaserin seems to affect body weight and glycemic control, it seems to be an agent for promoting or maintaining weight loss. However, future studies are needed to clarify the efficacy of lorcaserin in maintaining weight loss and blocking weight gain because of aging or use of other pharmacologic agents (eg, TZDs, insulin).

Naltrexone-bupropion

Naltrexone and bupropion have recently been combined (eg, Contrave) as a pharamacologic agent targeting the mesolimbic dopamine reward system and the hypothalamic melanocortin system to reduce food intake. Naltrexone-bupropion induces significant weight loss and proportional reductions in fat mass and visceral adiposity.[57] In addition, Hollander and colleagues[58] demonstrated that overweight/obese patients with T2D randomized to naltrexone-bupropion experienced significantly greater weight loss and improvements in HbA$_{1c}$ levels when compared with placebo. Although these results seem promising for combating obesity and hyperglycemia in the patient with T2D, there are reported side effects of constipation, headache, vomiting, and dizziness. Furthermore, a long-term cardiovascular outcomes trial is currently being held to understand the long-term safety and utility of this agent.

MANAGEMENT OF TYPE 2 DIABETES WITH BARIATRIC SURGERY

Several randomized trials have bolstered the claim of bariatric surgery being an effective treatment leading to T2D remission[59,60] together with durable weight loss.[61,62] Subsequently, bariatric surgery has illuminated the gastrointestinal system as a key pathophysiologic culprit in the development of T2D. Although the literature is inconsistent with the definition of T2D remission, Ribaric and colleagues[63] recently analyzed the remission criteria of each individual study to report an overall remission rate of patients with T2D who underwent bariatric surgery, and compared this with a rate of 15.6% with conventional therapy at a mean follow-up time of 17.3 months. The results of this work indicate that people undergoing bariatric surgery have 9.8 to 15.8 times the odds of reaching diabetes remission compared with conventional therapy. As a result of the collective impact of these studies and the literature, the American Diabetes Association and the International Diabetes Federation have identified bariatric surgery as an effective treatment of T2D.[64,65] Indeed, the literature supports the use of bariatric surgery as not only a weight loss treatment option, but also a "metabolic surgery" that restores glucose homeostasis in people with T2D. However, not all people remain in T2D remission 2 to 5 years postbariatric surgery and insulin resistance and β-cell dysfunction seem to be key factors explaining the relapse,[66–68] which has a direct relationship to years after surgery.[59] Most recently, a follow-up report to the Swedish Obese Subjects study showed that T2D remission rates decreased from 72.3% at 2 years to 30.4% at 15 years after surgery.[69] Moreover, long preoperative T2D duration, insulin use, poor glycemic control despite oral hypoglycemic agents, and microvascular complications are all additional indicators of inadequate β-cell function.[8] Thus, although bariatric surgery is a highly effective tool for promoting the reversal of T2D, it does not seem to be a treatment that "cures" the disease in all people, suggesting that continued monitoring of glycemic control is warranted.[44] Additional work is required to determine appropriate treatment plans with lifestyle modification[70] or pharmacologic therapy for preventing the relapse in T2D.

CLINICAL IMPLICATIONS AND CONCLUSIONS

The optimal treatment strategy for the obese person with T2D is likely going to vary between people based on the underlying pathophysiology. The complicated etiology of T2D highlights that several therapeutic options will likely be required to correct varying disturbances with tissues (eg, skeletal muscle, liver, adipose, gut, kidney) (**Fig. 1**). In this sense, it is prudent to select therapies based on the underlying cause of T2D rather than purely on blood glucose concentrations. Moreover, treatment earlier on in the disease is likely to preserve β-cell function and restore insulin sensitivity for long-term glycemic control and CVD risk reduction. The available evidence and clinical experience suggest that T2D is related to weight gain combined with the exhaustion of insulin-secreting pancreatic β-cells caused by insulin resistance in skeletal muscle, liver, and adipose tissue. Although there are still challenges with adhering to lifestyle modification over time, exercise and diet are successful approaches that maintain long-term weight loss and glycemic control. Thus, lifestyle modification should remain the first-line therapy for treatment of T2D. However, not all people are able to perform the necessary levels of physical activity needed to maintain metabolic health. As a result, pharmacologic intervention aimed at reducing weight and increasing insulin sensitivity (eg, metformin, TZDs, or canagliflozin), followed by treatments that promote insulin secretion, are appropriate treatment strategies. In addition, several of these pharmacologic agents (metformin, GLP1 agonists, SLGT2) promote modest weight loss in obese individuals with T2D. Importantly, the amount of weight loss following these pharmacologic treatment plans is modest (1–5 kg) relative to the amount needed for most obese people to achieve healthy weight status and/or optimal glycemic control and CVD risk reduction. Thus, any one pharmacologic agent is unlikely to be a sole antiobesity agent, and these drugs should only be considered as an adjunctive therapy to exercise plus diet. If these treatment strategies are

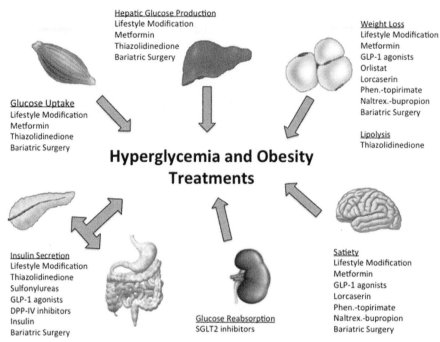

Fig. 1. Strategies to treat type 2 diabetes. Lifestyle modification has multiorgan effects to favorably impact glycemic control and weight management. Although pharmacologic agents may also act on different organs, they typically are designed to impact one central organ. Bariatric surgery is a newer treatment option for many obese individuals with type 2 diabetes compared with lifestyle modification and pharmacologic intervention and has proven antihyperglycemic effects. However, successful treatment for type 2 diabetes involves a highly personalized approach based on disease pathology. Thus, it is likely that a combination of therapies is needed to optimize weight regulation and glycemic control. Bariatric surgery primarily refers to Roux-en-Y gastric bypass and sleeve gastrectomy. Lifestyle modification refers to 150 min/wk of moderate to vigorous physical activity coupled with a low-fat diet. Naltrex, naltrexone; Phen, phentermine.

inadequate for the obese patient with T2D, then bariatric surgery represents a viable alternative with the potential of complete diabetes remission.

REFERENCES

1. Maruthur NM. The growing prevalence of type 2 diabetes: increased incidence or improved survival? Curr Diab Rep 2013;13(6):786–94.
2. Defronzo RA. Banting Lecture. From the triumvirate to the ominous octet: a new paradigm for the treatment of type 2 diabetes mellitus. Diabetes 2009;58(4): 773–95.
3. Malin SK, Kashyap SR, Hammel J, et al. Adjusting glucose-stimulated insulin secretion for adipose insulin resistance: an index of β-cell function in obese adults. Diabetes Care 2014;37(11):2940–6.
4. Hurt RT, Edakkanambeth Varayil J, Mundi MS, et al. Designation of obesity as a disease: lessons learned from alcohol and tobacco. Curr Gastroenterol Rep 2014;16(11):415.

5. Ebbert JO, Elrashidi MY, Jensen MD. Managing overweight and obesity in adults to reduce cardiovascular disease risk. Curr Atheroscler Rep 2014;16(10):445.

6. Tuomilehto J, Lindström J, Eriksson JG, et al. Prevention of type 2 diabetes mellitus by changes in lifestyle among subjects with impaired glucose tolerance. N Engl J Med 2001;344(18):1343–50.

7. Knowler WC, Barrett-Connor E, Fowler SE, et al. Reduction in the incidence of type 2 diabetes with lifestyle intervention or metformin. N Engl J Med 2002; 346(6):393–403.

8. Lee WJ, Hur KY, Lakadawala M, et al. Gastrointestinal metabolic surgery for the treatment of diabetic patients: a multi-institutional international study. J Gastrointest Surg 2012;16(1):45–51 [discussion: 51–2].

9. Houmard JA, Tanner CJ, Slentz CA, et al. Effect of the volume and intensity of exercise training on insulin sensitivity [Internet]. J Appl Physiol 2004;96(1):101–6.

10. Malin SK, Niemi N, Solomon TPJ, et al. Exercise training with weight loss and either a high- or low-glycemic index diet reduces metabolic syndrome severity in older adults. Ann Nutr Metab 2012;61(2):135–41.

11. Malin SK, Solomon TPJ, Blaszczak A, et al. Pancreatic beta cell function increases in a linear dose-response manner following exercise training in adults with prediabetes. Am J Physiol Endocrinol Metab 2013;305:E1248–54.

12. Rock CL, Flatt SW, Pakiz B, et al. Weight loss, glycemic control, and cardiovascular disease risk factors in response to differential diet composition in a weight loss program in type 2 diabetes: a randomized controlled trial. Diabetes Care 2014;37(6):1573–80.

13. Tay J, Luscombe-Marsh ND, Thompson CH, et al. A very low-carbohydrate, low-saturated fat diet for type 2 diabetes management: a randomized trial. Diabetes Care 2014;37(11):2909–18.

14. Solomon TPJ, Malin SK, Karstoft K, et al. Pancreatic β-cell function is a stronger predictor of changes in glycemic control after an aerobic exercise intervention than insulin sensitivity. J Clin Endocrinol Metab 2013;98(10):4176–86.

15. Umpierre D, Ribeiro PA, Kramer CK, et al. Physical activity advice only or structured exercise training and association with HbA1c levels in type 2 diabetes: a systematic review and meta-analysis. JAMA 2011;305(17):1790–9.

16. Malin SK, Haus JM, Solomon TPJ, et al. Insulin sensitivity and metabolic flexibility following exercise training among different obese insulin resistant phenotypes. Am J Physiol Endocrinol Metab 2013;305:E1292–8.

17. Solomon TPJ, Malin SK, Karstoft K, et al. The influence of hyperglycemia on the therapeutic effect of exercise on glycemic control in patients with type 2 diabetes mellitus. JAMA Intern Med 2013;173(19):1834–6.

18. Kitabchi AE, Temprosa M, Knowler WC, et al. Role of insulin secretion and sensitivity in the evolution of type 2 diabetes in the diabetes prevention program: effects of lifestyle intervention and metformin. Diabetes 2005;54(8):2404–14.

19. Li G, Zhang P, Wang J, et al. The long-term effect of lifestyle interventions to prevent diabetes in the China Da Qing Diabetes Prevention Study: a 20-year follow-up study. Lancet 2008;371(9626):1783–9.

20. Wing RR, Goldstein MG, Acton KJ, et al. Behavioral science research in diabetes: lifestyle changes related to obesity, eating behavior, and physical activity. Diabetes Care 2001;24(1):117–23.

21. Ali MK, Bullard KM, Saaddine JB, et al. Achievement of goals in U.S. diabetes care, 1999-2010. N Engl J Med 2013;368(17):1613–24.

22. Venditti EM, Bray GA, Carrion-Petersen ML, et al. First versus repeat treatment with a lifestyle intervention program: attendance and weight loss outcomes. Int J Obes (Lond) 2008;32(10):1537–44.

23. Look AHEAD Research Group, Wing RR, Bolin P, Brancati FL, et al. Cardiovascular effects of intensive lifestyle intervention in type 2 diabetes. N Engl J Med 2013; 369(2):145–54.

24. Malin SK, Braun B. Impact of metformin on exercise-induced metabolic adaptations to lower type 2 diabetes risk. Exerc Sport Sci Rev 2016;44(1):4–11.

25. Rhee M, Herrick K, Ziemer D, et al. Many Americans have pre-diabetes and should be considered for metformin therapy. Diabetes Care 2010;33(1):49–54.

26. Malin SK, Kashyap SR. Effects of metformin on weight loss: potential mechanisms. Curr Opin Endocrinol Diabetes Obes 2014;21(5):323–9.

27. Diabetes Prevention Program Research Group. Long-term effects of lifestyle intervention or metformin on diabetes development and microvascular complications over 15-year follow-up: the Diabetes Prevention Program Outcomes Study. Lancet Diabetes Endocrinol 2015;3(11):866–75.

28. Punthakee Z, Almeras N, Despres JP, et al. Impact of rosiglitazone on body composition, hepatic fat, fatty acids, adipokines and glucose in persons with impaired fasting glucose or impaired glucose tolerance: a sub-study of the DREAM trial. Diabet Med 2014;31(9):1086–92.

29. DeFronzo RA, Tripathy D, Schwenke DC, et al. Pioglitazone for diabetes prevention in impaired glucose tolerance. N Engl J Med 2011;364(12):1104–15.

30. Kahn SE, Cooper ME, Del Prato S. Pathophysiology and treatment of type 2 diabetes: perspectives on the past, present, and future. Lancet 2014;383(9922): 1068–83.

31. Matthews DR, Cull CA, Stratton IM, et al. UKPDS 26: sulphonylurea failure in non-insulin-dependent diabetic patients over six years. UK Prospective Diabetes Study (UKPDS) Group. Diabet Med 1998;15(4):297–303.

32. Bennett WL, Maruthur NM, Singh S, et al. Comparative effectiveness and safety of medications for type 2 diabetes: an update including new drugs and 2-drug combinations. Ann Intern Med 2011;154(9):602–13.

33. Holst J, Vilsbll T, Deacon C. The incretin system and its role in type 2 diabetes mellitus. Mol Cell Endocrinol 2009;297(1–2):127–36.

34. Gil-Lozano M, Mingomataj EL, Wu WK, et al. Circadian secretion of the intestinal hormone GLP-1 by the rodent L cell. Diabetes 2014;63(11):3674–85.

35. Davies MJ, Bergenstal R, Bode B, et al. Efficacy of liraglutide for weight loss among patients with type 2 diabetes: the SCALE diabetes randomized clinical trial. JAMA 2015;314(7):687–99.

36. Pi Sunyer X, Blackburn G, Brancati F, et al. Reduction in weight and cardiovascular disease risk factors in individuals with type 2 diabetes: one-year results of the look AHEAD trial. Diabetes Care 2007;30(6):1374–83.

37. Wadden TA, Hollander P, Klein S, et al. Weight maintenance and additional weight loss with liraglutide after low-calorie-diet-induced weight loss: the SCALE Maintenance randomized study. Int J Obes (Lond) 2013;37(11):1443–51.

38. Liu SC, Tu YK, Chien MN, et al. Effect of antidiabetic agents added to metformin on glycaemic control, hypoglycaemia and weight change in patients with type 2 diabetes: a network meta-analysis. Diabetes Obes Metab 2012;14(9):810–20.

39. Ryder RE. The potential risks of pancreatitis and pancreatic cancer with GLP-1-based therapies are far outweighed by the proven and potential (cardiovascular) benefits. Diabet Med 2013;30(10):1148–55.

40. Shah P, Ardestani A, Dharmadhikari G, et al. The DPP-4 inhibitor linagliptin restores beta-cell function and survival in human isolated islets through GLP-1 stabilization. J Clin Endocrinol Metab 2013;98(7):E1163–72.

41. Shah Z, Kampfrath T, Deiuliis J, et al. Long-term dipeptidyl-peptidase 4 inhibition reduces atherosclerosis and inflammation via effects on monocyte recruitment and chemotaxis. Circulation 2011;124(21):2338–49.

42. Malin SK, Huang H, Mulya A, et al. Lower dipeptidyl peptidase-4 following exercise training plus weight loss is related to increased insulin sensitivity in adults with metabolic syndrome. Peptides 2013;47:142–7.

43. Yanovski SZ, Yanovski JA. Long-term drug treatment for obesity: a systematic and clinical review. JAMA 2014;311(1):74–86.

44. Fenske WK, Pournaras DJ, Aasheim ET, et al. Can a protocol for glycaemic control improve type 2 diabetes outcomes after gastric bypass? Obes Surg 2012; 22(1):90–6.

45. Monami M, Nardini C, Mannucci E. Efficacy and safety of sodium glucose cotransport-2 inhibitors in type 2 diabetes: a meta-analysis of randomized clinical trials. Diabetes Obes Metab 2014;16(5):457–66.

46. Bailey CJ, Gross JL, Pieters A, et al. Effect of dapagliflozin in patients with type 2 diabetes who have inadequate glycaemic control with metformin: a randomised, double-blind, placebo-controlled trial. Lancet 2010;375(9733):2223–33.

47. Vasilakou D, Karagiannis T, Athanasiadou E, et al. Sodium-glucose cotransporter 2 inhibitors for type 2 diabetes: a systematic review and meta-analysis. Ann Intern Med 2013;159(4):262–74.

48. Verrotti A, Scaparrotta A, Agostinelli S, et al. Topiramate-induced weight loss: a review. Epilepsy Res 2011;95(3):189–99.

49. Garvey WT, Ryan DH, Look M, et al. Two-year sustained weight loss and metabolic benefits with controlled-release phentermine/topiramate in obese and overweight adults (SEQUEL): a randomized, placebo-controlled, phase 3 extension study. Am J Clin Nutr 2012;95(2):297–308.

50. Garvey WT, Ryan DH, Henry R, et al. Prevention of type 2 diabetes in subjects with prediabetes and metabolic syndrome treated with phentermine and topiramate extended release. Diabetes Care 2014;37(4):912–21.

51. Torgerson JS, Hauptman J, Boldrin MN, et al. XENical in the prevention of diabetes in obese subjects (XENDOS) study: a randomized study of orlistat as an adjunct to lifestyle changes for the prevention of type 2 diabetes in obese patients. Diabetes Care 2004;27(1):155–61.

52. Derosa G, Cicero AF, D'Angelo A, et al. Effects of 1-year orlistat treatment compared to placebo on insulin resistance parameters in patients with type 2 diabetes. J Clin Pharm Ther 2012;37(2):187–95.

53. Scheen AJ, Van Gaal LF. Combating the dual burden: therapeutic targeting of common pathways in obesity and type 2 diabetes. Lancet Diabetes Endocrinol 2014;2(11):911–22.

54. Martin CK, Redman LM, Zhang J, et al. Lorcaserin, a 5-HT(2C) receptor agonist, reduces body weight by decreasing energy intake without influencing energy expenditure. J Clin Endocrinol Metab 2011;96(3):837–45.

55. Hoy SM. Lorcaserin: a review of its use in chronic weight management. Drugs 2013;73(5):463–73.

56. O'Neil PM, Smith SR, Weissman NJ, et al. Randomized placebo-controlled clinical trial of lorcaserin for weight loss in type 2 diabetes mellitus: the BLOOM-DM study. Obesity (Silver Spring) 2012;20(7):1426–36.

57. Smith SR, Fujioka K, Gupta AK, et al. Combination therapy with naltrexone and bupropion for obesity reduces total and visceral adiposity. Diabetes Obes Metab 2013;15(9):863–6.
58. Hollander P, Gupta AK, Plodkowski R, et al. Effects of naltrexone sustained-release/bupropion sustained-release combination therapy on body weight and glycemic parameters in overweight and obese patients with type 2 diabetes. Diabetes Care 2013;36(12):4022–9.
59. Brethauer SA, Aminian A, Romero-Talamás H, et al. Can diabetes be surgically cured? Long-term metabolic effects of bariatric surgery in obese patients with type 2 diabetes mellitus. Ann Surg 2013;258(4):628–36.
60. Courcoulas AP, Belle SH, Neiberg RH, et al. Three-year outcomes of bariatric surgery vs lifestyle intervention for type 2 diabetes mellitus treatment: a randomized clinical trial. JAMA Surg 2015;150(10):931–40.
61. Kashayp SR, Bhatt D, Wolski K, et al. Metabolic effects of bariatric surgery in patients with moderate obesity and type 2 diabetes: analysis of a randomized control trial comparing surgery vs intensive medical treatment. Diabetes Care 2013;36:2175–82.
62. Malin SK, Samat A, Wolski K, et al. Improved acylated ghrelin suppression at 2 years in obese patients with type 2 diabetes: effects of bariatric surgery vs standard medical therapy. Int J Obes 2014;38:364–70.
63. Ribaric G, Buchwald JN, McGlennon TW. Diabetes and weight in comparative studies of bariatric surgery vs conventional medical therapy: a systematic review and meta-analysis. Obes Surg 2014;24(3):437–55.
64. Standards of medical care in diabetes-2015: summary of revisions. Diabetes Care 2015;38(Suppl):S4.
65. Dixon J, Zimmet P, Alberti KG, et al. Bariatric surgery: an IDF statement for obese type 2 diabetes. Surg Obes Relat Dis 2011;7(4):433–47.
66. Khanna V, Malin SK, Bena J, et al. Adults with long-duration type 2 diabetes have blunted glycemic and ß-cell function improvements after bariatric surgery. Obesity (Silver Spring) 2015;23(3):523–6.
67. Malin SK, Bena J, Abood B, et al. Attenuated improvements in adiponectin and fat loss characterize type 2 diabetes non-remission status after bariatric surgery. Diabetes Obes Metab 2014;16:1230–8.
68. Wang GF, Yan YX, Xu N, et al. Predictive factors of type 2 diabetes mellitus remission following bariatric surgery: a meta-analysis. Obes Surg 2015;25(2):199–208.
69. Sjostrom L, Peltonen M, Jacobson P, et al. Association of bariatric surgery with long-term remission of type 2 diabetes and with microvascular and macrovascular complications. JAMA 2014;311(22):2297–304.
70. Coen P, Tanner C, Helbling N, et al. Clinical trial demonstrates exercise following bariatric surgery improves insulin sensitivity. J Clin Invest 2015;125(1):248–57.

Behavioral Treatment of the Patient with Obesity

Naji Alamuddin, MD, BCh, MTR[a],*, Thomas A. Wadden, PhD[b]

KEYWORDS

- Obesity • Weight loss • Behavioral treatment • Lifestyle modification • Health

KEY POINTS

- Weight loss of 5% to 10% of initial body weight is produced by a comprehensive 16 to 26 week behavioral intervention, consisting of diet, exercise, and behavior therapy.
- Behavioral treatment can be combined with diets of varying macronutrient composition, all of which are successful if they induce an appropriate energy deficit.
- Physical activity alone is of limited benefit for inducing weight loss but is important for improving health and quality of life and for facilitating long-term weight management.
- Weight regain is common following behavioral treatment but can be prevented by providing patients twice monthly or monthly weight loss maintenance sessions.
- The Diabetes Prevention Program and the Look AHEAD study provide examples of comprehensive behavioral interventions that produced long-term improvements in weight-related comorbid conditions.

INTRODUCTION

Expert panels sponsored by the World Health Organization, the National Institutes of Health, and several professional societies have recommended that obese individuals lose approximately 10% of initial body weight to improve their health and quality of life.[1–3] This goal can be achieved using a comprehensive behavioral program that includes 3 principal components: diet, physical activity, and behavior therapy. This article describes behavioral treatment of obesity (also referred to as behavioral weight control or lifestyle modification), its short-term and long-term results of treatment, and new developments in the field.

Disclosure Statement: T.A. Wadden serves on advisory boards for Nutrisystem and Weight Watchers International, each of which provides behavioral weight loss programs. N. Alamuddin has no disclosures.
[a] Division of Endocrinology, Diabetes, and Metabolism; and Center for Weight and Eating Disorders, Perelman School of Medicine, University of Pennsylvania, 3535 Market Street, Suite 3025, Philadelphia, PA 19104, USA; [b] Department of Psychiatry, Center for Weight and Eating Disorders, Perelman School of Medicine, University of Pennsylvania, 3535 Market Street, Suite 3029, Philadelphia, PA 19104, USA
* Corresponding author.
E-mail address: Naji.alamuddin@uphs.upenn.edu

Endocrinol Metab Clin N Am 45 (2016) 565–580
http://dx.doi.org/10.1016/j.ecl.2016.04.008
0889-8529/16/$ – see front matter © 2016 Elsevier Inc. All rights reserved.

OVERVIEW OF BEHAVIORAL TREATMENT

The Diabetes Prevention Program (DPP) provides an excellent example of a comprehensive behavioral intervention.[4] It randomly assigned more than 3200 overweight or obese subjects with impaired glucose tolerance to placebo, metformin, or an intensive lifestyle intervention (ILI); the latter was designed to induce and maintain a 7 kg reduction in initial weight. The study's primary outcome was the reduction in the incidence of type 2 diabetes. Lifestyle participants attended 16 individual counseling sessions (with a registered dietitian) during the first 24 weeks and then had 1 contact at least every other month for the remainder of the 4-year study. Subjects were instructed to consume a low-fat, reduced-calorie diet (ie, 1200–2000 kcal/d, based on body weight), made up of conventional foods that they selected. The physical activity goal was 150 min/wk (principally of brisk walking). The study was stopped after a mean of 2.8 years, at which time lifestyle participants had achieved a mean loss of 5.6 kg, compared with significantly smaller losses of 2.1 kg for metformin and 0.1 kg for placebo. The lifestyle intervention, compared with the placebo and metformin groups, reduced the risk of developing type 2 diabetes by 58% and 31%, respectively, leading to the study's early termination to provide lifestyle modification to the other 2 groups. A 10-year follow-up assessment found that, compared with placebo, the lifestyle intervention maintained a 34% reduction in the risk of developing type 2 diabetes, even though the latter subjects had regained most of their lost weight.[5] Comparable favorable findings were observed in trials conducted in Finland and China.[6,7]

The following section provides a fuller description of the components of behavioral treatment as provided in the DPP and clinical practice. Detailed accounts are provided by treatment manuals such as the Lifestyle, Exercise, Attitudes, Relationships, Nutrition (LEARN) Program for Weight Control or the protocols developed for the DPP and Action for Health in Diabetes (Look AHEAD) trials.[4,8,9]

PRINCIPAL COMPONENTS OF BEHAVIORAL TREATMENT
Diet

Behavioral weight control typically prescribes a calorie target to induce an energy deficit of 500 to 1000 kcal/d.[8] The target is usually 1200 to 1500 kcal/d for women and 1500 to 1800 kcal/d for men.[10] Alternatively, numerous studies have prescribed calorie goals based on body weight, with 1200 to 1499 kcal/d for individuals less than 250 lb and 1500 to 1800 kcal/d for those greater than this weight.[11] A couple of weeks of calibration may be required for participants to identify the calorie level that produces the desired loss of 0.5 to 1 kg/wk.

Although the DPP prescribed a traditional low-fat, low-calorie diet, a variety of different interventions can be incorporated in behavioral treatment, including low-carbohydrate, low-glycemic, and Mediterranean-type diets. All diets will produce weight loss, regardless of their macronutrient composition, if a consistent caloric deficit is achieved. This was demonstrated by the 2-year Preventing Obesity Using Novel Dietary Strategies (POUNDS) Lost study, in which participants in 4 diets groups were all prescribed a 750 kcal/d deficit but were instructed to consume different percentages of protein (15% or 25%), fat (20% or 40%), and carbohydrate (ranging from 35% to 65% of daily calories).[12] Short-term and long-term weight losses did not differ significantly at any time among the 4 dietary interventions, all of which were combined with a comprehensive program of lifestyle modification. Foster and colleagues[13] similarly found no significant differences in short-term or long-term weight loss in subjects assigned to low-carbohydrate versus low-fat diets, each combined with intensive lifestyle modification. Although the macronutrient composition of the reducing diet does not seem to affect weight loss, it may contribute to improvements in cardiometabolic risk factors. A low-glycemic index diet, for example, produced greater improvements in hemoglobin A1c (HbA$_{1c}$) in overweight subjects with type 2 diabetes than did a traditional low-fat diet that induced comparable weight loss.[14] **Table 1** summarizes the results of selected randomized trials that examined the effects of macronutrient composition on changes in weight and health outcomes.[12–21]

Self-Monitoring

Recording the type and amount of foods and beverages consumed, along with their calorie content, is a critical component of behavioral treatment. Self-monitoring helps patients identify patterns in their eating (including times and places associated with consumption), select targets for reducing calorie intake, and track progress in meeting calorie goals. Self-monitoring records can be expanded to include the patient's thoughts and feelings associated with inappropriate eating. More frequent self-monitoring is associated with greater weight loss.[22,23]

Patients traditionally have used paper records and a calorie book to track their food intake but these have been largely replaced by on-line trackers and applications (apps), such as My Fitness Pal or Lose It. Self-monitoring of physical activity is similarly encouraged, using a paper log or a device such as a pedometer or accelerometer (as provided by a Fitbit or a smartphone). Patients also are instructed to weigh themselves regularly, usually once or twice per week during active weight loss and as often as daily during weight loss maintenance. Cellular-connected "smart" scales, which measure weight digitally and send participants a graph of their progress, may help to induce weight loss when used as a primary intervention.[24]

Stimulus Control

Stimulus control teaches patients to manage external cues, such as the sight or smell of food, as well as times, places, and events associated with eating.[8,11] By reducing exposure to problem foods, patients are less likely to overeat. For example, patients are advised to avoid venues (eg, fast-food restaurants or all-you-can-eat buffets) that increase the risk of excess eating. At home, they are instructed to store foods out of sight, to serve modest portion sizes, to keep the table free of serving dishes, and to clean plates immediately after eating. They similarly are taught to limit eating to 1 or 2 rooms in the home and to avoid snacking while engaging in other behaviors (eg, watching television).

Goal Setting

Behavioral treatment helps patients make objective, measurable changes in eating, activity, and related behaviors.[8,11] They are guided in setting specific targets for calorie intake, minutes of physical activity, and frequency of self-monitoring. Goal setting clearly identifies the behavior to be changed and stipulates when, where, and how it will be performed. Patients regularly review with their interventionist progress made in meeting goals, as recorded in their food and activity logs.

Problem-Solving

Behavioral weight control usually includes additional components, such as problem solving skills that help patients analyze challenges they have in adhering to their diet and activity prescriptions.[8,11,23] They are taught to identify several possible solutions to the problem, to pick the most promising, and then implement it. Patients also learn cognitive restructuring skills, such as identifying cognitive distortions (eg, "I'll

Table 1
Weight losses from randomized trials that compared diets with varying macronutrient compositions

Study	Number	Number of Lifestyle Sessions Provided	Dietary Intervention	Weight Change	mo	Comment or Other Results
Dansinger et al,[15] 2005	160 (51% F) 58% completed	4	Atkins Zone Weight Watchers Ornish	-2.1 kg[a] -3.2 kg[a] -3.0 kg[a] -3.3 kg[a]	12	All participants had hypertension, dyslipidemia, and/or fasting hyperglycemia Weight loss was associated with level of adherence Each diet decreased LDL to HDL ratio No significant effects on BP or blood glucose at 12 months
Das et al,[16] 2007*	34 (% F unknown) 85% completed	52	Low-glycemic load High-glycemic load	-7.8%[a] -8.0%[a]	12	No differences were observed between groups in change in CVD risk factors
Fabricatore et al,[14] 2011	79 (80% F) 63% completed	30	Low-glycemic load Low-fat	-4.5%[a] -6.4%[a]	9	All participants had type 2 diabetes Larger reductions in HbA$_{1c}$ in the low-glycemic load group†
Foster et al,[17] 2003	63 (68% F) 59% completed	3	Low-carbohydrate (high protein, high fat) Conventional (high-carbohydrate, low-fat)	-4.4%[a] -2.5%[a]	12	HDL cholesterol increased more and triglycerides decreased more in the low-carbohydrate group† Greater reductions in LDL and total cholesterol in the low-fat group at 3 mo† Diastolic BP decreased in both groups
Foster et al,[13] 2010	307 (68% F) 63% completed	38	Low-carbohydrate Low-fat	-6.3 kg[a] -7.4 kg[a]	24	Greater increase in HDL cholesterol in the low-carbohydrate group† Greater decrease in triglycerides at 3 and 6 mo in the low-carbohydrate group† Greater decrease in LDL at 3 and 6 mo in the low-fat group†
Gardner et al,[18] 2007	311 (100% F) 80% completed	8	Atkins (low-carbohydrate) Zone (even distribution) LEARN (calorie-restricted) Ornish (low-fat)	-4.7 kg[a] -1.6 kg[b] -2.2 kg[ab] -2.6 kg[ab]	12	Greater increase in HDL cholesterol larger in Atkins than Ornish group and greater decrease in triglyceride levels in Atkins than Zone group No differences in insulin or blood glucose between groups† Systolic BP decreased more in Atkins than in all other groups† Diastolic BP decreased more in Atkins group than in Ornish group† All participants had diabetes

Study	Sample	Diet	Weight change	Months	Results
Sacks et al,[12] 2009	811 (64% F) 80% completed	Low-fat, average protein (highest carbohydrate) Low-fat, high-protein High-fat, average-protein High-fat, high-protein (lowest carbohydrate)	−2.9 kg[a] −3.8 kg[a] −3.1 kg[a] −3.5 kg[a]	24	LDL cholesterol decreased significantly more in lowest fat to highest carbohydrate than in highest fat groups to lowest carbohydrate groups[†] HDL cholesterol increased more with lowest carbohydrate than with the highest carbohydrate diet[†] All diets decreased triglyceride levels similarly All diets, except the highest carbohydrate, decreased fasting insulin (greater decrease in the high protein vs average protein diets)
Shai et al,[19] 2008	322 (14% F) 85% completed	Low-fat Mediterranean Low-carbohydrate	−2.9 kg[a] −4.4 kg[b] −4.7 kg[b]	24	No significant change in LDL cholesterol in any group HDL cholesterol increased in all groups, significantly more in the low-carbohydrate than low-fat group Triglyceride levels decreased more in the low-carbohydrate than in the low-fat group[†] In diabetic participants, only the Mediterranean diet group had a decrease in fasting glucose Insulin decreased in all groups, for both diabetic and nondiabetic participants All groups had a significant decrease in BP
Stern et al,[20] 2004	132 (17% F) 66% completed	Low-carbohydrate Conventional (low-fat)	−5.1 kg[a] −3.1 kg[a]	12	Triglyceride levels decreased more in the low-carbohydrate group than in the low-fat group[†] HDL cholesterol decreased less in the low-carbohydrate group than in the low-fat group[†] Greater improvements in HbA1C in type 2 diabetics in the low-carbohydrate group[†]
Yancy et al,[21] 2004	120 (76% F) 66% completed	Low-fat diet Low-carbohydrate, ketogenic diet with nutritional supplements	−6.5%[a] −12.0%[b]	6	All participants were hyperlipidemic Low-carbohydrate group showed greater decreases in triglycerides and greater increases in HDL[†]

All studies were analyzed by use of an intention-to-treat population, with the exception as indicated by an asterisk (*).

Different letters (in superscript) indicate statistically significant differences in weight loss between groups.

Abbreviations: BP, blood pressure; CVD, cardiovascular disease; F, female; HDL, high-density lipoprotein; LDL, low-density lipoprotein; MR, meal replacements; VLDL, very low density lipoprotein.

* A completer's population was examined.

† Results reported as "greater," "larger," "increased more," and so forth represent statistically significant differences between treatment conditions.

never be able to lose weight because I ate that dessert") and replacing them with rational responses (eg, "The 150 calories in ice cream is not going to hinder my weight loss, particularly if I walk after dinner"). Relapse prevention training teaches patients to anticipate and respond to lapses (eg, slips in their diet or exercise adherence) and high-risk situations (eg, the winter eating holidays). Details of problem solving and relapse prevention have been provided by Perri and colleagues[25]

Physical Activity

Patients in behavioral weight control programs are instructed to gradually increase their physical activity to approximately 150 to 180 min/wk over the first 6 months.[10,11] Activity usually consists of brisk walking or other forms of moderate-intensity aerobic exercise. Short-term studies (<6 months) have shown that physical activity alone induces minimal reductions in body weight compared with losses produced by dieting (ie, caloric restriction). Wing and colleagues,[26] for example, found that physical activity alone, diet alone, and diet plus physical activity interventions produced mean losses of 2.1, 9.1, and 10.3 kg, respectively, in 6 months of weekly intervention. Many obese individuals are not able to engage, at least initially, in the high levels of physical activity required to reduce body weight by 1 lb per week (by exercise alone). Patients must walk approximately 35 miles per week to achieve this loss. Alternatively, they can lose 1 lb/wk by just reducing their food intake by 500 kcal/d (the equivalent of eliminating 2 20 oz sugared sodas per day). Thus, patients must be cautioned not to expect significant weight loss from exercising alone or to try to use physical activity as a means of offsetting dietary indiscretions.

High levels of physical activity are required to facilitate the maintenance of lost weight (see later discussion). Patients, however, should be encouraged to exercise in the near term to improve their cardiovascular health. Several investigations have found that high levels of cardiorespiratory fitness significantly attenuate the risk of cardiovascular disease (CVD) mortality in overweight and obese individuals. A 10-study meta-analysis that assessed the combined effects of cardiorespiratory fitness and obesity on mortality found that, compared with normal weight and fit individuals, unfit individuals had twice the mortality rate, regardless of body mass index (BMI).[27] Obese but fit individuals had similar rates of survival as individuals of average weight (ie, BMI <25 kg/m^2). Similarly, Lee and colleagues[28] found in a longitudinal study of 25,000 men that obese but fit individuals had lower rates of CVD death than lean but unfit men. Even in the absence of weight loss, regular aerobic activity reduces blood pressure (BP), lipid concentrations, and visceral fat, while ameliorating glucose intolerance and insulin resistance in nondiabetic individuals, and improving glycemic control in persons with type 2 diabetes.[29]

STRUCTURE AND FREQUENCY OF BEHAVIORAL WEIGHT CONTROL

Behavioral treatment typically is delivered by a registered dietitian, psychologist, or other health professional, in an individual or group format.[11,30] Visits are usually held weekly for 16 to 24 weeks, followed by every-other-week or monthly meetings. Sessions begin with patients being weighed in private, which provides an important opportunity for accountability and prompts participants to examine the relationship between their changes in weight and behavior.[30] After the weigh-in, they report on their progress in meeting their calorie and physical activity goals and use problem solving skills to address difficulties encountered. The remainder of the meeting focuses on discussing a new weight management skill, as described in the structured curriculum. The session concludes with goals and assignments for the coming week.

Group sessions usually include 10 to 20 members and run 60 to 90 minutes, with individual meetings lasting about half that time.[11,30] Group treatment, in addition to being less costly than individual care, has the advantage of providing social support, empathy, and a healthy dose of competition for patients.[30] A randomized controlled trial found that a group-delivered intervention produced approximately 2 kg greater weight loss than individual treatment.[31]

SHORT-TERM AND LONG-TERM WEIGHT LOSSES
Short-Term Efficacy

Structured lifestyle modification programs (see previous discussion) produce an average loss of 7 to 10 kg in the first 6 months, equal to a reduction of 7% to 10% of initial weight.[3,11] Weight losses are largest when at least 14 intervention sessions are provided during this time; lower intensity treatment is not as effective.[3] Approximately 50% to 70% of patients achieve a 5% or greater reduction in initial weight, a criterion for clinically meaningful weight loss.[3] Individuals with the best attendance and greatest consistency in keeping self-monitoring records achieve the largest weight losses.[22,23]

The previously described study by Foster and colleagues[13] provides an excellent example of a state-of-the-art lifestyle intervention for the first year. Subjects in both the low-fat and low-carbohydrate diet groups were provided 20 weekly group sessions, 10 every-other-week sessions (through week 40), and then every-other-month sessions through 2 years. As shown in **Fig. 1**, participants in both groups lost approximately 11.8 kg at 6 months and maintained a loss of approximately this size at 12 months (10.8 kg for both groups).

Long-Term Efficacy

Gradual weight regain is common following behavioral treatment, as illustrated by Foster and colleagues[13] study at month 24. In the absence of further treatment, participants typically regain 3 to 4 kg in the first year following intervention, with 1 to 2 kg per year thereafter. Five years after treatment, about half of the participants have returned to their baseline weight.[11,30] Decreased adherence to diet and exercise

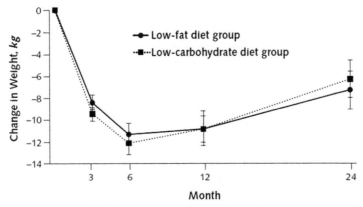

Fig. 1. Change in body weight for participants in low-fat and low-carbohydrate diet groups after 24 months, based on random-effects linear model. (*From* Foster GD, Wyatt HR, Hill JO, et al. Weight and metabolic outcomes after 2 years on a low-carbohydrate versus low-fat diet: a randomized trial. Ann Intern Med 2010;153:147–57; with permission.)

prescriptions and a return to previous habits contribute to weight regain,[30] as do unfavorable changes in appetite hormones (eg, ghrelin, leptin) and energy expenditure (both resting and nonresting).[32] Caloric restriction and weight loss induce decreases in leptin (a hormone that facilitates satiety), and increases in ghrelin (a hormone that stimulates hunger). Thus, decreased leptin and increased ghrelin promote overfeeding and weight regain. Sumithran and colleagues[32] demonstrated that these changes are not transient but continue even when patients stop losing weight and start to regain it, suggesting that these compensatory biological responses regrettably defend the body against weight reduction.

IMPROVING THE MAINTENANCE OF LOST WEIGHT
Weight Loss Maintenance Sessions

The most effective method for preventing weight regain is to provide patients continued behavioral support on an every-other-week or monthly basis following the initial weight loss program. Perri and colleagues[33] found that participants who attended group sessions every other week for 1 year after weight reduction maintained 13 kg of their 13.2 kg end-of-treatment weight loss. Those who received no further care regained 5.1 kg during the year. Wing and colleagues[23] similarly demonstrated that monthly weight loss maintenance sessions attenuated weight regain over 18 months. The most successful patients monitored their weight weekly or more frequently and responded quickly to small increases in weight. **Table 2** summarizes what the authors believe are the key components of lifestyle modification for both inducing and maintaining a weight loss of 7% to 10% of initial body weight.[11]

Weight loss maintenance sessions provide patients important support and accountability.[30] In addition, participants are instructed in the cardinal behaviors practiced by individuals in the National Weight Control Registry, all of whom have lost at least 13.6 kg (30 lb) and kept the weight off for 1 year or more.[34] Registry members engage in high levels of physical activity (eg, 225–300 min/wk), eat a low-fat, low-calorie diet (1200–1300 kcal/d for women), and weigh themselves frequently (once a week or more).

High Levels of Physical Activity

Numerous studies have demonstrated the critical role of increased physical activity in facilitating the maintenance of lost weight. Jeffery and colleagues,[35] for example, randomly assigned subjects to expend either 1000 kcal/wk or 2500 kcal/wk (principally through walking). Both groups also received a comprehensive program of lifestyle modification. There were no significant differences in weight loss between the 2 groups at month 6 (8.1 and 9.0 kg, respectively), consistent with the previous discussion of the limited effects of exercise on short-term weight loss. However, at month 18, subjects in the high activity group maintained a loss of 6.7 kg, compared with a significantly smaller 4.1 kg for the low-activity group. In a secondary analysis of a randomized controlled trial, Jakicic and colleagues[36] similarly demonstrated that women who exercised more than 200 min/wk maintained greater weight loss than those who exercised 150 to 199 min/wk, or less than 150 min/wk. The American College of Sports Medicine recommends physical activity of 60 minutes/d (ie, brisk walking or its equivalent) to facilitate the maintenance of lost weight.[37]

Physical activity may improve long-term weight loss by multiple mechanisms, including exercise's positive effects on mood, body composition, and resting metabolic rate.[38] Compelling findings indicate that high levels of physical activity are needed to compensate for increased energy efficiency following weight loss. Rosenbaum and colleagues[39] had obese individuals lose 10% of initial weight and found

Table 2
Key components of comprehensive behavioral weight loss interventions to achieve and maintain a 7% to 10% weight loss

Component	Weight Loss	Weight Loss Maintenance
Frequency and duration of treatment contact	Weekly contact, in person, or by telephone, for 20–26 wk. (Internet or e-mail contact yields smaller weight loss) Group or individual contact	Every-other-week contact for 52 wk (or longer) Monthly contact may be adequate Group or individual contact
Dietary prescription	Low-calorie diet (1200–1499 kcal for those <250 lb; 1500–1800 kcal for those ≥250 lb) Typical macronutrient composition: ≤30% fat (≤7% saturated fat); 15%–25% protein; remainder from carbohydrate (diet composition may vary based on individual needs or preferences)	Consumption of a hypocaloric diet to maintain reduced body weight Typical macronutrient composition: similar to that for weight loss
Physical activity prescription	180 min/wk of moderately vigorous aerobic activity (eg, brisk walking); strength training also desirable	200–300 min/wk of moderately vigorous aerobic activity (eg, brisk walking); strength training also desirable
Behavior therapy prescription	Daily monitoring of food intake and physical activity by use of paper or electronic diaries Weekly monitoring of weight Structured curriculum of behavior change (eg, DPP) Regular feedback from an interventionist	Occasional to daily monitoring of food intake and physical activity by use of similar diaries Twice weekly to daily monitoring of weight. Curriculum of behavior change, including relapse prevention and individualized problem solving Periodic feedback from an interventionist

From Wadden TA, Webb VL, Moran CH, et al. Lifestyle modification for obesity: new developments in diet, physical activity, and behavior therapy. Circulation 2012;125:1157–70; with permission.

that maintenance of a reduced body weight was associated with a decrease in total energy expenditure (TEE) that was approximately 300 to 500 kcal/d greater than that predicted by changes in body weight and composition. The decrease in TEE was due predominately to reduced energy expended during physical activity (ie, non-resting energy expenditure), reflecting increased work efficiency of skeletal muscle. Thus, paradoxically, successful weight losers may have to approximately double their amount of physical activity to compensate for their increased (undesired) energy efficiency.

Practitioners should emphasize that for weight control this activity can be performed at a moderate intensity and in short bouts, as brief as 10 minutes. When included as part of a comprehensive weight loss program, multiple short bouts of activity (throughout the day) are as effective as 1 long bout (>40 min) in achieving weight control.[40,41] Additional studies have shown that lifestyle activity, which involves increasing energy expenditure throughout the course of the day, without concern for the intensity or duration of the activity, is as effective for weight control as more traditional programmed activity (eg, jogging, swimming, or biking).[42,43] Pedometers and a new generation of activity trackers (eg, Fitbit, Jawbone, smartphones) provide some of the most convenient methods of monitoring lifestyle activity.[44] The ultimate goal is to walk approximately 10,000 steps daily, the equivalent of 4 to 5 miles, as practiced by members of the National Weight Control Registry.

HEALTH BENEFITS OF LIFESTYLE MODIFICATION FOR OBESITY

An extensive literature has demonstrated that losses of 5% or more of initial body weight are associated with both short-term and long-term improvements in cardiometabolic health, cardiorespiratory fitness, physical function, quality of life, mood, and sleep apnea (only a partial list of the benefits).[1–3] The Look AHEAD trial has provided the most extensive assessment of the health consequences of a lifestyle intervention, including its effects on cardiovascular morbidity and mortality over a 10-year period.[9] More than 5100 overweight or obese individuals with type 2 diabetes mellitus were randomly assigned to a diabetes support and education (DSE) group or an ILI group. The DSE participants received medical care from their own health professional who were encouraged to provide state-of-the-art care to manage comorbid conditions. Participants in ILI also received medical care from their own providers. In addition, they were provided a high-intensity lifestyle intervention, described previously, which was designed to help subjects achieve (and maintain) at least at 7% reduction in initial weight and 175 min/wk of physical activity.[45]

At the end of year 1, ILI participants lost a mean of 8.6% of initial weight, compared with a significantly smaller 0.7% in the DSE group.[46] The ILI group was superior to DSE in improvements in BP, blood glucose, HbA_{1c}, fitness, quality of life, physical function, sleep apnea, and other outcomes. A secondary analysis of selected outcomes, shown in **Fig. 2**, revealed the strong linear relationship between weight loss and improvements in selected cardiometabolic outcomes.[47] Losses as little as 2% to 4.9% of initial weight were sufficient to improve systolic BP and triglyceride levels, while reductions of 5% to 9.9% also improved HbA_{1c}, diastolic BP, and high-density lipoprotein (HDL) cholesterol. These findings are useful in underscoring to patients the benefits of losing as few as 5 to 10 lb (2.3–4.6 kg). The results also clearly demonstrated that larger weight losses generally were associated with greater improvements in cardiometabolic risk factors. Thus, patients should be encouraged to achieve a loss of 10% or more of initial weight when feasible.

Look AHEAD's primary outcome was a composite of cardiovascular morbidity and mortality (ie, fatal and nonfatal stroke and myocardial infarction, plus hospitalization for angina). The study was terminated after a mean follow-up of 9.6 years when statistical analyses revealed no significant differences between the ILI and DSE groups on the primary outcome, and investigators determined that extending the period of follow-up was unlikely to reveal any.[9] This was an unexpected result that led some commentators to suggest that weight loss was not beneficial. To the contrary, the ILI, compared with DSE, was associated with greater reductions in HbA_{1c}; decreased use of medications to treat diabetes, hypertension, and hyperlipidemia; lower medical costs; and reduced risk of developing very-high risk chronic kidney disease.[9,48,49] It was also associated with reduced hospitalization and other medical costs. Investigators currently are examining whether the ILI resulted in reduced all-cause mortality.

NEW DEVELOPMENTS IN THE DELIVERY OF LIFESTYLE MODIFICATION

New methods of delivering lifestyle modification are emerging with the rapid growth in digital means of communication (eg, Internet, e-mail, text messaging, Facebook,

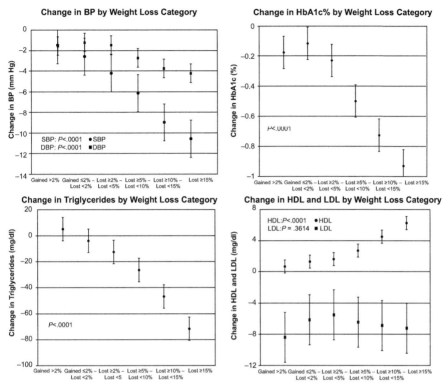

Fig. 2. Change in risk factors by weight loss categories for the Look AHEAD cohort. Data in all figures are presented as least square means and 95% confidence intervals adjusted for clinical sites, age, sex, race or ethnicity, baseline weight, baseline measurement of the outcome variable, and treatment group assignment. HDL, high-density lipoprotein; LDL, low-density lipoprotein. (*Adapted from* Wing RR, Lang W, Wadden TA, et al. Benefits of modest weight loss in improving cardiovascular risk factors in overweight and obese individuals with type 2 diabetes. Diabetes Care 2011;34:1481.)

Twitter), with their potentially greater convenience and reduced cost. This section briefly examines efforts to deliver lifestyle modification by telephone and the Internet.

Telephone-Delivered Programs

Participants treated by Donnelly and colleagues[50] received a 12-week weight loss program (ie, a 1200–1500 kcal/d diet of meal replacements and conventional foods) followed by a 14-week weight maintenance program. Half of the participants received all instruction via group conference calls and the other half attended on-site groups. Median weight losses at 12 weeks were −10.6 kg and −12.7 kg, respectively ($P<.05$) and at 26 weeks were 12.8 kg and 12.5 kg, respectively (not significantly different).

Perri and colleagues[51] demonstrated the effectiveness of telephone-based counseling for maintaining lost weight. Obese women who had lost an average of 10 kg during a 6-month run-in period were randomly assigned to receive a twice-monthly weight loss maintenance program that was delivered by telephone or on site. Women in a third group received newsletters only. Participants in the 2 weight loss maintenance interventions regained only 1.2 kg in the year of treatment compared with a significantly greater gain of 3.7 kg for those in the newsletter group. Appel and colleagues[52] also reported excellent maintenance of weight loss at 2 years with a principally telephone-delivered intervention. These findings suggest that lifestyle modification could be effectively delivered by call centers, as currently used for smoking cessation, diabetes management, and other conditions. Cost-effectiveness analyses are needed to compare further the benefits of on-site versus telephone-delivered interventions.

Digitally-Delivered Programs

In a first-generation study, Tate and colleagues[53] randomly assigned participants to 1 of 2 6-month programs delivered by Internet. The educational (control) intervention provided a directory of Internet resources for weight management (but no specific instruction in changing eating and activity habits). The behavior therapy intervention included this directory but also 24 weekly lessons conducted by e-mail in which participants submitted their food and activity records on-line and received feedback from an interventionist. Participants in the behavior therapy group lost significantly more weight than those in the educational group (4.1 vs 1.6 kg). In a 1-year follow-up study, Tate and colleagues[54] randomly assigned individuals at risk of type 2 diabetes to a low-intensity Internet intervention or to the same program with the addition of weekly behavioral counseling, delivered by e-mail. Participants in the latter group lost significantly more weight at 1 year (2.0 vs 4.4 kg). These 2 studies underscore the importance of patients keeping records of their food intake, physical activity, and other behavioral assignments. Educational instruction (ie, information) alone is not sufficient to induce clinically meaningful weight loss. This point was underscored by a recent study by Svetkey and colleagues[55] of young adults who used a smartphone-delivered program without the support of an interventionist. Similarly, despite their popularity, little is known about the effectiveness of smartphone apps for weight management. A randomized controlled trial that compared differences in weight loss in overweight patients who received either a MyFitnessPal app, along with usual primary care, or usual primary care only, revealed essentially no weight loss over 6 months.[56] Most participants used the app for the first month; however, logins decreased significantly after that with few participants using the app at 6 months.

The first head-to-head comparison of an Internet versus on-site delivered intervention was conducted by Harvey-Berino and colleagues.[57] They provided obese adults in the 2 groups the same 24-session intervention (delivered by different modalities). Participants in the Internet program lost 5.5 kg in 6 months, compared with a significantly greater 8.0 kg for those who received on-site treatment. Collectively, these studies suggest that the most successful Internet programs, in which therapists provide weekly e-mail feedback to participants, will induce weight losses of approximately two-thirds the size of those achieved by traditional on-site behavioral programs.[11] The reduced efficacy of Internet programs, however, is offset by the potentially greater accessibility and affordability of this approach, compared with traditional face-to-face behavioral treatment.

SUMMARY

Obese individuals can lose 7% to 10% of initial weight with a comprehensive behavioral weight control program consisting of caloric restriction, physical activity, and behavioral therapy. This weight loss produces clinically important improvements in CVD risk factors and quality of life. The main challenges facing researchers, practitioners, and patients are improving the maintenance of lost weight and making behavior weight control more available to the millions of individuals who would benefit from it.

ACKNOWLEDGMENTS

The authors thank Zayna M. Bakizada for her editorial assistance.

REFERENCES

1. World Health Organization. Obesity: preventing and managing the global epidemic. Geneva (Switzerland): World Health Organization; 1998.
2. National Institutes of Health/National Heart, Lung, and Blood Institute. Clinical guidelines on the identification, evaluation, and treatment of overweight and obesity in adults. Obes Res 1998;6:51S–210S.
3. Jensen MD, Ryan DH, Apovian CM, et al. 2013 AHA/ACC/TOS guideline for the management of overweight and obesity in adults: a report of the American College of Cardiology/American Heart Association Task Force on Practice Guidelines and The Obesity Society. J Am Coll Cardiol 2014;63:2985–3023.
4. Knowler WC, Barrett-Connor E, Fowler SE, et al. Reduction in the incidence of type 2 diabetes with lifestyle intervention or metformin. N Engl J Med 2002;346: 393–403.
5. Diabetes Prevention Program Research Group, Knowler WC, Fowler SE, Hamman R, et al. 10-year follow-up of diabetes incidence and weight loss in the Diabetes Prevention Program Outcomes Study. Lancet 2009;374:1677–86.
6. Tuomilehto J, Lindstrom J, Eriksson JG, et al. Prevention of type 2 diabetes mellitus by changes in lifestyle among subjects with impaired glucose tolerance. N Engl J Med 2001;344:1343–50.
7. Pan XR, Li GW, Hu YH, et al. Effects of diet and exercise in preventing NIDDM in people with impaired glucose tolerance: the Da Qing IGT and Diabetes Study. Diabetes Care 1997;20:537–44.
8. Brownell KD. The LEARN program for weight management. Dallas (TX): American Health Publishing Company; 2004.
9. Look AHEAD Research Group, Wing RR, Bolin P, Brancati FL, et al. Cardiovascular effects of intensive lifestyle intervention in type 2 diabetes. N Engl J Med 2013; 369:145–54.
10. The Diabetes Prevention Program Research Group. The Diabetes Prevention Program (DPP): description of lifestyle intervention. Diabetes Care 2002;25:2165–71.
11. Wadden TA, Webb VL, Moran CH, et al. Lifestyle modification for obesity: new developments in diet, physical activity, and behavior therapy. Circulation 2012;125: 1157–70.
12. Sacks FM, Bray GA, Carey VJ, et al. Comparison of weight-loss diets with different compositions of fat, protein, and carbohydrates. N Engl J Med 2009; 360:859–73.
13. Foster GD, Wyatt HR, Hill JO, et al. Weight and metabolic outcomes after 2 years on a low-carbohydrate versus low-fat diet: a randomized trial. Ann Intern Med 2010;153:147–57.
14. Fabricatore AN, Wadden TA, Ebbeling CB, et al. Targeting dietary fat or glycemic load in the treatment of obesity and type 2 diabetes: a randomized controlled trial. Diabetes Res Clin Pract 2011;92:37–45.

15. Dansinger ML, Gleason JA, Griffith JL, et al. Comparison of the Atkins, Ornish, Weight Watchers, and Zone diets for weight loss and heart disease risk reduction: a randomized trial. J Am Med Assoc 2005;293:43–53.

16. Das SK, Gilhooly CH, Golden JK, et al. Long-term effects of 2 energy-restricted diets differing in glycemic load on dietary adherence, body composition, and metabolism in CALERIE: a 1-y randomized controlled trial. Am J Clin Nutr 2007;85:1023–30.

17. Foster GD, Wyatt HR, Hill JO, et al. A randomized trial of a low-carbohydrate diet for obesity. N Engl J Med 2003;348:2082–90.

18. Gardner CD, Kiazand A, Alhassan S, et al. Comparison of the Atkins, Zone, Ornish, and LEARN diets for change in weight and related risk factors among overweight premenopausal women: the A TO Z weight loss study: a randomized trial. JAMA 2007;297:969–77.

19. Shai I, Schwarzfuchs D, Henkin Y, et al. Weight loss with a low-carbohydrate, Mediterranean, or low-fat diet. N Engl J Med 2008;359:229–41.

20. Stern L, Iqbal N, Seshadri P, et al. The effects of low-carbohydrate versus conventional weight loss diets in severely obese adults: one-year follow-up of a randomized trial. Ann Intern Med 2004;140:778–85.

21. Yancy WS Jr, Olsen MK, Guyton JR, et al. A low-carbohydrate, ketogenic diet versus a low-fat diet to treat obesity and hyperlipidemia: a randomized, controlled trial. Ann Intern Med 2004;140:769–77.

22. Wadden TA, Berkowitz RI, Womble LG, et al. Randomized trial of lifestyle modification and pharmacotherapy for obesity. N Engl J Med 2005;353:2111–20.

23. Wing RR, Tate DF, Gorin AA, et al. A self-regulation program for maintenance of weight loss. N Engl J Med 2006;355:1563–71.

24. Steinberg DM, Tate DF, Bennett GG, et al. The efficacy of a daily self-weighing weight loss intervention using smart scales and e-mail. Obesity (Silver Spring) 2013;21:1789–97.

25. Perri MG, Shapiro RM, Ludwig WW, et al. Maintenance strategies for the treatment of obesity: an evaluation of relapse prevention training and posttreatment contact by mail and telephone. J Consult Clin Psychol 1984;52:404–13.

26. Wing RR, Venditti E, Jakicic JM, et al. Lifestyle intervention in overweight individuals with a family history of diabetes. Diabetes Care 1998;21:350–9.

27. Barry VW, Baruth M, Beets MW, et al. Fitness vs. fatness on all-cause mortality: a meta-analysis. Prog Cardiovasc Dis 2014;56:382–90.

28. Lee CD, Blair SN, Jackson AS. Cardiorespiratory fitness, body composition, and all-cause and cardiovascular disease mortality in men. Am J Clin Nutr 1999;69: 373–80.

29. Gaesser GA, Angadi SS, Sawyer BJ. Exercise and diet, independent of weight loss, improve cardiometabolic risk profile in overweight and obese individuals. Phys Sportsmed 2011;39:87–97.

30. Wadden TA, Butryn ML, Wilson C. Lifestyle modification for the management of obesity. Gastroenterology 2007;132:2226–38.

31. Renjilian DA, Perri MG, Nezu AM, et al. Individual versus group therapy for obesity: effects of matching participants to their treatment preferences. J Consult Clin Psychol 2001;69:717–21.

32. Sumithran P, Prendergast LA, Delbridge E, et al. Long-term persistence of hormonal adaptations to weight loss. N Engl J Med 2011;365:1597–604.

33. Perri MG, McAllister DA, Gange JJ, et al. Effects of four maintenance programs on the long-term management of obesity. J Consult Clin Psychol 1988;56:529–34.

34. Wing RR, Hill JO. Successful weight loss maintenance. Annu Rev Nutr 2001;21: 323–41.

35. Jeffery RW, Wing RR, Sherwood NE, et al. Physical activity and weight loss: does prescribing higher physical activity goals improve outcome? Am J Clin Nutr 2003; 78:684–9.

36. Jakicic JM, Marcus BH, Gallagher KI, et al. Effect of exercise duration and intensity on weight loss in overweight, sedentary women: a randomized trial. JAMA 2003;290:1323–30.

37. Donnolly JE, Blair SN, Jakicic JM, et al. American College of Sports Medicine Position Stand. Appropriate physical activity intervention strategies for weight loss and prevention of weight regain for adults. Med Sci Sports Exerc 2009;41: 459–71.

38. Wadden TA, Vogt RA, Andersen RE, et al. Exercise in the treatment of obesity: effects of four interventions on body composition, resting energy expenditure, appetite, and mood. J Consult Clin Psychol 1997;65:269–77.

39. Rosenbaum M, Goldsmith R, Bloomfield D, et al. Low-dose leptin reverses skeletal muscle, autonomic, and neuroendocrine adaptations to maintenance of reduced weight. J Clin Invest 2005;115:3579–86.

40. Murphy MH, Blair SN, Murtagh EM. Accumulated versus continuous exercise for health benefit: a review of empirical studies. Sports Med 2009;39:29–43.

41. Jakicic JM, Donnelly JE, Pronk NP, et al. Prescription of exercise intensity for the obese patient: the relationship between heart rate, VO2 and perceived exertion. Int J Obes Relat Metab Disord 1995;19:382–7.

42. Andersen RE, Wadden TA, Bartlett SJ, et al. Effects of lifestyle activity vs structured aerobic exercise in obese women: a randomized trial. JAMA 1999;281: 335–40.

43. Epstein LH, Wing RR, Koeske R, et al. A comparison of lifestyle exercise, aerobic exercise, and calisthenics on weight loss in obese children. Behav Ther 1985;16: 345–56.

44. Bravata DM, Smith-Spangler C, Sundaram V, et al. Using pedometers to increase physical activity and improve health: a systematic review. JAMA 2007;298: 2296–304.

45. Look AHEAD Research Group, Wadden TA, West DS, Delahanty L, et al. The Look AHEAD study: a description of the lifestyle intervention and the evidence supporting it. Obesity (Silver Spring) 2006;14:737–52.

46. Look AHEAD Research Group, Pi-Sunyer X, Blackburn G, Brancati FL, et al. Reduction in weight and cardiovascular disease risk factors in individuals with type 2 diabetes: one-year results of the Look AHEAD trial. Diabetes Care 2007; 30:1374–83.

47. Wing RR, Lang W, Wadden TA, et al. Benefits of modest weight loss in improving cardiovascular risk factors in overweight and obese individuals with type 2 diabetes. Diabetes Care 2011;34:1481–6.

48. Espeland MA, Glick HA, Bertoni A, et al. Impact of an intensive lifestyle intervention on use and cost of medical services among overweight and obese adults with type 2 diabetes: the action for health in diabetes. Diabetes Care 2014;37: 2548–56.

49. Look AHEAD Research Group. Effect of a long-term behavioural weight loss intervention on nephropathy in overweight or obese adults with type 2 diabetes: a secondary analysis of the Look AHEAD randomised clinical trial. Lancet Diabetes Edocrinol 2014;2:801–9.

50. Donnelly JE, Smith BK, Dunn L, et al. Comparison of a phone vs clinic approach to achieve 10% weight loss. Int J Obes (Lond) 2007;31:1270–6.

51. Perri MG, Limacher MC, Durning PE, et al. Extended-care programs for weight management in rural communities: the treatment of obesity in underserved rural settings (TOURS) randomized trial. Arch Intern Med 2008;68:2347–54.

52. Appel LJ, Clark JM, Yeh HC, et al. Comparative effectiveness of weight-loss interventions in clinical practice. N Engl J Med 2011;365:1959–68.

53. Tate DF, Wing RR, Winett RA. Using Internet technology to deliver a behavioral weight loss program. JAMA 2001;285:1172–7.

54. Tate DF, Jackvony EH, Wing RR. Effects of Internet behavioral counseling on weight loss in adults at risk for type 2 diabetes: a randomized trial. JAMA 2003;289:1833–6.

55. Svetkey LP, Batch BC, Lin PH, et al. Cell phone intervention for you (CITY): A randomized, controlled trial of behavioral weight loss intervention for young adults using mobile technology. Obesity (Silver Spring) 2015;23:2133–41.

56. Laing BY, Mangione CM, Tseng CH, et al. Effectiveness of a smartphone application for weight loss compared with usual care in overweight primary care patients: a randomized, controlled trial. Ann Intern Med 2014;161:S5–12.

57. Harvey-Berino J, West D, Krukowski R, et al. Internet delivered behavioral obesity treatment. Prev Med 2010;51:123–8.

The Role of Macronutrient Content in the Diet for Weight Management

 CrossMark

George A. Bray, MD*, Patty W. Siri-Tarino, PhD

KEYWORDS

- Very-low-calorie diets • Low carbohydrate diets • High-protein diets • Low-fat diets
- Balanced-deficit diets • Mediterranean diets • Weight loss • Macronutrients

KEY POINTS

- Diets for the treatment of weight loss have been used for more than 2500 years, but have only been rigorously tested in randomized controlled trials in the last 20 years.
- Negative energy balance through caloric restriction is necessary for weight loss with diets, and all diets on average induce weight loss.
- Weight loss is highly variable with all diets, some people losing a lot of weight and others gaining weight; differences in macronutrient composition do not convincingly favor any one diet.
- Lower-fat diets are associated with lower low-density lipoprotein cholesterol levels, and higher-fat diets are associated with lower triglyceride and higher high-density lipoprotein levels in most longer-term weight loss studies; these effects on lipids are generally related to the magnitude of the weight loss.
- Higher protein intake and lower fat intake may benefit in maintaining weight loss.

INTRODUCTION
Historical Introduction

There is an entrenched belief that there is a magic weight loss diet that helps people to lose weight and keep it off. This widespread belief has stimulated numerous studies that have focused on different amounts of dietary fat, protein, or carbohydrate and even dietary supplements. The idea that uniquely composed diets might miraculously solve the problem of obesity goes back a long way in history.[1] Hippocrates 2500 years ago treated obesity with diet and exercise. Diet was also used by Galen in Roman times and by Avicenna in the tenth century AD when Arabic medicine was the dominant

Disclosure: Dr Bray is on the Herbalife Nutrition Advisory Board; the Medifast Advisory Board; and is a consultant to Novo-Nordisk. Dr Siri-Tarino has nothing to disclose.
Atherosclerosis Research Program, Children's Hospital Oakland Research Institute, 5700 Martin Luther King Drive, Oakland, CA 94609, USA
* Corresponding author. 300 Third Street, Suite 618, San Francisco, CA 94107.
E-mail address: bray@pbrc.edu

medical tradition. At the start of the eighteenth century a scientific basis for understanding obesity began to accumulate. The oxygen theory of metabolism was formulated by Lavoisier in 1787. This theory was followed 50 years later by the First Law of Thermodynamics and the concept of energy balance, which was shown to apply to animals and human beings during the later part of the nineteenth century.[1]

Modern diets can be dated to 1863 when William Banting,[2] an undertaker, published his 50-pound (23-kg) weight loss (**Fig. 1**) using a low-carbohydrate diet prescribed by his physician William Harvey.[2] His publication of "A Letter on Corpulence Addressed to the Public" first appeared in 1863, printed privately at Mr Banting's own expense, to tell the public that he had lost 50 pounds in 1 year with this diet and that many of his weight-related handicaps had resolved.[2] His book was so popular that it went through many editions and was translated into several languages. Carl van Noorden, a leading teacher and scholar in the late nineteenth and early twentieth centuries, recommended reduced-calorie diets in which fat was limited. The initial step of his approach was a 20% reduction in calories (eg, consuming 2000 rather than 2500 calories for a 70-kg man). Greater reductions in calories were advised for more significant weight loss. Thus toward the end of the nineteenth century both low-carbohydrate diets and low-fat diets had entered the realm of medically prescribed programs for patients with obesity.

At the beginning of the twentieth century the life insurance industry began to warn that excess weight was associated with shortened life expectancy.[1] The principal causes of death in the first half of the twentieth century continued to be infection, tuberculosis, and then heart disease. As the century progressed, the patterns of disease shifted steadily until, by the end of World War II, chronic diseases such as heart disease, cancer, hypertension, and diabetes had moved to the top of the list. Gradually the importance of excess weight as a factor in the development of these problems became clear.

The 1970s might be viewed as a watershed for diet and health. First the United States Senate Select Committee on Nutrition held hearings of hunger and published reports that highlighted the detrimental effects of the American Diet on the increasing incidence of noninfectious chronic diseases such as heart disease, diabetes, and cancer. Second, the "diet-heart" hypothesis was widely used to explain how eating too

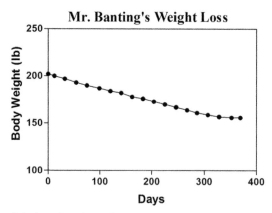

Fig. 1. Banting's weight loss diet. (*Data from* Banting W. Letter on corpulence, addressed to the public. 3rd edition. London: Harrison; 1864. vi, 7–50; [includes 2 addenda and appendix].)

much dietary saturated fat and cholesterol was responsible for the increasing rate of heart disease.[3] In addition, the increasing number of diet books that had begun with Mr Banting reached a new high, and Consumer Reports began a short-lived publication called "Rating the Diets."[4] Dr Atkins Diet Revolution, a popular diet, was published in 1972,[5] and led to an uproar from the medical profession about the potential hazards of a diet that recommended unlimited amounts of meat and fat, but very little carbohydrate.[4] This response is reminiscent of the criticism that Mr Banting had received from the medical profession 100 years earlier when he published his famous diet. Dr Atkins Diet Revolution, like most other popular diets, was published without clinical trials showing its effectiveness and safety. It would take another 30 years before such trials were done. This article reviews diets for weight loss and weight maintenance from the perspective of their macronutrient compositions.

Diets for Weight Loss

Although energy reduction is the sine qua non for weight loss, there are several other factors involved in selecting a diet for weight loss. In the Diabetes Prevention Program (DPP), reduction in calorie intake was the major predictor of weight loss.[6] However, reducing fat intake was the second predictor, and physical activity was only an important predictor if the calorie intake was not reduced.[6]

How can energy intake be reduced? People can use a prescribed diet and weigh out the foods they eat. They can purchase and use prepared foods with defined calorie levels. They can use nutrition labels on foods and on menus in restaurants to keep track of calories. With an effective program for lifestyle modification and diet, weight loss may be up to 8% of baseline body weight.[7] **Table 1** is a list of some of the popular diets that have been published to test the idea that there is a magic formula for weight loss. The increasing pandemic of obesity makes it clear that none of these diets have cured or even delayed it.

A calorie deficit of 500 kcal/d produces a weekly deficit of about 3500 kcal, which is equivalent to the energy in 450 g (1 pound) of fat tissue.[8] With this degree of calorie restriction, the rate of weight loss can be estimated (**Fig. 2**). As a general rule, weight loss is often calculated as though it were linear, but in reality it is not linear and is initially more rapid and then decreases in a logarithmic fashion as weight is lost until it reaches a new plateau. Computer-derived weight loss from 3 different models along with the linear estimates are shown in **Fig. 2**.[9–12] Note that for the first 3 to 6 months weight loss is almost linear but gradually tapers off until a new plateau is reached many months later.[10] Most weight loss diets produce a decline in energy expenditure with a decrease in triiodothyronine and leptin intake.[13,14] Treatment with leptin partially corrects these changes.[15]

There is a range of weight loss with all diets. This range is shown for the Look AHEAD study[16] and the POUNDS Lost study (Bray, Obesity POUNDS Lost, personal communication, 2015) in **Fig. 3**. Some people lose a considerable amount of weight, some lose the average amount, and some even gain weight. At least 2 factors predict this difference in response. The first is the initial rate of weight loss.[17] In the Look AHEAD study, individuals in the highest tertile of initial weight loss at 1 and 2 months had nearly twice the weight loss at 4 and 8 years as those in the lowest tertile of weight loss. Thus it is desirable to achieve as much weight loss in the early stages of weight management as possible, but the ability to accomplish this may be related to both the individuals' adherence to the diet as well as to their biological responsiveness to the dietary intervention.

Adherence to any dietary program is a critical factor in its success, an observation that has been consistently documented.[18–20] For example, in the POUNDS Lost study, the more sessions the participants attended, the more weight they lost (**Fig. 4**).

Table 1
Comparison of diet programs and eating plans with the typical American diet

Type of Diet	Example	General Dietary Characteristics	Comments	AHA/ACC/TOS Evaluation and Others
Typical American diet	—	Carbohydrate: 50% Protein: 15% Fat: 35% Average of 2200 kcal/d	Low in fruits and vegetables, dairy, and whole grains High in saturated fat and unrefined carbohydrates	—
Balanced-nutrient, moderate-calorie approach	DASH Diet or diet based on MyPyramid food guide; commercial plans such as Diet Center, Jenny Craig, NutriSystem, Physician's Weight Loss, Shapedown Pediatric Program, Weight Watchers, Setpoint Diet, Sonoma Diet, Volumetrics	Carbohydrate: 55%–60% Protein: 15%–20% Fat: 20%–30% Usually 1200–1800 kcal/d	Based on set pattern of selections from food lists using regular grocery store foods or prepackaged foods supplemented by fresh food items Low in saturated fat and ample in fruits, vegetables, and fiber Recommended reasonable weight-loss goal of 225–900 g/wk (0.5–2.0 lb/wk) Prepackaged plans may limit food choices Most recommend exercise plan Many encourage dietary record keeping Some offer weight-maintenance plans/support	Meta-analysis showing DASH approach better than control or healthy diets (WMD 0.87–1.5 kg)
Low-fat and very-low-fat, high-carbohydrate approach	Ornish Diet (Eat More, Weigh Less), Pritikin Diet, T-factor Diet, Choose to Lose, Fit or Fat	Carbohydrate: 65% Protein: 10%–20% Fat: ≤10–19% Limited intake of animal protein, nuts, seeds, other fats	Long-term compliance with some plans may be difficult because of low level of fat Can be low in calcium. Some plans restrict healthful foods (seafood, low-fat dairy, poultry) Some encourage exercise and stress management techniques	Same weight loss at 6 mo comparing <30% fat with >40% fat Strength of evidence: moderate

Low energy density	Volumetrics	Carbohydrate: 55% Protein: 10%–25% Fat: 20%–35% Focus on fruits, vegetables and soups	Four food categories: 1. Very low density: nonstarchy fruits and vegetables, nonfat milk, broth-based soups 2. Low density: starchy fruits/vegetables, grains, breakfast cereal, low-fat meats and mixed dishes 3. Medium density: meat, cheese, pizza, fries, dressings, bread, and so forth 4. High density: desserts, nuts, butter, oils Focus on categories 1 and 2, some from 3, minimum from 4	More weight loss at 6 mo with low-energy diet: RCT
Portion controlled	Use of meal replacements, both liquid and solid meals	—	—	Weight loss at 1 y in Look AHEAD trial related to frequency of consuming portion-control meals
Mediterranean-style diets	—	Carbohydrate: 35%–40% Protein: 12%–20% Fat: 40%–50% Approximately 25%–30% of energy from monounsaturated fat	Eat primarily plant-based foods (fruits, vegetables, whole grains, legumes, and nuts) Healthy oils (olive) instead of saturated fats Limit red meat to a few times a month Eat fish and poultry at least twice a week Red wine in moderation, if you choose to drink alcohol Be active and enjoy meals with family and friends	—
Low-carbohydrate, high-protein, high-fat approach	Atkins New Diet Revolution, Protein Power, Stillman Diet (The Doctor's Quick Weight Loss Diet), the Carbohydrate Addict's Diet, Scarsdale Diet	Carbohydrate: ≤20% Protein: 25%–40% Fat: ≥55%–65% Strictly limits carbohydrate to <100–125 g/d	Promotes quick weight loss (much is water loss rather than fat loss) Ketosis causes loss of appetite Can be too high in saturated fat Low in carbohydrates, vitamins, minerals, and fiber Not practical for long-term use because of rigid diet or restricted food choices	Same weight loss at 6 mo comparing <30 g/d vs 55% carbohydrate/15% protein with 40% carbohydrate/30% protein Strength of evidence: low

(continued on next page)

Table 1
(continued)

Type of Diet	Example	General Dietary Characteristics	Comments	AHA/ACC/TOS Evaluation and Others
Higher-protein, moderate-carbohydrate, moderate-fat approach	The Zone Diet, Sugar Busters, South Beach Diet	Carbohydrate: 40%–50% Protein: 25%–40% Fat: 30%–40%	Diet rigid and difficult to maintain Enough carbohydrates to avoid ketosis Low in carbohydrate; can be low in vitamins and minerals	Same weight loss at 6 mo comparing 25%–30% vs 15% protein Strength of evidence: high
Glycemic load	The Glycemic-Load Diet	Carbohydrate: 40–>55% Protein: 15%–30% Fat: 30%	Focus on low-glycemic-load foods	Same weight loss at 6 mo comparing high vs low glycemic load Strength of evidence: low
Low-sugar or non–sugar-sweetened beverages	Not diet but a call to reduce sugar-sweetened beverage intake as a preventive strategy	No recommendation other than to reduce/remove sugar-sweetened beverages from people's overall diet plans	Meta-analyses show that consumption of sugar-sweetened beverages is related to risk of obesity, diabetes, and heart disease	Weight loss less in adolescents comparing artificial vs sugar-sweetened drinks Strength of evidence: RCT comparing artificial sweeteners vs sugar-sweetened beverages
Novelty diets	Immune Power Diet, Rotation Diet, Cabbage Soup Diet, Beverly Hills Diet, Dr Phil	Most promote certain foods, or combinations of foods, or nutrients as having allegedly magical qualities	No scientific basis for recommendations	—
Very-low-calorie diets	Health Management Resources, Medifast, Optifast	<800 kcal/d	Requires medical supervision For clients with BMI ≥30 or ≥27 with other risk factors; may be difficult to transition to regular meals	—
Online weight-loss diets	Cyberdiet, DietWatch, eDiets, Nutrio.com	Meal plans and other tools available online	Recommend reasonable weight loss of 225–900 g/wk (0.5–2.0 lb/wk) Most encourage exercise Some offer weight-maintenance plans/support	—

Abbreviations: BMI, body mass index; DASH, Dietary Approaches to Stop Hypertension; RCT, randomized controlled trial; WMD, weighted mean difference.

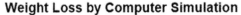
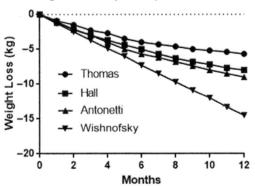

Fig. 2. Prediction of weight loss by computer with a 500 kcal/d deficit. The straight line uses the Wishnofsky projection that a 500-kcal/d deficit will produce a 3500-kcal deficit per week and that 1 kg of adipose tissue is equivalent to 7700 kcal. The other lines use computer-generated weight loss adjusting for reduced weight and changes in metabolism. (*Data from* Thomas DM, Gonzalez MC, Pereira AZ, et al. Time to correctly predict the amount of weight loss with dieting. J Acad Nutr Diet 2014;114:857–61.)

Genetic variation can also influence weight loss and biological response to a diet, as has been shown for both the DPP[21,22] and the POUNDS Lost trial.[23–30] **Table 2** summarizes the effects of several genes on weight change, change in body composition, and changes in cardiometabolic variables in response to the high-fat versus low-fat diets or high-protein versus average-protein diets in the POUNDS Lost study. **Fig. 5** shows that individuals with the A genotype of the *FTO* gene lost significantly more weight on the high-protein diet in a gene-dose–dependent fashion, but that the *FTO* genotype did not affect the response to the low-protein diet.[25] Using genetic profiles

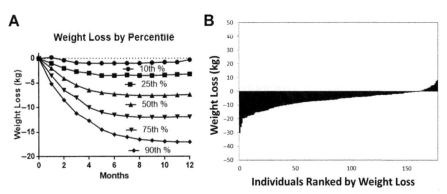

Fig. 3. Variability of weight loss. (*A*) Weight loss during the first year of the Look AHEAD trial was divided into groups losing less than 10%, less than 25%, less than 50%, less than 75%, and less than 90%. (*B*) Weight change from baseline to 6 months in patients prescribed a low-fat diet in the POUNDS Lost study listed individually from highest weight loss to weight gain. (*Data from* [A] Espeland MGA, Neiberg BR, Rejeski WJ, et al. Describing patterns of weight changes using principal components analysis: results from the action for health in diabetes (Look AHEAD) study group. Ann Epidemiol 2009;19(10):701–10; and [B] Bray, GA unpublished observations from POUNDS Lost.)

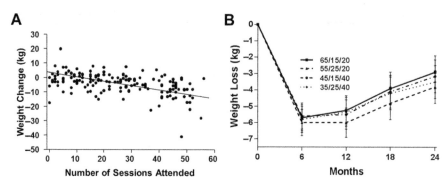

Fig. 4. Effect of adherence to the lifestyle program and weight loss for each diet group in the POUNDS Lost study. (*A*) Weight loss according to the number of behavioral sessions that were attended. Subjects who attended more sessions lost more weight. (*B*) Weight loss using imputed data over 2 years in men and women assigned to 1 of 4 diets with compositions as listed. There were no significant differences as a function of assignment to low or high fat, or high or average protein. (*Data from* Sacks FM, Bray GA, Carey V, et al. Comparison of weight-loss diets with different compositions of fat, carbohydrate and protein. N Engl J Med 2009;360(9):859–73.)

may thus be of value in the future in developing personalized dietary regimens for management of obesity.

Macronutrient Composition of Diets and Their Effects on Weight Loss

There is an entrenched belief that there is a magic weight loss diet, but is there any basis for this belief? A wide range of macronutrients have been proposed in various diets (see **Table 1**). This article examines this proposition from 2 perspectives: weight loss with diets of different macronutrient compositions, and the effect of these diets on cardiometabolic parameters.

As a basis for comparing the cardiometabolic effects of the diets listed in **Table 1**, this article starts with the effect on cardiometabolic parameters of the Look AHEAD[31] study and the DPP,[32,33] two large randomized trials with greater than 90% follow-up, which have examined the effect of an intensive lifestyle program in healthy individuals with prediabetes (DPP) or in people with diabetes (Look AHEAD). These two large trials provide an opportunity to examine the effects of weight loss on lipids and blood pressure in a setting of significant weight loss. The DPP showed significant weight reductions in the intensive lifestyle group compared with the metformin or placebo groups over 8, but not 10, years. In line with the significant reductions in weight observed within 3 years of randomization, improvements in cardiometabolic parameters in the same period were observed, including decreased systolic and diastolic blood pressure and triglyceride levels along with increased high-density lipoprotein (HDL) cholesterol concentrations.[32] Although total and low-density lipoprotein (LDL) cholesterol concentrations were not improved with weight loss, the prevalence of LDL pattern B was decreased, in line with the observed improvement with triglycerides and HDL cholesterol, as part of the well-established pattern of atherogenic dyslipidemia. Similarly, the Look AHEAD study showed significant improvements in cardiometabolic parameters with significantly greater weight loss (−6.15% vs −0.88%; P<.0001) in the intensive lifestyle intervention group at 4 years, including greater reductions in systolic and diastolic blood pressure, increases in HDL cholesterol levels (+1.70 mg/dL), and reductions in triglyceride levels (−5.81 mg/dL) (Look AHEAD 2010). After adjusting for

Table 2
Genetic markers in the POUNDS Lost study that modified response to a low-carbohydrate or low-fat diet

Author, Year	Gene	Changes Observed
Qi et al,[23] 2012	GIPR	The glucose-dependent insulinotropic polypeptide receptor that stimulates insulin release potently in the presence of increased glucose level. The T allele (rs2287019) in those assigned the low-fat diet was associated with more weight loss and greater decreases in fasting glucose, fasting insulin, and HOMA-IR. Thus GIPR rs2287019 T-allele carriers may obtain more weight loss and improvement of glucose homeostasis than those without this allele by choosing a low-fat diet
Zhang et al,[24] 2012	APOA5	Apolipoprotein A5 is an important determinant of plasma triglyceride levels. In the low-fat diet (20% energy as fat), carriers of the G allele showed greater reductions in total cholesterol and LDL-cholesterol levels than noncarriers. In the high-fat diet group (40% fat energy), participants with the G allele had a greater increase in HDL cholesterol than did participants without this allele. Thus there was more improvement in lipid profiles from long-term low-fat diet intake in the APOA5 G-risk allele
Zhang et al,[25] 2012	FTO	The fat mass and obesity-associated (FTO) gene is associated with obesity. There were significant modifications of 2-year changes in fat-free mass, whole-body % fat mass, total adipose tissue mass, visceral adipose tissue mass, and superficial adipose tissue mass by FTO genotype and dietary protein. Carriers of the risk allele had a greater reduction in weight, body composition, and fat distribution in response to a high-protein diet, whereas there was an opposite genetic effect in the low-protein diet. There were also significant interactions observed at 6 mo. Thus, a high-protein diet may be beneficial for weight loss and improvement of body composition and fat distribution in individuals with the risk allele of the FTO variant rs1558902 (see **Fig. 5**)
Qi et al,[26] 2013	IRS-1	The insulin receptor substrate is a link between the insulin receptor an intracellular activity. Among participants with the A allele, the reversion rates of the metabolic syndrome were higher in the high-fat diet group than in the low-fat diet group over the 2-year intervention ($P = .002$), whereas no significant difference between diet groups was observed among those without the A allele ($P = .27$). High-fat weight-loss diets might be more effective in the management of the metabolic syndrome
Xu et al,[27] 2013	PPM1K	This factor is essential for the regulation and nutrient-induced activation of the branched-chain alpha-keto acid dehydrogenase complex (BCKD or BCKDC), which catalyzes the breakdown of BCAA. In the high-fat diet group, the C allele was related to less weight loss and smaller decreases in serum insulin level and HOMA-IR, whereas an opposite effect of genotype on changes in insulin level and HOMA-IR was observed in the low-fat diet group. At 2 y, the gene-diet interactions remained significant for weight loss ($P = .008$) but became null for changes in serum insulin level and HOMA-IR because of weight regain. The C allele of BCAA/AAA ratio may benefit less in weight loss and improvement of insulin resistance than the lack of this allele when eating a high-fat diet

(continued on next page)

Table 2 (continued)		
Author, Year	Gene	Changes Observed
Mirzaei et al,[28] 2014	CRY2 MTNR1B	Both cryptochrome 2 and melatonin-2 receptor 1B are involved in the circadian rhythms of plants and animals. We found significant associations of CRY2 rs11605924 genotype with changes of RQ, RMR, and RMR/Kg; and of the MTNR1B rs10830963 genotype with RQ by the 2-year intervention. In addition, we observed significant modification effects of dietary fat on RQ changes for both SNPs. Our data indicate that the genotype of glucose and circadian-related loci CRY2 and MTNR1B might affect long-term change in energy expenditure, and that dietary fat intake might modify the genetic effects (www.clinicaltrials.gov; NCT00072995)
Zheng et al,[29] 2015	FTO	The fat mass and obesity-associated (FTO) gene is associated with obesity. The A allele was associated with a greater decrease in food cravings among the participants with high-protein diet ($P = .027$), but not in the low-protein diet group ($P = .384$). Weight regain from 6 mo to 24 mo attenuated the gene-protein interactions. Protein intakes did not modify the FTO genotype effects on other appetite measures. Individuals with the FTO A allele might obtain more reduction in food cravings by choosing a hypocaloric, higher-protein weight-loss diet
Lin et al,[30] 2015	NPY	NPY is a potent stimulator of food intake. The C allele (rs16147) was associated with a greater reduction in WC at 6 mo. In addition, the genotypes showed a statistically significant interaction with dietary fat in relation to WC and subcutaneous adipose tissue: the association was stronger in individuals with high-fat intake than in those with low-fat intake. At 24 mo, the association remained statistically significant for WC in the high-fat diet group ($P = .02$), although the gene–dietary fat interaction became nonsignificant. In addition, we found statistically significant genotype–dietary fat interaction on the change in total abdominal adipose tissue, visceral adipose tissue, and subcutaneous adipose tissue at 24 mo: the rs16147 T allele seemed to associate with more adverse changes in abdominal fat deposition in the high-fat diet group than in the low-fat diet group. The NPY rs16147 genotypes affect the change in abdominal adiposity in response to dietary interventions, particularly in the context of high fat diets

Abbreviations: AAA, aromatic amino acid; BCAA, branched chain amino acid; CRY2, cryptochrome 2; FTO, fat mass and obesity-associated gene; GIPR, glucose-dependent insulinotropic polypeptide receptor; HDL, high-density lipoprotein; HOMA-IR, homeostatic measurement of insulin resistance; IRS-1, insulin receptor substrate-1; LDL, low-density lipoprotein; MC4R, melanocortin-4 receptor; MTNR1B, melatonin receptor 1B; NPY, neuropeptide Y; PPM1K, protein phosphatase Mg/Mn 1K; RMR, resting metabolic rate; RMR/Kg, resting metabolic rate per kg body weight; RQ, respiratory quotient; SNPs, single-nucleotide polymorphisms; WC, waist circumference.

medication use, LDL cholesterol was not different between the treatment and control groups (without adjustment, LDL cholesterol was higher in the intervention group).

Very-low-calorie diets

Very-low-calorie diets (VLCDs; also called very-low-energy diets) have energy levels between 200 and 800 kcal/d. In a review comparing low-calorie diets with VLCDs, Tsai and Wadden[33] identified 6 randomized controlled trials (RCTs) that included a follow-up of at least 1 year. VLCDs produced significantly greater short-term weight

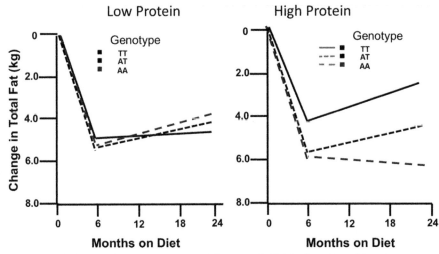

Fig. 5. Weight loss in the POUNDS Lost trial among individuals eating either the average-protein (15%) or the high-protein (25%) diets according to their genotype with the FTO gene. (*Data from* Zhang X, Qi Q, Zhang C, et al. FTO genotype and 2-year change in body composition and fat distribution in response to weight-loss diets: the POUNDS LOST Trial. Diabetes 2012;61(11):3005–11.)

loss (16.1%) than the low-calorie comparison diets (9.7%) but similar longer-term weight losses.[34]

Carbohydrate, low-carbohydrate diets, and sugar-sweetened beverages

Carbohydrates in the diet are provided by starches and added sugars and can be ingested in solid food or in beverages. Carbohydrate as a cause for obesity is based on the belief that insulin is the driving force for becoming obese and that, if carbohydrate is absent, the body oxidizes fat. In 1972, Atkins[5] published one of the most popular recent low-carbohydrate-diet books, but it was 30 years before any controlled studies of this diet were done. Two of these trials are shown in **Fig. 6**. It is clear that for the first few months the low-carbohydrate diet produced more weight loss but that this disappeared as the diet was continued.[35–38] In a meta-analysis, Nordmann and colleagues[39] found that weight loss was greater at 6 months with the low-carbohydrate diet (weighted mean difference −3.3 kg; 95% confidence interval [CI], −5.3 to − 1.4), but not at 12 months (−1.0; 95% CI, −3.5 to 1.5). Blood pressure was not affected, but changes in triglyceride levels (−22.1 mg/dL; 95% CI, −38.1 to −5.3) and HDL cholesterol levels (4.6 mg/dL; 95% CI, 1.5–8.1) favored the low-carbohydrate diet, whereas cholesterol levels at 6 and 12 months (10.1 mg/dL; 95% CI, 3.5–16.2 at 12 months) and LDL cholesterol (7.7 mg/dL; 95% CI, 1.9–13.9 at 12 months) changed more favorably with the low-fat diet. When the effect of named diets like those in **Table 1** were compared in a meta-analysis there was no significant difference between them in terms of weight loss. That is, the low-carbohydrate diets were not better than the low-fat diets,[40] a conclusion supported by the obesity guidelines.[7] However, several longer-term studies using low-carbohydrate (<20 g/d)[41] or high-protein diets[42] as the intervention over at least 1 year showed reduced triglyceride and/or increased HDL cholesterol levels even with comparable reductions in weight relative to the control diets, suggesting potential cardiovascular benefit from the macronutrients and not the weight loss. Note that studies over the long term are

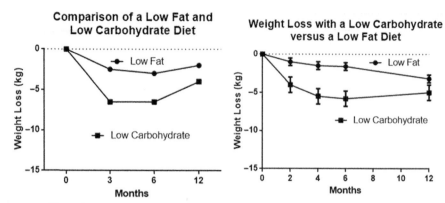

Fig. 6. Effect of low carbohydrate diets (Atkins Diet) versus low-fat diets. (*Left*) Weight loss was greater with the low carbohydrate diet at 3 and 6 months, but not 12 months. (*Right*) Weight was greater at 2, 4 and 6 months, but not 12 months in this Veterans Administration hospital study. (*Data from* Refs.[34,36,37])

hindered by the ability of participants to consistently comply with prescribed dietary regimens, often limiting the achievable differences in targeted macronutrient composition and possibly also effects on weight and other outcomes.

Carbohydrate, as sugar or high-fructose corn syrup in beverages, provides an additional challenge to the weight loss diet, because some of these calories are "invisible" or undetectable when ingested in beverages and people usually do not reduce the intake of other energy-containing foods by the amount of energy in the beverage.[43] Thus sugar-containing beverages (soft drinks, fruit drinks, and fruit juices) can be viewed as add-on calories. A randomized clinical trial that substituted artificially sweetened beverages given to some children over 18 months found that children consuming the artificially sweetened beverages gained less weight, and that in the upper half of the weight group the caloric compensation was inadequate, thus accounting for a relative weight loss.[44]

Dietary fat, energy density, and low-fat diets

Low-fat diets are a standard strategy to help patients lose weight because fat has more energy per unit weight than either protein or carbohydrate (ie, it has higher energy density).[45] Thus reducing dietary fat reduces fat intake and reduces the energy density of the diet. A meta-analysis of 594 participants in 6 trials covered an intervention period that varied from 3 to 18 months with follow-up from 6 to 18 months.[46] There were no significant differences between low-fat diets ranging from 20 to 30 g/d or 20% of total energy versus other weight-reducing diets in terms of sustained weight loss. Weight loss at 6 months was 5.5 kg for the low-fat group and 6.5 kg for the comparison group. The overall weight loss at the 12-month to 18-month follow-up in all studies was very small (2–4 kg) (**Fig. 7**A).

A second strategy for reducing energy density, besides reducing dietary fat, is to use foods with higher water content, which was done in a trial comparing a reduced-fat diet with a diet with extra fruits and vegetables, which reduces energy density (**Fig. 7**B). In this trial the addition of fruits and vegetables enhanced weight loss compared with reducing fat only,[47] leading to the Volumetrics diet.[48]

Low glycemic-index diets

The glycemic index is based on the increase in blood glucose level in response to the test food compared with the increase after eating a 50-g portion of white bread;

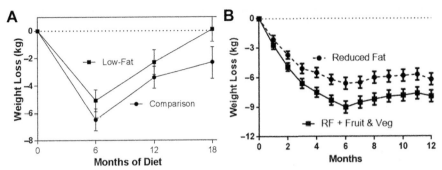

Fig. 7. Effect of low-fat diets on body weight. (*A*) Meta-analysis of low-fat diets and comparison in which the low-fat diet produced weight loss that was not different from control. (*B*) Weight loss comparing a reduced-fat diet (N = 36) with a reduced-fat (RF) plus fruits and vegetables diet (n = 35) over 12 months. (*Data from* [*A*] Pirozzo S, Summerbell C, Cameron C, et al. Should we recommend low-fat diets for obesity? Obes Rev 2003;4(2):83–90; and [*B*] Ello-Martin JA, Roe LS, Ledikwe JH, et al. Dietary energy density in the treatment of obesity: a year-long trial comparing 2 weight-loss diets. Am J Clin Nutr 2007;85(6):1465–77.)

glycemic load is the product of glycemic index and amount of carbohydrate in the food.[49,50] The effect of low-glycemic-index diets on weight loss has been studied in several randomized clinical trials in adults. In a meta-analysis by Schwingshackl and Hoffmann,[51] the only difference between diets with low glycemic index/load and high glycemic index/load was in plasma insulin levels (−5.16 pmol/L; 95% CI, −8.45 to −1.88) favoring low glycemic index/load. Thomas and colleagues[52] in another meta-analysis identified 6 studies including 202 participants who met their inclusion criteria. Three of these studies compared low-glycemic-index diets with higher-glycemic-index diets, whereas the other 3 compared an ad-lib reduced-glycemic-load diet with a conventional energy-restricted reduced-fat diet, or an energy-restricted low-glycemic-index diet with a normal energy-restricted diet. Interventions were short, ranging from 5 weeks to 6 months. There was a small significant difference in body weight of 1.1 kg (95% CI, −2.0 to −0.2) that favored the low-glycemic-index diets. The body mass decreased by 1.1 kg (*P*<.05) and fat mass by a similar amount compared with the change of weight in the control diet group. Both total and LDL cholesterol levels decreased more with the low-glycemic-index diets.[52]

High-protein diets

High-protein diets have also been claimed to be beneficial in managing weight loss.[53] The left panel of **Fig. 8** shows that individuals assigned to a high-protein diet who adhered to that diet during the 2 years of the POUNDS Lost study lost progressively more weight.[20] A second 2-year study compared 12% and 25% protein diets eaten as part of a 30% fat diet.[54,55] Weight loss over 36 weeks was substantially greater with the higher-protein diet and this difference was maintained at 56 weeks but not at 104 weeks (see **Fig. 8**). A meta-analysis of energy-restricted, high-protein, low-fat diets compared with standard-protein low-fat diets by Wycherly and colleagues[56] showed a borderline significant effect of the higher-protein diets on body weight in trials lasting more than 12 weeks (−0.97 kg; 95% CI, −2.07 to 0.13) and in trials lasting less than 12 weeks (−0.79 kg; 95% CI, −1.34 to 0.37). However, fat mass declined significantly more in the high-protein groups in trials lasting less than 12 weeks and in those lasting more than 12 weeks (−0.83 kg; 95% CI, −1.31 to −0.34), favoring

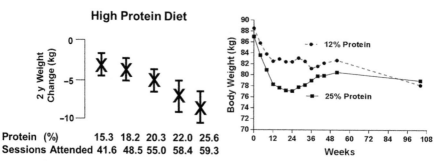

Fig. 8. Effect of dietary protein on weight loss. (*Left*) Weight loss at 2 years according to adherence to dietary protein determined from 3 dietary recalls. (*Right*) Weight loss with 12% or 25% protein in individuals eating a 30% fat diet followed for 1 year and then reevaluated after 2 years. (*Data from* Skov AR, Toubro S, Rønn B, et al. Randomized trial on protein vs carbohydrate in ad libitum fat reduced diet for the treatment of obesity. Int J Obes Relat Metab Disord 1999;23(5):528–36; and Due A, Toubro S, Skov AR, et al. Effect of normal-fat diets, either medium or high in protein, on body weight in overweight subjects: a randomised 1-year trial. Int J Obes Relat Metab Disord 2004;28(10):1283–90.)

high-protein diets. The decrease in triglyceride levels also favored the higher-protein diets (0.23 mmol/L; 95% CI, −0.36 to −0.11), as did the increase in HDL cholesterol levels (0.61 mmol/L; 95% CI, 0.20–1.02). An increase in resting energy expenditure also occurred in the trials lasting less than 12 weeks (595 kJ/d; 95% CI, 66.95–1124.05), favoring the high-protein diet. This finding is similar to the effects observed with the measurement of energy expenditure during overfeeding in response to different levels of dietary protein.[57] In a second meta-analysis by Schwingshackl and Hoffmann[58] comparing the long-term effects of low-fat diets with either low or high protein, fasting insulin level was again the main difference in response (−0.71 µU/mL; 95% CI, −1.36 to −0.05), favoring diets with low glycemic index/load.

Mediterranean diets
Mediterranean diets are characterized by their emphasis on high intake of legumes and whole-grain cereals, an abundance of fruits and vegetables, a high ratio of mono-unsaturated to polyunsaturated fatty acids, moderate alcohol consumption, and low consumption of meat and dairy products. In diabetic individuals this diet produced a significantly greater weight loss over 4 years than the comparison diet[59–61] (**Fig. 9**). In addition, this dietary pattern is associated with a reduction in risk of myocardial infarction[62] and in all-cause mortality.[63] In diabetic individuals the Mediterranean-style diets improved glycemic control and body weight (−0.29 kg; 95% CI, −0.55 to −0.04) favoring the Mediterranean diet.[62] Another meta-analysis[63] found that the Mediterranean diet compared with low-fat diets improved weight loss (−2.2 kg; 95% CI, −3.9 to −0.6) and improved systolic and diastolic blood pressure, fasting plasma glucose levels (−3.83 mg/dL; 95% CI, −7.04 to −0.62), total cholesterol levels (−7.35 mg/dL; 95% CI, −10.3 to −4.30), and high-sensitivity C-reactive protein levels (−0.97 mg/dL; 95% CI, −1.49 to −0.46) but the diet did not affect HDL cholesterol or fasting insulin.

Diets that reduce carbohydrate, protein, and fat, the so-called balanced-deficit diets or prudent diets, have been widely used in treating obesity. In a meta-analysis of studies classified as 600 kcal/d deficit or low-fat diets, Avenell and colleagues[64] found that after 12 months on the diet there was a weighted mean difference in weight loss of −5.31 kg (95% CI, −5.86 to −4.77) compared with the usual-care control setting.

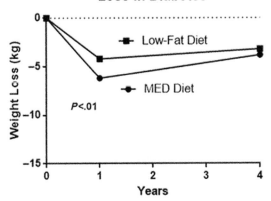

Fig. 9. Effect of a Mediterranean-style diet (MED) on body weight loss in patients with diabetes. (*Data from* Esposito K, Maiorino MI, Ciotola M, et al. Effects of a Mediterranean-style diet on the need for antihyperglycemic drug therapy in patients with newly diagnosed type 2 diabetes: a randomized trial. Ann Intern Med 2009;151(5):306–14.)

When 12-month weight changes from studies with imputed values were compared with studies with no assumed values, the weight changes were −4.52 kg (95% CI, −5.67 to −4.94) favoring the 600 kcal/d deficit diet. At 12 months, diastolic and systolic blood pressure, lipid levels, and fasting plasma glucose levels were all significantly improved compared with the control group.[64]

Portion-controlled diets or meal replacements are one way of achieving a balanced caloric deficit. This deficit can be achieved most simply by using individually packaged foods. Frozen low-calorie meals containing 250 to 350 kcal/package can be a convenient way to do this, except for the high salt content of many of these foods. In a 6-month intervention, the daily use of a commercially available portion-control plate was effective in inducing weight loss in obese, type 2 diabetic patients versus a usual-care dietary teaching group (1.8% vs 0.1%; $P = .006$), resulting in a decrease in necessary hypoglycemic medications.[65] A meta-analysis of 6 studies using meal replacements showed more weight loss at 3 months and in those completing the trials than in the low-calorie comparison diets.[66] In addition, a recent but small and shorter-term trial conducted over 18 months provides data to support the concept that portion control can increase diet quality while maintaining significant weight loss.[67]

Comparison of Diets with Different Macronutrient Compositions

Several randomized clinical trials lasting 1 year[18,68] or 2 years[20,39,69] have compared diets head to head. In the first, 169 obese individuals were randomized to one of 4 popular diets, including the Atkins Diet,[5] The Ornish Diet,[70] the Weight Watchers diet,[71] and the Zone Diet.[72] At the end of 12 months, each diet produced weight loss of about 5 kg, but there was no difference between diets (**Fig. 10A**). Adherence to the diet was the single most important criterion of success in this trial and the Atkins and Ornish diets were apparently more difficult to adhere to. In a second 1-year study by Gardner and colleagues[69] comparing the Atkins, Zone, Ornish, and LEARN (Lifestyle, Exercise, Attitudes, Relationships and Nutrition) diets, the Atkins Diet led to the greatest weight loss and associated improvements in cardiometabolic parameters (not shown). This study was conducted in premenopausal women, which may

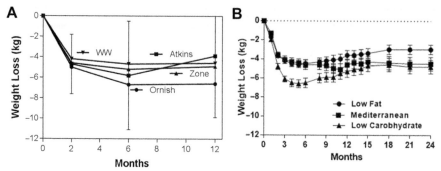

Fig. 10. Comparison of weight loss with diets. (*A*) Data from Dansinger and colleagues[18] comparing the Atkins Diet, the Ornish Diet, the Zone Diet, and the Weight Watchers (WW) diet over 12 months. The wide range of weight loss is shown by the vertical lines for standard deviation. The best predictor of weight loss was adherence to the diet, and not the diet itself. (*B*) Comparison of the Mediterranean diet, the Atkins Diet, and a low-fat diet over 2 years in a predominantly male Israeli working population. Note the reacceleration of weight loss in the Mediterranean group after the weight loss plateau had been reached. (*Data from* Dansinger ML, Gleason JA, Griffith JL, et al. Comparison of the Atkins, Ornish, Weight Watchers, and Zone diets for weight loss and heart disease risk reduction: a randomized trial. JAMA 2005;293(1):43–53; and Shai I, Schwarzfuchs D, Henkin Y, et al; Dietary Intervention Randomized Controlled Trial (DIRECT) Group. Weight loss with a low-carbohydrate, Mediterranean, or low-fat diet. N Engl J Med 2008;359(3):229–41.)

represent a cohort with a metabolic response that differs significantly from men and older women. In a 2-year study (**Fig. 10**B) a low-fat diet was compared with a low-carbohydrate diet (Atkins Diet) and a Mediterranean-style diet.[69] This trial was conducted in Israel and the participants were primarily men. At about 8–9 months, something unexpected and unexplained happened in the group eating the Mediterranean diet. After stabilizing, their body weights began to decrease to reach the level of the low-carbohydrate diet by 12 months. There are no other trials known to these authors that have had a resurgence of weight loss after the plateau; it almost always increases. There is no explanation for this unexpected phenomenon and it raises concern about protocol maintenance.[69]

The POUNDS Lost study shown in **Fig. 4** was more than twice as large as the 2 studies presented in **Fig. 10**. It was conducted at 2 sites in the United States.[20] A total of 811 men and women were randomized to 1 of 4 diets and 80% of them provided weights at the end of 2 years. The diets were (1) 20% fat, 15% protein; (2) 20% fat, 25% protein; (3) 49% fat, 15% protein; or (4); 40% fat, 25% protein. The foods used for all 4 diets were the same, just the quantities were varied. At the end of 6 months, 12 months, or 2 years, the weight loss was similar for all 4 diets (**Fig. 4**B). The weight loss and the effect of adherence on weight loss are shown in **Fig. 4**A.

Commercial Programs for Weight Loss

Several commercial weight loss programs have now published enough data to make comparison possible. Two of these studies are shown in **Fig. 11**.[73,74] In a meta-analysis, Gudzune and colleagues[75] reported that, at 12 months, Weight Watchers participants achieved at least 2.6% greater weight loss than those assigned to control/education. Jenny Craig resulted in at least 4.9% greater weight loss at 12 months than control/education and counseling. Nutrisystem resulted in at least 3.8% greater

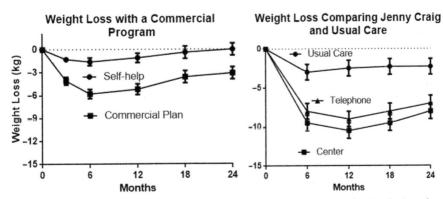

Fig. 11. Weight loss comparing 2 commercial weight loss programs. (*Left*) Weight Watchers program and usual care over 12 months. (*Right*) Comparison of usual care with the Jenny Craig program delivered either by participants coming to the center or by telephone. (*Data from* Heshka S, Anderson JW, Atkinson RL, et al. Weight loss with self-help compared with a structured commercial program: a randomized trial. JAMA 2003;289(14):1792–8; and Rock CL, Flatt SW, Sherwood NE, et al. Effect of a free prepared meal and incentivized weight loss program on weight loss and weight loss maintenance in obese and overweight women: a randomized controlled trial. JAMA 2010;304(16):1803–10.)

weight loss at 3 months than control/education and counseling. Very-low-calorie programs (Health Management Resources, Medifast, and Optifast) resulted in at least 4.0% greater short-term weight loss than counseling, but some attenuation of effect occurred beyond 6 months when reported. Atkins resulted in 0.1% to 2.9% greater weight loss at 12 months than counseling.[75] Although the differences in weight loss were small, it is possible that macronutrient composition may have had effects of cardiovascular risk factors.

Association of Dietary Macronutrients with Successful Maintenance of Long-term Weight Loss

In all treatments for obesity, weight loss slows over time and eventually stops. In most cases weight subsequently increases in most people toward baseline levels. This tendency is shown most clearly in the 2 large randomized trials discussed throughout this article: the DPP[76] and the Look AHEAD trial (**Fig. 12**).[53] The 8-year weight loss data for both trials are shown in **Fig. 12**. After the initial loss of weight, which reached a nadir between 6 and 12 months, there was a gradual increase to a level below baseline for both trials, but still a substantial weight regain.

Although there is little to choose between diets for weight loss, it is conceivable that some macronutrient combinations may be better in helping to maintain weight loss. Two of these are briefly reviewed here: protein and fat.

Higher-protein diets and the maintenance of weight loss

Higher-protein diets may enhance weight maintenance.[53,77] Following weight loss with a VLCD for 4 weeks, 148 male and female subjects were stratified by age, body mass index, body weight, restrained eating, and resting energy expenditure, and randomized to a control condition or a supplement of 48.2 g/d of additional protein. At the end of 3 months, the group receiving the protein supplement to bring protein to 18% had a 50% reduction in body weight regain (**Fig. 13**). The differential effect on fat mass and fat-free mass suggests that the higher protein intake was helping to conserve lean body mass.

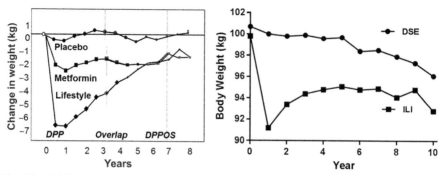

Fig. 12. Weight Loss over 8 years in the DPP/DPP Outcome Study (DPPOS) and the Look AHEAD study. (*Left*) Weight loss in the lifestyle group reaches a nadir at 6 to 12 months with weight regain thereafter, with weight remaining 2 kg below control levels out to 8 years. (*Right*) Weight loss in the lifestyle group reached a nadir at 12 months with regain after that. Beginning at about 5 years, the weight of the control group began to decline more rapidly toward the treated group, narrowing the therapeutic difference. DSE, diabetes, support and education; ILI, intensive lifestyle intervention. (*Data from* Venditti EM, Bray GA, Carrion-Peterson ML, et al; for the Diabetes Prevention Research Group. First versus repeat treatment with a lifestyle intervention program: attendance and weight loss outcomes. Int J Obes 2008;32,1537–64; and The Look AHEAD Research Group, Wing RR, Bolin P, Brancati FL, et al. Cardiovascular effects of intensive lifestyle intervention in type 2 diabetes. N Engl J Med 2013;369(2):145–54.)

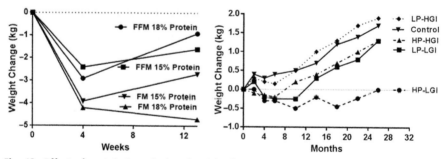

Fig. 13. Effect of protein in reducing the risk of regaining weight. (*Left*) One-hundred and forty-eight men and women who lost weight on a very-low-calorie diet were then randomly assigned to a protein supplement or not for 4 months. (*Right*) Adding protein to the low glycemic index diet enhanced the ability to maintain weight loss compared with the diets in a randomized controlled dietary intervention study investigating the effects of dietary protein and glycemic index on weight gain/regain and metabolic and cardiovascular risk factors in obese and overweight families in 8 European centers. A total of 891 families with at least 1 overweight/obese parent underwent screening. The parents started an initial 8-week low-calorie diet and families with minimum 1 parent attaining a weight loss of greater than or equal to 8%, were randomized to 1 of 5 energy ad libitum, low-fat (25–30 E%) diets for 6 or 12 months. The median weight loss on the low-calorie diet was 10.3 kg. A total of 773 adults and 784 children were randomized to the 6-month weight gain/regain prevention phase. FFM, fat free mass; FM, fat mass; HP-HGI, high protein-high glycemic index; HP-LGI, high protein-low glycemic index; LP-HGI, low protein-high glycemic index; LP-LGI, low protein-low glycemic index. (*Data from* Westerterp-Plantenga MS, Lejeune MP, Nijs I, et al. High protein intake sustains weight maintenance after body weight loss in humans. Int J Obes Relat Metab Disord 2004;28(1):57–64; and Larsen TM, Dalskov SM, van Baak M, et al; Diet, Obesity, and Genes (Diogenes) Project. Diets with high or low protein content and glycemic index for weight-loss maintenance. N Engl J Med 2010;363(22):2102–13.)

The other study was a large multicenter trial in Europe in which individuals were randomized to one of 5 diets after an initial weight loss. It is clear that the group with the higher protein intake regained very little weight, in contrast with all of the other groups.

Low-fat diets and the Mediterranean diet for the maintenance of weight loss

Reduced dietary fat intake may be of value for long-term weight maintenance.[78,79] In the Women's Health Initiative, a large clinical trial of low-fat versus control diets as a potential for prevention of cancer conducted in 48,835 women, the low-fat diet group was significantly lighter than the normal-fat diet group after an average of 7.5 years of follow-up.[78] There was a positive association between the self-reported decrease in percentage of fat consumed and the amount of weight loss ($P<.001$ for trend). These results are corroborated by a 2012 meta-analysis by Hooper and colleagues,[79] which evaluated 33 RCTs (this included the Women's Health Initiative) conducted for at least 6 months and for as long as 8 years. The analysis showed a small but statistically significant 1.57-kg mean reduction in body weight over the study period in the reduced-fat versus usual-fat arms using data from 73,589 participants who had a baseline fat intake between 28% and 43% of energy. Subgroup analyses showed no differences in weight after 5 years, but confirmed an association between reduced fat intake and greater weight loss when studies in which different levels of attention were given to the treatment versus control arms were eliminated. It is probable that the prescriptions to reduce fat intake were associated with an overall reduced caloric intake over the long term. A meta-analysis of 13 RCTs with 1569 participants with 1 to 2 years of follow-up showed greater reductions in weight with very-low-carbohydrate, ketogenic diets (<50 g/d) compared with low-fat diets.[80] This weight loss was associated with decreased triglyceride levels and diastolic blood pressure and increased HDL and LDL cholesterol levels. Longer-term studies documenting the sustainability of very-low-carbohydrate ketogenic diets and their effects on cardiovascular disease are lacking.

Adhering to a Mediterranean diet may also be beneficial in maintaining weight loss. In a study of 10,376 Spanish men and women who were university graduates, diet was

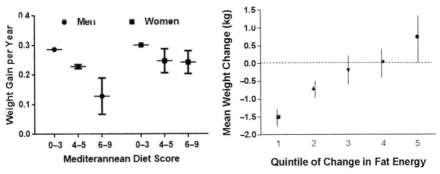

Fig. 14. Effect of Mediterranean or low-fat diet on maintenance of weight loss. (*Left*) Spanish men and women adhering to more components of the Mediterranean diet were more successful in preventing weight gain. (*Right*) Seven-year weight change in relation to fat intake in the Women's Health Initiative. The lower the reported fat intake, the less weight was regained. (*Data from* Howard BV, Manson JE, Stefanick ML, et al. Low-fat dietary pattern and weight change over 7 years: the Women's Health Initiative Dietary Modification Trial. JAMA 2006;295(1):39–49; and Beunza JJ, Toledo E, Hu FB, et al. Adherence to the Mediterranean diet, long-term weight change, and incident overweight or obesity: the Seguimiento Universidad de Navarra (SUN) cohort. Am J Clin Nutr 2010;92(6):1484–93.)

assessed at baseline with a 136-item, previously validated food-frequency question-naire and weight was assessed at baseline and twice a year during follow-up.[81] Par-ticipants with the lowest adherence ($\leq$3 points) to the Mediterranean dietary score showed the highest average yearly weight gain, whereas participants with the highest adherence showed the lowest weight gain (**Fig. 14**).

FUTURE CONSIDERATIONS/SUMMARY

Several macronutrient dietary strategies can be used to induce weight loss. Weight reduction occurs most rapidly in the first 3 to 6 months, with a plateau or weight regain occurring by 1 to 2 years. In 2 major long-term follow-up studies with intensive lifestyle interventions, the DPP and Look AHEAD trial, weight differences remained significant for 8 years in the DPP study. In the Look AHEAD study, body weight remained signif-icantly lower in the intervention than in the control group throughout the 10-year study. Improvements in lipid levels and blood pressure were observed in the early years of the DPP study and the Look AHEAD trial, but no differences remained in these param-eters at the end of 10 years. Long-term weight loss maintenance may be influenced mostly by the ability to adhere to diets, and behavioral support significantly affects outcomes. There are marked individual differences in the response to each diet. Consideration for genetic variability in the dietary response to weight loss offers the possibility of personalized dietary regimens improving the efficacy of long-term weight-loss regimens.

REFERENCES

1. Bray GA. The Battle of the Bulge. Pittsburgh (PA): Dorrance Publishing; 2007.
2. Banting W. Letter on corpulence, addressed to the public. 3rd edition. London: Harrison; 1864. p. vi, 7–50 (includes 2 addenda and appendix).
3. Keys A, Aravanis C, Blackburn HW, et al. Epidemiological studies related to cor-onary heart disease: characteristics of men aged 40–59 in seven countries. Acta Med Scand Suppl 1966;460:1 392.
4. Berland T, Consumer Guide, editors. Rating the diets. New York: Beekman House; 1979.
5. Atkins RC. Dr. Atkins' diet revolution: the high calorie way to stay thin forever. New York: David McKay; 1972.
6. Hamman RF, Wing RR, Edelstein SL, et al. Effect of weight loss with lifestyle inter-vention on risk of diabetes. Diabetes Care 2006;29:2102–7.
7. Jensen MD, Ryan DH, Donato KA, et al. Guidelines (2013) for managing over-weight and obesity in adults. Obesity 2014;22(S2):S1–410.
8. Bray GA. The obese patient. In: Smith LH, editor. Major problems in internal med-icine, vol. 9. Philadelphia: WB Saunders; 1976. p. 1–450.
9. Antonetti V. The computer diet. New York: M Evans; 1973.
10. Thomas DM, Gonzalez MC, Pereira AZ, et al. Time to correctly predict the amount of weight loss with dieting. J Acad Nutr Diet 2014;114:857–61.
11. Thomas DM, Weedermann M, Fuemmeler BF, et al. Dynamic model predicting overweight, obesity, and extreme obesity prevalence trends. Obesity 2014; 22(2):590–7.
12. Hall KD, Sacks G, Chandramohan D, et al. Quantification of the effect of energy imbalance on bodyweight. Lancet 2011;378(9793):826–37.
13. Schwartz A, Doucet E. Relative changes in resting energy expenditure during weight loss: a systematic review. Obes Rev 2010;11:531–47.

14. Sumithran P, Prendergast LA, Delbridge E, et al. Long-term persistence of hormonal adaptations to weight loss. N Engl J Med 2011;365(17):1597–604.
15. Rosenbaum M, Goldsmith R, Bloomfield D, et al. Low-dose leptin reverses skeletal muscle, autonomic, and neuroendocrine adaptations to maintenance of reduced weight. J Clin Invest 2005;115(12):3579–86.
16. Espeland M, Bray GA, Neiberg R, et al. Describing patterns of weight changes using principal components analysis: results from the Action for Health in Diabetes (Look AHEAD) study group. Ann Epidemiol 2009;19(10):701–10.
17. Unick JL, Neiberg RH, Hogan PE, et al, Look AHEAD Research Group Obesity. Weight change in the first 2 months of a lifestyle intervention predicts weight changes 8 years later. Obesity (Silver Spring) 2015;23:1353–6.
18. Dansinger ML, Gleason JA, Griffith JL, et al. Comparison of the Atkins, Ornish, Weight Watchers, and Zone diets for weight loss and heart disease risk reduction: a randomized trial. JAMA 2005;293(1):43–53.
19. Alhassan S, Kim S, Bersamin A, et al. Dietary adherence and weight loss success among overweight women: results from the A to Z weight loss study. Int J Obes 2008;32:985–91.
20. Sacks FM, Bray GA, Carey V, et al. Comparison of weight-loss diets with different compositions of fat, carbohydrate and protein. N Engl J Med 2009;360(9): 859–73.
21. Delahanty LM, Pan Q, Jablonski KA, et al, Diabetes Prevention Program Research Group. Genetic predictors of weight loss and weight regain after intensive lifestyle modification, metformin treatment, or standard care in the Diabetes Prevention Program. Diabetes Care 2012;35(2):363–6.
22. Papandonatos GD, Pan Q, Pajewski NM, et al, Diabetes Prevention Program and the Look AHEAD Research Groups. Genetic predisposition to weight loss & regain with lifestyle intervention: analyses from the Diabetes Prevention Program & the Look AHEAD randomized controlled trials. Diabetes 2015;64(12):4312–21.
23. Qi Q, Bray GA, Hu FB, et al. Weight-loss diets modify glucose-dependent insulinotropic polypeptide receptor rs2287019 genotype effects on changes in body weight, fasting glucose, and insulin resistance: the Preventing Overweight Using Novel Dietary Strategies trial. Am J Clin Nutr 2012;95(2):506–13.
24. Zhang X, Qi Q, Bray GA, et al. APOA5 genotype modulates 2-year changes in lipid profile in response to weight-loss diet intervention: the Pounds Lost Trial. Am J Clin Nutr 2012;96(4):917–22.
25. Zhang X, Qi Q, Zhang C, et al. FTO g8notype and 2-year change in body composition and fat distribution in response to weight-loss diets: the POUNDS LOST Trial. Diabetes 2012;61(11):3005–11.
26. Qi Q, Xu M, Wu H, et al. IRS1 genotype modulates metabolic syndrome reversion in response to 2-year weight-loss diet intervention: the POUNDS LOST trial. Diabetes Care 2013;36(11):3442–7.
27. Xu M, Qi Q, Liang J, et al. Genetic determinant for amino acid metabolites and changes in body weight and insulin resistance in response to weight-loss diets: the POUNDS LOST Trial. Circulation 2013;127(12):1283–9.
28. Mirzaei K, Xu M, Qibin Qi Q, et al. Glucose and circadian related genetic variants affect response of energy expenditure to weight-loss diets: the POUNDS LOST Trial. Am J Clin Nutr 2014;99(2):392–9.
29. Zheng Y, Huang T, Zhang X, et al. Dietary fat modifies the effects of FTO Genotype on changes in insulin sensitivity. J Nutr 2015;145(5):977–82.
30. Lin X, Qi Q, Zheng Y, et al. Neuropeptide Y genotype, central obesity and abdominal fat distribution: the POUNDS Lost trial. Am J Clin Nutr 2015;102(2):514–9.

31. Look AHEAD Research Group, Wing RR. Long term effects of a lifestyle intervention on weight and cardiovascular risk factors in individuals with type 2 diabetes: four year results of the look AHEAD trial. Arch Intern Med 2010;170(17):1566–75.

32. Ratner R, Goldberg R, Haffner S, et al, Diabetes Prevention Program Research Group. Impact of intensive lifestyle and metformin therapy on cardiovascular disease risk factors in the diabetes prevention program. Diabetes Care 2005;28(4): 888–94.

33. Tsai AG, Waddden TA. The evolution of very-low-calorie diets: an update and meta-analysis. Obesity (Silver Spring) 2006;14:1283–93.

34. Foster GD, Wyatt HR, Hill JO, et al. A randomized trial of a low-carbohydrate diet for obesity. N Engl J Med 2003;348(21):2082–90.

35. Brehm BJ, Seeley RJ, Daniels SR, et al. A randomized trial comparing a very low carbohydrate diet and a calorie-restricted low fat diet on body weight and cardiovascular risk factors in healthy women. J Clin Endocrinol Metab 2003;88(4): 1617–23.

36. Samaha FF, Iqbal N, Seshadri P, et al. A low-carbohydrate as compared with a low-fat diet in severe obesity. N Engl J Med 2003;348(21):2074–81.

37. Stern L, Iqbal N, Seshadri P, et al. The effects of low-carbohydrate versus conventional weight loss diets in severely obese adults: one-year follow-up of a randomized trial. Ann Intern Med 2004;140(10):778–85.

38. Westman EC, Mavropoulos J, Yancy WS, et al. A review of low-carbohydrate ketogenic diets [review]. Curr Atheroscler Rep 2003;5(6):476–83.

39. Nordmann AJ, Nordmann A, Briel M, et al. Effects of low-carbohydrate vs low-fat diets on weight loss and cardiovascular risk factors: a meta-analysis of randomized controlled trials. Arch Intern Med 2006;166(3):285–93.

40. Johnston BC, Kanters S, Bandayrel K, et al. Comparison of weight loss among named diet programs in overweight and obese adults: a meta-analysis. JAMA 2014;312(9):923–33.

41. Foster GD, Wyatt HR, Hill JO, et al. Weight and metabolic outcomes after 2 years on a low-carbohydrate versus low-fat diet: a randomized trial. Ann Intern Med 2010;153(3):147–57.

42. Layman DK, Evans EM, Erickson D, et al. A moderate-protein diet produces sustained weight loss and long-term changes in body composition and blood lipids in obese adults. J Nutr 2009;139(3):514–21.

43. Bray GA, Popkin BM. Dietary sugar and body weight: have we reached a crisis in the epidemic of obesity and diabetes?: health be damned! Pour on the sugar. Diabetes Care 2014;37(4):950–6.

44. de Ruyter JC, Olthof MR, Seidell JC, et al. A trial of sugar-free or sugar-sweetened beverages and body weight in children. N Engl J Med 2012;367(15):1397–406.

45. Astrup A, Grunwald GK, Melanson EL, et al. The role of low-fat diets in body weight control: a meta-analysis of ad libitum dietary intervention studies. Int J Obes Relat Metab Disord 2000;24(12):1545–52.

46. Pirozzo S, Summerbell C, Cameron C, et al. Should we recommend low-fat diets for obesity? Obes Rev 2003;4(2):83–90.

47. Ello-Martin JA, Roe LS, Ledikwe JH, et al. Dietary energy density in the treatment of obesity: a year-long trial comparing 2 weight-loss diets. Am J Clin Nutr 2007; 85(6):1465–77.

48. Rolls BJ, Barnett RA. Volumetrics: feel full on fewer calories. New York: HarperCollins; 2000.

49. Ebbeling CB, Leidig MM, Sinclair KB, et al. A reduced-glycemic load diet in the treatment of adolescent obesity. Arch Pediatr Adolesc Med 2003;157(8):773–9.

50. Ebbeling CB, Leidig MM, Feldman HA, et al. Effects of a low-glycemic load vs low-fat diet in obese young adults: a randomized trial. JAMA 2007;297(19): 2092–102.
51. Schwingshackl L, Hoffmann G. Long-term effects of low glycemic index/load vs. high glycemic index/load diets on parameters of obesity and obesity-associated risks: a systematic review and meta-analysis. Nutr Metab Cardiovasc Dis 2013; 23(8):699–706.
52. Thomas DE, Elliott EJ, Baur L. Low glycemic index or low glycemic load diets for overweight and obesity [review]. Cochrane Database Syst Rev 2007;(3):CD005105.
53. Westerterp-Plantenga MS, Lejeune MP, Nijs I, et al. High protein intake sustains weight maintenance after body weight loss in humans. Int J Obes Relat Metab Disord 2004;28(1):57–64.
54. Skov AR, Toubro S, Rønn B, et al. Randomized trial on protein vs carbohydrate in ad libitum fat reduced diet for the treatment of obesity. Int J Obes Relat Metab Disord 1999;23(5):528–36.
55. Due A, Toubro S, Skov AR, et al. Effect of normal-fat diets, either medium or high in protein, on body weight in overweight subjects: a randomised 1-year trial. Int J Obes Relat Metab Disord 2004;28(10):1283–90.
56. Wycherley TP, Moran LJ, Clifton PM, et al. Effects of energy-restricted high-protein, low-fat compared with standard-protein, low-fat diets: a meta-analysis of randomized controlled trials. Am J Clin Nutr 2012;96(6):1281–98.
57. Bray GA, Smith SR, de Jonge L, et al. Effect of dietary protein content on weight gain, energy expenditure, and body composition during overeating: a randomized controlled trial. JAMA 2012;307(1):47–55.
58. Schwingshackl L, Hoffmann G. Long-term effects of low-fat diets either low or high in protein on cardiovascular and metabolic risk factors: a systematic review and meta-analysis. Nutr J 2013;12:48.
59. Esposito K, Maiorino MI, Ciotola M, et al. Effects of a Mediterranean-style diet on the need for antihyperglycemic drug therapy in patients with newly diagnosed type 2 diabetes: a randomized trial. Ann Intern Med 2009;151(5):306–14.
60. Estruch R, Rios E, Salas-Salvedo J, et al. Primary prevention of cardiovascular disease with a Mediterranean diet. N Engl J Med 2013;368(14):1279–90.
61. Sofi F, Cesari F, Abbate R, et al. Adherence to Mediterranean diet and health status: meta-analysis [review]. BMJ 2008;337:a1344.
62. Huo R, Du T, Xu Y, et al. Effects of Mediterranean-style diet on glycemic control, weight loss and cardiovascular risk factors among type 2 diabetes individuals: a meta-analysis. Eur J Clin Nutr 2014. http://dx.doi.org/10.1038/ejcn.2014.243.
63. Nordmann AJ, Suter-Zimmermann K, Bucher HC, et al. Meta-analysis comparing Mediterranean to low-fat diets for modification of cardiovascular risk factors. Am J Med 2011;124(9):841–51.
64. Avenell A, Broom J, Brown TJ, et al. Systematic review of long-term effects and economic consequences of treatments for obesity and implications for health improvement. Health Technol Assess 2004;8(21):i–ix, 1–458.
65. Pedersen SD, Kang J, Kline GA. Portion control plate for weight loss in obese patients with type 2 diabetes mellitus: a controlled clinical trial. Arch Intern Med 2007;167(12):1277–83.
66. Heymsfield SB, van Mierlo CA, Knaap HC, et al. Weight management using a meal replacement strategy: meta and pooling analysis from six studies. Int J Obes 2003;27:537–49.

67. Ptomey LT, Willis EA, Goetz JR, et al. Portion-controlled meals provide increases in diet quality during weight loss and maintenance. J Hum Nutr 2015. http://dx. doi.org/10.1111/jhn.12296.

68. Gardner CD, Kiazand A, Alhassan S, et al. Comparison of the Atkins, Zone, Ornish, and LEARN Diets for change in weight and related risk factors among overweight premenopausal women. JAMA 2007;297:969–77.

69. Shai I, Schwarzfuchs D, Henkin Y, et al, Dietary Intervention Randomized Controlled Trial (DIRECT) Group. Weight loss with a low-carbohydrate, Mediterranean, or low-fat diet. N Engl J Med 2008;359(3):229–41.

70. Ornish D. Eat more, weigh less: Dr. Dean Ornish's life choice program for losing weight safely while eating abundantly. New York: HarperCollins; 1993.

71. Nidetch J, Heilman JR. The story of weight watchers. New York: New American Library; 1972.

72. Sears B. The zone: a revolutionary life plan to put your body in total balance for permanent weight loss. New York: HarperCollins Publishers; 1995. 7th printing.

73. Heshka S, Anderson JW, Atkinson RL, et al. Weight loss with self-help compared with a structured commercial program: a randomized trial. JAMA 2003;289(14): 1792–8.

74. Rock CL, Flatt SW, Sherwood NE, et al. Effect of a free prepared meal and incentivized weight loss program on weight loss and weight loss maintenance in obese and overweight women: a randomized controlled trial. JAMA 2010;304(16): 1803–10.

75. Gudzune KA, Doshi RS, Mehta AK, et al. Efficacy of commercial weight-loss programs: an updated systematic review. Ann Intern Med 2015;162(7):501–12.

76. The Look AHEAD Research Group, Wing RR, Bolin P, Brancati FL, et al. Cardiovascular effects of intensive lifestyle intervention in type 2 diabetes. N Engl J Med 2013;369(2):145–54.

77. Larsen TM, Dalskov SM, van Baak M, et al, Diet, Obesity, and Genes (Diogenes) Project. Diets with high or low protein content and glycemic index for weight-loss maintenance. N Engl J Med 2010;363(22):2102–13.

78. Howard BV, Manson JE, Stefanick ML, et al. Low-fat dietary pattern and weight change over 7 years: the Women's Health Initiative Dietary Modification Trial. JAMA 2006;295(1):39–49.

79. Hooper L, Abdelhamid A, Moore HJ, et al. Effect of reducing total fat intake on body weight: systematic review and meta-analysis of randomised controlled trials and cohort studies. BMJ 2012;345:e7666.

80. Bueno NB, de Melo IS, de Oliveira SL, et al. Very-low-carbohydrate ketogenic diet vs. low-fat diet for long-term weight loss: a meta-analysis of randomised controlled trials. Br J Nutr 2013;110:1178–87.

81. Beunza JJ, Toledo E, Hu FB, et al. Adherence to the Mediterranean diet, long-term weight change, and incident overweight or obesity: the Seguimiento Universidad de Navarra (SUN) cohort. Am J Clin Nutr 2010;92(6):1484–93.

Brown and Beige Adipose Tissue

Therapy for Obesity and Its Comorbidities?

Anny Mulya, PhD[a], John P. Kirwan, PhD[a,b,c],*

KEYWORDS

- Brown adipose tissue • Beige adipose tissue • Energy expenditure • Thermogenesis
- Obesity • Type 2 diabetes • Lifestyle intervention

KEY POINTS

- Our understanding of the role of brown (BAT)/beige adipose tissues on body weight in obese humans is evolving.
- Unanswered questions include the abundance of beige adipocytes, "browning" of white adipose tissue, contribution of BAT thermogenesis to homeostasis, and the extent to which thermogenesis can be upregulated to have sufficient impact on weight loss.
- Resolution of these issues will determine the future for BAT as a therapeutic target in obesity and obesity-related comorbidities.

INTRODUCTION

Overweight and obesity are now among the greatest health challenges in both developed and developing countries. In 2013, worldwide estimates for the percentage of overweight/obese adults was 36.9% for men and 38% for women, and the prevalence in children and adolescents—23.8% for boys and 22.6% for girls is equally alarming.[1] The situation in the United States is even more dire, where 65% of US adults are overweight/obese, and 32.2% and 25.3% of children (aged 2–19 years) are overweight and obese, respectively. Obesity is associated with a number of comorbidities, including the metabolic syndrome, insulin resistance, cardiovascular diseases, type 2 diabetes, and cancer, all of which impact the social and economic burden on the population, and is contributing to the substantial increase in direct and indirect cost of health care. Thus, there is an urgent need to identify new therapeutic strategies to combat obesity and its comorbidities.

Disclosure: The authors have received funding for NIH, R01 DK089547.
[a] Department of Pathobiology, Lerner Research Institute, Cleveland Clinic, 9500 Euclid Avenue, NE40, Cleveland, OH 44195, USA; [b] Department of Nutrition, School of Medicine, Case Western Reserve University, 10900 Euclid Avenue, Cleveland, OH 44106, USA; [c] Metabolic Translational Research Center, Endocrine and Metabolism Institute, Cleveland Clinic, 9500 Euclid Avenue, Cleveland, OH 44195, USA
* Corresponding author.
E-mail address: kirwanj@ccf.org

Endocrinol Metab Clin N Am 45 (2016) 605–621
http://dx.doi.org/10.1016/j.ecl.2016.04.010
0889-8529/16/$ – see front matter © 2016 Elsevier Inc. All rights reserved.

Obesity is a chronic condition caused by excess energy intake relative to energy expenditure, creating positive energy balance and weight gain. Much of this extra energy is stored in the form of triacylglycerols in white adipose tissue (WAT). One of the strategies to reverse obesity is to generate "negative energy balance" with a focus on decreasing energy intake and increasing energy expenditure.[2] Understanding the physiologic, cellular, and molecular mechanisms of energy intake, storage, and expenditure to achieve whole body energy homeostasis may allow us to identify effective and durable (treatment) strategies for treating and managing obesity. One of the exciting possibilities of brown adipose tissue (BAT) is that it can oxidize fatty acids and glucose, and thus could in theory, dissipate energy in the form of heat via uncoupling mechanisms. This approach is supported by the strong negative association between BAT and body weight, body fat, and visceral fat.[3–5] Thus, further understanding of the genetic, molecular, and physiologic attributes of BAT may generate empirical data to support the idea that upregulation of BAT activity could lead to the discovery of a novel, effective, and durable therapy for treating and managing obesity. However, the significance and viability of this approach is the subject of some skepticism. In this review, we focus on how brown/beige fat cell activation may impact obesity therapy and its potential to mitigate obesity-related comorbidities.

FEATURE CHARACTERISTICS, AND PHYSIOLOGIC AND METABOLIC PHENOTYPE OF THERMOGENIC ADIPOCYTES

In mammals, thermogenic adipocytes are classified into BAT and the recently discovered "brownlike"/"beige"/"brite" adipocytes.[6] BAT is highly vascularized, is characterized by a light pink color, and is densely innervated by the sympathetic nervous system. Brown adipocytes are packed with multilocular small vacuoles that are rich in mitochondria that contain dense cristae.[7] In rodents and small mammals, the most classical brown fat presentation is around the upper back (interscapular), the kidney (perirenal), and heart (periaortic) regions. In humans, active BAT was traditionally thought to be restricted to newborns and the early childhood period, and was viewed as a natural defense mechanism against hypothermia.[8–10] More recently, several groups of investigators have reported functional active BAT in healthy adult humans using a combination of radiolabeled glucose tracers, 2-deoxy-2-[^{18}F]-fluoro-D-glucose ([^{18}F]-FDG), and PET and computed tomographic (CT) scanning technology.[3,4,11,12] These data show that BAT is present in the upper trunk, including the cervical, supraclavicular, paravertebral, and pericardial regions, and to a lesser extent in the mediastinal and mesenteric areas.[3,4,11] Glucose uptake and perfusion of the tissue are both increased in human BAT in response to cold, indicating active thermogenesis.[13] The amount of active BAT in humans is heterogeneous, but the exact mass has never been measured precisely. Estimates suggest that healthy humans have about 50 g of active BAT (approximately 0.1% of body mass).[14,15]

Beige adipocytes have similar morphologic features to classical brown adipocytes, with central nuclei, multilocular lipid droplets, and are rich in mitochondria.[16] Beige adipocytes arise upon external cues, such as stimulation of sympathetic activity during chronic cold exposure or administration of β3-adrenergic receptor agonists, or exercise. Unlike brown adipocytes, which seem to have a discrete anatomic location, beige adipocytes reside within the WAT depot, mainly in inguinal WAT in rodents. In humans, there remains uncertainty regarding the presence of both the precursor of white adipocytes committed to "browning" or functional beige adipocytes, and whether trans-differentiation of white into beige adipocytes is indeed a real physiologic phenomenon. Several reports suggest that human BAT, particularly from the neck region, represent both the classical brown as well as beige adipocytes found in mice.[6,17–19] Recent findings, using a combination of both RNA sequencing and genome-wide expression analysis of a preadipoycte lineage derived from supraclavicular BAT of nonobese individuals, found a smaller population (10.8%) of uncoupling protein (UCP)[+] human adipocytes that were representative of beige adipocytes.[20] To support this observation, they also reported the presence of potassium channel K3 and mitochondrial tumor suppressor 1, which are molecular markers of beige adipocyte differentiation and thermogenic function. Nonetheless, the study of beige adipocytes in humans remains challenging because (1) [^{18}F]-FDG-PET/CT scans do not distinguish brown versus beige adipocytes, and (2) investigations on the biological stimulation and thermogenic features of inducible brown adipocytes in humans is difficult owing to the requirement of more than minimally invasive intervention to assess the mass and activity.

Classical brown and beige adipocytes originate from distinct cellular lineages. Classical brown adipocytes share the same cellular lineage as skeletal myocytes. During embryonic development, classical brown adipocytes arise from Engrailed-1 (En1)-expressing cells in the central dermomyotome,[21] and a myf5[+] cell lineage, which is a similar progenitor as that of skeletal muscle myocytes. Transcriptional profile data from recent microarray experiments support the view that brown preadipocytes and myocytes share a common lineage.[22] In addition, high-resolution quantitative mass spectrometry has been used to show that the mitochondrial proteomic profile of brown fat is more similar to skeletal muscle than to white fat cells.[23] The transcriptional coregulator PRD1-BF-1-RIZ1 homologous domain-containing protein-16 (PRDM16) acts as a switch that controls the bidirectional cell fate between myoblasts and brown preadipocytes.[24] Loss of PRDM16 from brown preadipocytes favors a muscle cell differentiation program, whereas ectopic expression of PRDM16 in myoblasts induces programming that leads to brown fat cell differentiation.[24] The cellular origin of beige adipocytes is also complex. It is thought that, depending on the metabolic milieu, beige adipocytes emerge from a myf5[−] lineage of precursor cells similar to white adipocytes.[25] However, it has been shown that a subset of beige adipocytes can also originate from myf5[+] cells.[26] Recently, Long and colleagues[27] used a ribosomal profiling approach to demonstrate that a subset of beige adipocytes (about 10%–15%) originated from a smooth muscle-like precursor driven by Myh11. Clonal analysis of adipogenic cell lines from the inguinal WAT in rodents led to the realization that beige and white adipocytes are distinct cell types with distinctive molecular profiles.[6] Distinct cellular origin and molecular signatures at the precursor stage between brown/beige and white adipocytes have also been found in adult humans.[20,28] These data suggest that (1) brown fat cells originate differently from beige or white fat cells, (2) brown adipocytes share a similar developmental program with myocytes, and (3) beige adipocytes may be derived from an heterogeneous population of cell lineage.[3]

Another unique biochemical and molecular feature of brown and beige adipocytes is the expression of thermogenic proteins. A key thermogenic protein is UCP1 (also called thermogenin), a 33-kDa protein located in the inner mitochondrial membrane that functions as a proton and anion transporter.[29] The role of UCP1 in BAT has been elegantly demonstrated by Nicholls and colleagues.[30] Activation of UCP1 is mediated by free fatty acids (FFAs), particularly long-chain fatty acids.[31,32] Beige adipocytes resemble white adipocytes in that they have an extremely low basal expression of UCP1, but after full differentiation, beige adipocytes turn into UCP1[+] cells, which is similar to classical brown adipocytes. Consequently, beige adipocytes are classified as nonclassical/inducible brown adipocytes.[6] Of note, the process of generating beige adipocytes is called "beiging" or "browning."

White (WAT) and brown (BAT) adipose tissue have distinct physiologic functions and this is particularly evident when we consider whole body energy homeostasis. Under conditions of increased energy intake, WAT maintains energy homeostasis by storing extra energy in the form of triacylglycerols and by breaking down this stored energy into FFA and glycerol to generate energy in the form of adenosine triphosphate when energy demands increase. In contrast, BAT predominantly promotes energy expenditure. It can dissipate chemical energy by oxidizing glucose and lipids for heat generation via uncoupled mitochondrial respiration mediated by UCP1 in a process called adaptive thermogenesis. The number of visceral white fat cells increases when there is a positive energy balance, whereas new brown fat cells are generated in response to cold temperature. Beige adipocytes are thought to be associated with the maintenance of energy balance, and this may be similar for classical brown adipocytes.

THE MECHANISM OF BROWN ADIPOSE TISSUE ACTIVATION AND BROWNING OF WHITE ADIPOSE TISSUE

The thermogenic activity of BAT is stimulated by cold exposure and activation of the sympathetic nervous system via β3-adrenergic agonism.[32] Upon cold exposure norepinephrine binds to β3-adrenergic receptors that are coupled with G-proteins on the cell surface of brown adipocytes. This leads to activation of adenylate cyclase, catalyzing the formation of cyclic adenosine monophosphate (cAMP), which in turn activates the cAMP–protein kinase A signaling pathway. β3-Adrenergic stimulation generates both acute and chronic effects on BAT. Acutely, stimulation of β3-receptors results in activation of UCP1. In brief, stimulation of the cAMP–protein kinase A pathway induces hormone-sensitive lipase, adipose triglyceride lipase, and monoacylglycerol lipase, enzymes that regulate the hydrolysis of triacylglycerols, diacylglycerols, and monoacylglycerides, respectively, leading to the release of FFAs.[32] These FFAs are imported into the mitochondria where they bind and activate UCP1[33,34] and are oxidized through cellular respiration, amplifying the free flow of protons across the inner mitochondrial membrane,[35] and the rapid release of chemical energy as heat.[30,32] Besides activation of lipolysis, norepinephrine also increases glucose transporter and lipase expression to increase glucose and FFA uptake, and thus provide the substrate that is needed for thermogenesis to proceed. The long-term effect of β3-adrenergic stimulation results in upregulation of the thermogenic gene program (UCP1), mitochondrial biogenesis, and both hyperplasia and hypertrophy of BAT,[36] resulting in increased total BAT mass. In humans, long-term effects can occur through cold acclimation and this results in a 37% increase in BAT volume, comparable changes are observed in rodents.[37] The mechanism requires upregulation of the cAMP-protein kinase A pathway, followed by activation of the transcription factor CREB, which is bound to the CRE promoter within the thermogenic program (UCP1),[32] or upregulation of the mitogen-activated protein kinase and extracellular signal-regulated kinases 1/2 pathways that control mitochondrial biogenesis and oxidative phosphorylation genes, such as PGC-1α.[38]

The mechanism of browning of WAT was recently reviewed by Warner and Mittag.[39] They concluded that browning of WAT can be achieved by different mechanisms. First by the activation of the central nervous system through modulation of sympathetic output to WAT. This mechanism is primarily mediated by neurons in the hypothalamus, including proopiomelanocortin[40] and agouti-related peptide[41] producing neurons. Second, browning of WAT can be achieved by the recruitment and activation of immune cells (such as eosinophils and the interleukin [IL]-14/13 signaling pathway,[42] or ILC2 immune cells[43,44]) to WAT; or lastly by direct action of stimuli on beige adipocyte precursor cells. Current nonpharmacologic and pharmacologic strategies for WAT browning was reviewed by Lee and Greenfield,[45] and can be categorized into sympathomimetics (β3-adrenergic receptor agonists), nonadrenergic cold mimetics (eg, fibroblast growth factor [FGF]21 and irisin), peroxisome proliferator activated receptor-γ agonists, or capsaicin/capsinoidlike compounds.

MODULATION OF BEIGE ADIPOCYTE FORMATION IN HUMAN INTERVENTION TRIALS
Exercise Intervention

Exercise is associated with numerous health benefits, but from a metabolic perspective one of the most important is whole-body glucose homeostasis via adaptation in insulin-sensitive tissues, including fat, liver, and skeletal muscle. Although adaptation in skeletal muscle is perhaps the most widely studied, changes in the structure and function of adipose tissue is also important. In WAT, exercise decreases adipocyte size[46,47] and lipid content, which reduces adiposity. At the cellular level, exercise increases mitochondrial protein abundance and activity, and these responses are mediated by endothelial nitric oxide synthase and PGC-1α.[48–51] Recent data suggest that exercise may also induce "beiging" of subcutaneous WAT. When previously sedentary mice increase physical activity, there is an increased expression in the "beige" adipocyte marker genes including UCP1, Prdm16, Cidea, Elovl3, PGC-1α, PPARγ, Tbx1, and other related markers of BAT or beige adipocytes.[49,50,52,53] This increased gene expression is also associated with increased UCP1 immunofluorescence.

The mechanism responsible for exercise-induced "beiging" of subcutaneous WAT may be related to irisin (gene: FNDC5), an exercise-induced myokine that works through the PGC-1α pathway. Boström and colleagues[52] reported that irisin stimulates the expression of UCP-1 in white adipocytes, stimulates beige adipocyte formation and improves metabolic outcomes. However, the role of irisin in "beige" adipocyte development in humans remains controversial. Although some research groups have reported that circulating irisin is increased acutely after exercise,[54,55] several groups have not been able to detect or confirm a role for irisin in humans, and there has been a failure to demonstrate a positive correlation between plasma irisin levels following exercise training and the browning of fat in humans.[56–60] Moreover, genomic sequencing of human *FNDC5* reveals that humans have an alternative start codon for *FNDC5* (ATA), whereas rodents have a highly conserved ATG start codon.[61] Thus, humans may have a lower translational efficiency for the gene, and this is verified by in vitro data showing that only 1% of the full-length FNDC5 protein is translated with an ATA start codon. This difference may explain some of the contradictory observations on circulating irisin levels in humans and rodents.[61] In addition to the confusion surrounding the detection of circulating irisin levels and the response to exercise training, recent findings also challenge the view that irisin may play a beneficial role in obesity therapy. It seems that irisin is not only a myokine, but it is also an adipokine,[62] and plasma irisin levels are unexpectedly higher in obese humans.[63,64] Furthermore, Viitasalo and colleagues[65] found a positive and unfavorable correlation between plasma FFAs and irisin in overweight children. More reliable and sensitive detection methods and greater in depth study of the mechanistic regulation of irisin are required to establish whether irisin is indeed a mediator of pathways that propagate obesity, or whether irisin has potential as a therapeutic target for treating or managing obesity.

In addition to irisin, there are several other proteins that may mediate exercise-induced beige adipocyte biogenesis. IL-6 is a myokine that is released from contracting skeletal muscle cells,[66] and it may impact metabolism in adipose tissue.[67] Knudsen and colleagues[68] found that exercise training increased the expression of IL-6 in inguinal WAT, and upregulated UCP1 messenger RNA expression in wild-type control mice, but not in IL-6 knockout mice. However, cold exposure failed to stimulate the expression of genes responsible for brown fat activation in this model. In 2014, Rao and colleagues[69] reported that muscle PGC-1α4 overexpression in mice induces the expression of a protein that they named meteorin-like hormone. This protein was linked to the promotion of "beige" adipocyte formation via eosinophil-dependent M2 macrophage activation. Other metabolites secreted from skeletal muscle after exercise, such as lactate[70] and β-aminoisobutyric acid[71] have also been associated with the "beiging" of subcutaneous adipose tissue.

Dietary Intervention

Food ingestion leads to an increase in body temperature. This physiologic response is called diet-induced thermogenesis (DIT) and is associated with an increase in energy metabolism and activation of taste and smell senses by the intraoral sensory nervous system, as well as an increase in energy for food digestion and absorption.[72] Using an overfeeding rat model (cafeteria diet), Rothwell and Stock[15] performed seminal studies that established the role of DIT in energy balance. They found that overfeeding stimulates an adaptive response mechanism that serves to eliminate excess calories by activating the thermogenesis pathway. The responses include increased body temperature, energy expenditure, and resting oxygen consumption, and these responses are directed through BAT thermogenesis.

All macronutrients (lipid, carbohydrates, and protein) stimulate thermogenesis. However, the effect of high-fat feeding on BAT activation in rodents remains controversial. Some data suggest that increased fat consumption reprograms BAT,[15,73] whereas other data conclude that there is no, or only a marginal increase in BAT mass after a high-fat diet.[74] Despite the controversy regarding BAT mass, there is general agreement that high-fat feeding upregulates UCP1 expression in BAT in rodents,[74] whereas in humans, high-fat feeding seems to increase BAT activity.[75] The source of dietary fat is an important determinant of the effects of diet on UCP1 upregulation; polyunsaturated fatty acids have the most potent effect.[74,76] There are several reports that DIT is a significant mechanism for weight loss induced by a high-protein diet. This is supported by the observation that a high protein diet has a higher thermic response and higher energy expenditure than a high carbohydrate diet.[77] Moreover, protein type also impacts DIT, with whey protein having a greater thermic effect compared with casein or soy.[77] Although a protein rich diet stimulates DIT, the effect of a high protein diet on BAT activation is less clear. When a high protein diet was compared against a high-fat diet, the protein diet did not affect UCP1 messenger RNA expression in BAT.[78] In addition to the major nutrients, several food ingredients have been shown to activate the thermogenic response in BAT through stimulation of transient receptor potential (TRP) channels (such as TRPV1, TRPM8, and TRPA1) that release norepinephrine.[79] Capsaicin, and its pungent analogs (capsinoids; capsiate, dihydrocapsiate, and nordihydrocapsiate) found in red peppers, has been shown to increase energy expenditure and promote weight reduction in individuals who have greater amounts of BAT than in BAT⁻ subjects.[80] Other food ingredients that have been reported to affect BAT activation include green tea extract,[81] curcumin,[82,83] and ginger extract.[84]

Bariatric Surgery

Physical reconstruction of the gastrointestinal tract through bariatric surgery is the most effective therapy for weight loss and the remission of type 2 diabetes. The mechanisms that facilitate these improvements are unclear. However, there are data to suggest that gastric bypass surgery improves energy expenditure in rodent models as well as in humans.[85–89] Whether the improvement in energy expenditure is due to increased BAT activation after surgery is unknown. Vijgen and colleagues[90] used [^{18}F]-FDG-PET/CT imaging to assess BAT activation and found greater activation 1 year after laparoscopic adjustable gastric binding surgery; however, the number of patients was small and definitive conclusions require larger studies. The mechanisms that determine how bariatric surgery may promote higher BAT activation remain elusive. One possible mechanism may act through bile acids, nutrient-responsive hormones that modulate energy balance. Obese subjects have a lower postprandial excursion of conjugated bile acids than lean individuals. Roux-en-Y gastric bypass surgery essentially normalizes the meal-induced increase in conjugated bile acids in morbidly obese subjects. The effect is evident within 2 weeks after surgery[91] and is sustained for at least 40 weeks.[92] Another possible mechanism is activation of the sympathetic nervous system signaling pathway by natriuretic peptides. Roux-en-Y gastric bypass surgery increases B-type natriuretic peptide expression in humans,[93] and Neinast and colleagues[94] have shown that Roux-en-Y gastric bypass increased natriuretic peptide receptors 1 and 2, B-type natriuretic peptide, and β-adrenergic receptor messenger RNA expression in gonadal adipose tissue. This adaptation was associated with increased UCP1 expression, which is consistent with increased BAT and a greater capacity for energy dissipation through thermogenesis.

FAT MASS AND OBESITY GENES AND BROWNING OF ADIPOSE TISSUE

Genome-wide association studies have helped to identify fat mass and obesity (FTO)-associated polygene variants in chromosome 16 as the most relevant to date for human obesity.[96,97] Several investigators report a strong correlation between genetic variance within the FTO gene and body weight regulation and fat mass, primarily in single nucleotide polymorphism variants located at the first intron of FTO.[95,98] Frayling and colleagues[95] found that 16% of adults who were homozygous for the risk allele A, weigh an average of 3 kg more, and have a 1.67-fold increased risk of obesity compared with those not inheriting a risk allele. Furthermore, Dina and colleagues[98] demonstrated that the T allele of single nucleotide polymorphism rs1121980 located in the first intron of the FTO gene was strongly associated with severe adult obesity. The FTO gene is widely expressed throughout multiple tissues and organs, so how FTO plays a role in the development of obesity is unclear. The first mechanistic study using loss of function of the FTO gene in mice showed resistance to diet-induced obesity owing to an increase in daily energy expenditure without changes in BAT mass and brown fat UCP1 expression.[99] In contrast, mice overexpressing the FTO gene have increased body and fat mass, but with no difference in energy expenditure.[100] Additional studies in FTO deficient mice have shown upregulation of UCP1 expression in gonadal and inguinal WAT, and this is associated with increased WAT browning and uncoupled respiration in white adipocytes, suggesting that FTO is significant for the induction of a brown adipocyte phenotype.[101] Recent data by Claussnitzer and colleagues[102] show that the single nucleotide variants rs1421085 of the FTO allele is associated with a reduction in mitochondrial thermogenesis. T-to-C single nucleotide variants within the ARID5B repressor were identified, which led to an increase IRX3 and IRX5 expression, causing a developmental shift from energy-dissipating beige adipocytes to energy-storing white adipocytes, with a reduction in mitochondrial thermogenesis by a factor of 5 and an increase in lipid storage capacity. Manipulation of the ARID5B-rs1421085-IRX3/5 regulatory axis by knocking down IRX3/IRX5 in primary adipocytes from participants with the risk allele reversed the obesity signature as observed by an increase in thermogenesis.[102] All of these findings suggest that the role of FTO in the control of energy homeostasis and body composition may be mediated by its role in regulating white adipocyte browning.

CONTRIBUTION OF BROWN ADIPOSE TISSUE THERMOGENESIS TO ENERGY EXPENDITURE

Energy balance is composed of 2 main variables: energy intake, which is derived from ingested food, and energy expenditure in the form of heat and physical work. An imbalance between either of these 2 variables results in storage of excess energy in the form of fat (positive balance; ie, weight gain), or burning of fat storage (negative balance; ie, weight loss). From the total of energy ingested in human, about 4% to 8% of energy is lost during digestion and 3% to 5% leaves the body in the form of urine and through the skin.[103] Thus, approximately 90% of the ingested energy is metabolized[14,104] and can be used as an expendable energy source. van Marken Lichtenbelt and Schrauwen[14] categorized this metabolizable energy into obligatory and facultative. The obligatory energy expenditure is vital, and covers the energy spent preserving normal cellular, tissue, and organ function (maintaining whole body temperature, respiration, protein turnover and other basic functions of tissues), DIT (energy for digestion and metabolism of ingested nutrients), and physical activity. Facultative energy expenditure covers adaptive thermogenesis, including cold-induced shivering and nonshivering thermogenesis, as well as exercise and nonexercise activity thermogenesis. The amount of expandable energy varies from person to person and is affected by age, gender, weight, height, body composition, environmental temperature, hormonal status, genes, and stress level.[105] Energy spent maintaining whole body metabolism accounts for the greatest amount of the total daily resting metabolic rate, about 55% to 65%.[14] Physical activity is the most variable and easily altered component, and depends on an individual's body mass and the intensity, duration, and frequency of exercise, as well as how efficient the individual is in performing the activity. Physical activity usually accounts for about 25% to 35% of the total daily metabolic rate, with a sedentary person expending less and a physically active person expending more energy.

Adaptive thermogenesis is defined as the process of heat production in response to environmental cues, such as changes in temperature or diet to protect the organism from cold exposure, or to regulate energy balance in response to change in calorie intake.[36] Maintenance of body temperature in small mammals or hibernating animals is achieved primarily by the ability of BAT and skeletal muscle to generate heat.[14] BAT thermogenic activity is minimal in a thermoneutral environment. With cold exposure the BAT thermogenic program is activated and this physiologic response is evident both in animals as well as humans.[37] In mice, the maximal heat producing capacity of BAT is approximately 300 W/kg, and this is the highest metabolic rate among mouse tissues.[32] In contrast, exposure to more comfortable warmer temperatures leads to a suppression of thermogenesis, owing primarily to a reduction in sympathetic drive to BAT.[37]

The potential contribution of BAT thermogenesis to whole body energy expenditure in humans was elegantly reviewed by van Marken Lichtenbelt and Schrauwen.[14] It is estimated that there is 40 to 60 g of BAT (approximately 0.1% of body mass) in a healthy human.[3,11] Rothwell and Stock[15] estimated that BAT activity may contribute up to 20% of daily energy expenditure in a lean healthy human. However, this estimate is based on assumptions that BAT can be maximally activated, and allometric relations were not taken into account when extrapolating energy expenditure in tissues/bodies of animals that differ in size.[14] When allometric corrections are included, Wang and colleagues[106] have estimated that BAT energy expenditure in humans is 80 W/kg, and with a 20% contribution from daily energy expenditure, a lean healthy human would need about 200 to 360 g of BAT (approximately 0.3 to 0.5% of body mass in a 70-kg human),[14] which is considerably higher than the first estimate. Based on [^{18}F]-FDG-PET/CT or ^{15}O-PET imaging observations,[3,11,14,107] a BAT mass of 40 to 60 g is likely for a healthy human. Thus, when fully activated BAT could account for approximately 2% to 5% of basal metabolic rate in a human.[14] Recently, Muzik and colleagues[107] examined the role of BAT on whole body energy expenditure in BAT^{+} and BAT^{-} human subjects. During thermoneutrality, whole body energy expenditure was similar for the 2 groups. Exposure to cold increased total energy expenditure in the BAT^{+} group. It was estimated that human BAT contributed up to 25 Kcal/d, which represents approximately 1% of total energy expenditure in an average person. By extrapolation, if 1% of daily energy expenditure represents an energy consumption of 100 Kcal/d, this translates into a loss of approximately 0.25 kg of fat per year.[11] Such a negligible amount is unlikely to impact the overweight and obesity problem that is facing the US population.

When these estimates are combined with physiologic and biochemical observations in humans and mice, the case for BAT and beige adipose tissue in the management or treatment of obesity in humans becomes challenging. Based on the observations reported, arguments against BAT and beige adipose tissue as current therapeutic targets for humans include (1) the presence of beige adipose tissue and the conversion of white fat cells into beige fat cells in humans is inconclusive at this point, (2) the capacity of BAT to contribute significantly to total daily energy expenditure is minimal and assumptions in favor of the alternative are based in part on a condition of continuous maximal activation, (3) obese people have modest BAT mass compared with lean individuals, and (4) pharmacologic stimulation of BAT in a thermoneutral environment would increase core body temperature, which may create an uncomfortable state including increases in respiration and/or perspiration.

THE ROLE OF BROWN ADIPOSE TISSUE BEYOND ENERGY BALANCE

Apart from its role in promoting energy expenditure for body weight regulation, activation of BAT may contribute to whole body physiologic and metabolic processes unrelated to weight modulation, but with a positive modulating impact on obesity-related comorbidities. Recent findings comparing BAT^{+} and BAT^{-} adults reveal that the BAT^{+} group has lower hemoglobin A_{1c}, total cholesterol, low-density lipoprotein cholesterol, and liver enzymes (alanine aminotransferase and aspartate aminotransferase).[5,108] These data suggest that activation of BAT may contribute to regulation of whole body glucose and lipid homeostasis, preventing states of insulin resistance, liver steatosis, cardiovascular disease, and immune system-related diseases. Possible mechanisms for these effects may be linked to the ability of BAT to channel blood glucose and lipid toward oxidation, or to secrete novel adipokines that target important metabolic tissues including the liver, skeletal muscle and pancreas.

There is considerable interest in the potential role of BAT as a mediator of glucose homeostasis and insulin resistance, and this is an area of active research. This work is primarily motivated by the need to find new therapies for treatment and prevention of type 2 diabetes. Because a reduction in fat mass typically improves insulin sensitivity, there is the potential that targeting BAT may uncover a new treatment approach. Recent reports from Chondronikola and colleagues[109] and Lee and colleagues[110] are supportive of this line of work and the data suggest that glucose metabolism in BAT in adult humans is associated with improved peripheral glucose homeostasis and insulin sensitivity. Peirce and Vidal-Puig[111] reviewed the potential mechanism of action whereby BAT activation regulates glucose homeostasis. One likely scenario is that BAT activation facilitates an increase in glucose disposal. One human study in which the hyperinsulinemic–euglycemic clamp was used to assess insulin-mediated glucose disposal found an acute bout of mild cold exposure for 5 hours increased glucose disposal in BAT$^+$ subjects, but this did not occur in subjects with undetectable BAT activation.[109] Based on empirical data, it was predicted that continuously activated BAT (approximately 70 mL) could clear approximately 20 to 30 g of glucose from the circulation over a 24-hour period.[109,112] In mice, the transcriptome profile of BAT was assessed using digital gene expression profiling and it was determined that cold exposure induced genes related to glucose metabolism,[113] suggesting that the use of glucose was upregulated in these animals and this may contribute to increased whole body glucose disposal. This improvement in whole body glucose metabolism would attenuate glucotoxicity and may also reduce β-cell dysfunction.[111] In addition, the effect of BAT activation on glucose homeostasis may be mediated by proteins secreted from brown fat cells. One such protein is FGF21, which is highly upregulated in BAT during prolonged cold exposure.[114] FGF21 is recognized as a metabolic regulator owing to its glucose lowering effects[115] and its role in promoting enhanced insulin sensitivity.[116]

The presence of BAT is also associated with a lower risk of nonalcoholic fatty liver disease (NAFLD) in human adults. Yilmaz and colleagues[117] performed whole body PET-CT scans on 1832 patients and found that the odds ratio for having NAFLD was significantly higher in BAT$^-$ subjects, and that the maximal standardized uptake values of [^{18}F]-FDG into BAT was significantly correlated with the ratio of mean liver attenuation to spleen attenuation. It is speculated that the role of BAT on attenuation of liver steatosis is mediated through brown fat adipokines, namely neuregulin (Nrg4). Nrg4 is a member of the epidermal growth factor family of extracellular ligands that are highly enriched in brown fat and expression and secretion is markedly increased during cold exposure and during brown adipocyte differentiation.[118,119] Analysis of serum Nrg4 level in humans has shown that NAFLD patients have significantly lower Nrg4 than non-NAFLD patients.[120] Gain-of-function and loss-of-function studies in mice have shown that Nrg4 protects against diet-induced insulin resistance and hepatosteatosis.[119] The protective role of Nrg4 may be mediated by binding with the extracellular domain of receptor tyrosine kinase ErbB3 (Erb-B2 receptor tyrosine kinase 3) and ErbB4 (Erb-B2 receptor tyrosine kinase 4) in hepatocytes. This binding downregulates hepatic de novo lipogenesis, which is mediated by the transcription factors LXR and SREBP1c through *Acc1*, *Scd1*, and *Fasn*.[119]

SUMMARY

Our understanding of the role of brown/beige adipose tissues on body weight in obese humans is evolving. Several unanswered questions remain, including the abundance of beige adipocytes, the mechanism of "WAT browning," the contribution of BAT thermogenesis to whole body homeostasis, and the extent to which thermogenesis can be upregulated to have sufficient impact on weight loss in humans. Resolution of these issues will determine the future for BAT as a therapeutic target in obesity and obesity-related comorbidities.

REFERENCES

1. Ng M, Fleming T, Robinson M, et al. Global, regional, and national prevalence of overweight and obesity in children and adults during 1980-2013; a systematic analysis for the Global Burden of Disease Study 2013. Lancet 2014;384(9945): 766–81.
2. Hill JO, Wyatt HR, Peters JC. Energy balance and obesity. Circulation 2012; 126(1):126–32.
3. van Marken Lichtenbelt WD, Vanhommerig JW, Smulders NM, et al. Cold-activated brown adipose tissue in healthy men. N Engl J Med 2009;360(15): 1500–8.
4. Cypess AM, Lehman S, Williams G, et al. Identification and importance of brown adipose tissue in adult humans. N Engl J Med 2009;360(15):1509–17.
5. Matsushita M, Yoneshiro T, Aita S, et al. Impact of brown adipose tissue on body fatness and glucose metabolism in healthy humans. Int J Obes (Lond) 2014; 38(6):812–7.
6. Wu J, Bostrom P, Sparks LM, et al. Beige adipocytes are a distinct type of thermogenic fat cell in mouse and human. Cell 2012;150(2):366–76.
7. Justo R, Oliver J, Gianotti M. Brown adipose tissue mitochondrial subpopulations show different morphological and thermogenic characteristics. Mitochondrion 2005;5(1):45–53.
8. Aherne W, Hull D. Brown adipose tissue and heat production in the newborn infant. J Pathol Bacteriol 1966;91(1):223–34.
9. Heaton JM. The distribution of brown adipose tissue in the human. J Anat 1972; 112(Pt 1):35–9.
10. Lean ME. Brown adipose tissue in humans. Proc Nutr Soc 1989;48(2):243–56.
11. Virtanen KA, Lidell ME, Orava J, et al. Functional brown adipose tissue in healthy adults. N Engl J Med 2009;360(15):1518–25.
12. Nedergaard J, Bengtsson T, Cannon B. Unexpected evidence for active brown adipose tissue in adult humans. Am J Physiol Endocrinol Metab 2007;293(2): E444–52.
13. Orava J, Nuutila P, Lidell ME, et al. Different metabolic responses of human brown adipose tissue to activation by cold and insulin. Cell Metab 2011;14(2): 272–9.
14. van Marken Lichtenbelt WD, Schrauwen P. Implications of nonshivering thermogenesis for energy balance regulation in humans. Am J Physiol Regul Integr Comp Physiol 2011;301(2):R285–96.
15. Rothwell NJ, Stock MJ. A role for brown adipose tissue in diet-induced thermogenesis. Nature 1979;281(5726):31–5.
16. Harms M, Seale P. Brown and beige fat: development, function and therapeutic potential. Nat Med 2013;19(10):1252–63.
17. Sharp LZ, Shinoda K, Ohno H, et al. Human BAT possesses molecular signatures that resemble beige/brite cells. PLoS One 2012;7(11):e49452.
18. Lee P, Werner CD, Kebebew E, et al. Functional thermogenic beige adipogenesis is inducible in human neck fat. Int J Obes (Lond) 2014;38(2):170–6.

19. Jespersen NZ, Larsen TJ, Peijs L, et al. A classical brown adipose tissue mRNA signature partly overlaps with brite in the supraclavicular region of adult humans. Cell Metab 2013;17(5):798–805.

20. Shinoda K, Luijten IH, Hasegawa Y, et al. Genetic and functional characterization of clonally derived adult human brown adipocytes. Nat Med 2015;21(4): 389–94.

21. Atit R, Sgaier SK, Mohamed OA, et al. Beta-catenin activation is necessary and sufficient to specify the dorsal dermal fate in the mouse. Dev Biol 2006;296(1): 164–76.

22. Timmons JA, Wennmalm K, Larsson O, et al. Myogenic gene expression signature establishes that brown and white adipocytes originate from distinct cell lineages. Proc Natl Acad Sci U S A 2007;104(11):4401–6.

23. Forner F, Kumar C, Luber CA, et al. Proteome differences between brown and white fat mitochondria reveal specialized metabolic functions. Cell Metab 2009;10(4):324–35.

24. Seale P, Bjork B, Yang W, et al. PRDM16 controls a brown fat/skeletal muscle switch. Nature 2008;454(7207):961–7.

25. Petrovic N, Walden TB, Shabalina IG, et al. Chronic peroxisome proliferator-activated receptor gamma (PPARgamma) activation of epididymally derived white adipocyte cultures reveals a population of thermogenically competent, UCP1-containing adipocytes molecularly distinct from classic brown adipocytes. J Biol Chem 2010;285(10):7153–64.

26. Sanchez-Gurmaches J, Hung CM, Sparks CA, et al. PTEN loss in the Myf5 lineage redistributes body fat and reveals subsets of white adipocytes that arise from Myf5 precursors. Cell Metab 2012;16(3):348–62.

27. Long JZ, Svensson KJ, Tsai L, et al. A smooth muscle-like origin for beige adipocytes. Cell Metab 2014;19(5):810–20.

28. Xue R, Lynes MD, Dreyfuss JM, et al. Clonal analyses and gene profiling identify genetic biomarkers of the thermogenic potential of human brown and white pre-adipocytes. Nat Med 2015;21(7):760–8.

29. Ricquier D, Casteilla L, Bouillaud F. Molecular studies of the uncoupling protein. FASEB J 1991;5(9):2237–42.

30. Nicholls DG, Locke RM. Thermogenic mechanisms in brown fat. Physiol Rev 1984;64(1):1–64.

31. Matthias A, Ohlson KB, Fredriksson JM, et al. Thermogenic responses in brown fat cells are fully UCP1-dependent. UCP2 or UCP3 do not substitute for UCP1 in adrenergically or fatty scid-induced thermogenesis. J Biol Chem 2000;275(33): 25073–81.

32. Cannon B, Nedergaard J. Brown adipose tissue: function and physiological significance. Physiol Rev 2004;84(1):277–359.

33. Fedorenko A, Lishko PV, Kirichok Y. Mechanism of fatty-acid-dependent UCP1 uncoupling in brown fat mitochondria. Cell 2012;151(2):400–13.

34. Silva JE. Thermogenic mechanisms and their hormonal regulation. Physiol Rev 2006;86(2):435–64.

35. Nicholls DG. Hamster brown-adipose-tissue mitochondria. Purine nucleotide control of the ion conductance of the inner membrane, the nature of the nucleotide binding site. Eur J Biochem 1976;62(2):223–8.

36. Lowell BB, Spiegelman BM. Towards a molecular understanding of adaptive thermogenesis. Nature 2000;404(6778):652–60.

37. van der Lans AA, Hoeks J, Brans B, et al. Cold acclimation recruits human brown fat and increases nonshivering thermogenesis. J Clin Invest 2013; 123(8):3395–403.

38. Cao W, Daniel KW, Robidoux J, et al. p38 mitogen-activated protein kinase is the central regulator of cyclic AMP-dependent transcription of the brown fat uncoupling protein 1 gene. Mol Cell Biol 2004;24(7):3057–67.

39. Warner A, Mittag J. Breaking BAT: can browning create a better white? J Endocrinol 2016;228(1):R19–29.

40. Dodd GT, Decherf S, Loh K, et al. Leptin and Insulin act on POMC neurons to promote the browning of white fat. Cell 2015;160(1–2):88–104.

41. Ruan HB, Dietrich MO, Liu ZW, et al. O-GlcNAc transferase enables AgRP neurons to suppress browning of white fat. Cell 2014;159(2):306–17.

42. Qiu Y, Nguyen KD, Odegaard JI, et al. Eosinophils and type 2 cytokine signaling in macrophages orchestrate development of functional beige fat. Cell 2014; 157(6):1292–308.

43. Brestoff JR, Kim BS, Saenz SA, et al. Group 2 innate lymphoid cells promote beiging of white adipose tissue and limit obesity. Nature 2015;519(7542):242–6.

44. Lee MW, Odegaard JI, Mukundan I, et al. Activated type 2 innate lymphoid cells regulate beige fat biogenesis. Cell 2015;160(1–2):74–87.

45. Lee P, Greenfield JR. Non-pharmacological and pharmacological strategies of brown adipose tissue recruitment in humans. Mol Cell Endocrinol 2015; 418(Pt 2):184–90.

46. Gollisch KS, Brandauer J, Jessen N, et al. Effects of exercise training on subcutaneous and visceral adipose tissue in normal- and high-fat diet-fed rats. Am J Physiol Endocrinol Metab 2009;297(2):E495–504.

47. Craig BW, Hammons GT, Garthwaite SM, et al. Adaptation of fat cells to exercise: response of glucose uptake and oxidation to insulin. J Appl Physiol Respir Environ Exerc Physiol 1981;51(6):1500–6.

48. Stallknecht B, Vinten J, Ploug T, et al. Increased activities of mitochondrial enzymes in white adipose tissue in trained rats. Am J Physiol 1991;261(3 Pt 1): E410–4.

49. Stanford KI, Middelbeek RJ, Townsend KL, et al. A novel role for subcutaneous adipose tissue in exercise-induced improvements in glucose homeostasis. Diabetes 2015;64(6):2002–14.

50. Sutherland LN, Bomhof MR, Capozzi LC, et al. Exercise and adrenaline increase PGC-1{alpha} mRNA expression in rat adipose tissue. J Physiol 2009;587(Pt 7): 1607–17.

51. Trevellin E, Scorzeto M, Olivieri M, et al. Exercise training induces mitochondrial biogenesis and glucose uptake in subcutaneous adipose tissue through eNOS-dependent mechanisms. Diabetes 2014;63(8):2800–11.

52. Boström P, Wu J, Jedrychowski MP, et al. A PGC1-alpha-dependent myokine that drives brown-fat-like development of white fat and thermogenesis. Nature 2012;481(7382):463–8.

53. Cao L, Choi EY, Liu X, et al. White to brown fat phenotypic switch induced by genetic and environmental activation of a hypothalamic-adipocyte axis. Cell Metab 2011;14(3):324–38.

54. Lee P, Linderman JD, Smith S, et al. Irisin and FGF21 are cold-induced endocrine activators of brown fat function in humans. Cell Metab 2014;19(2):302–9.

55. Daskalopoulou SS, Cooke AB, Gomez YH, et al. Plasma irisin levels progressively increase in response to increasing exercise workloads in young, healthy, active subjects. Eur J Endocrinol 2014;171(3):343–52.

56. Hew-Butler T, Landis-Piwowar K, Byrd G, et al. Plasma irisin in runners and non-runners: no favorable metabolic associations in humans. Physiol Rep 2015;3(1): e12262.

57. Norheim F, Langleite TM, Hjorth M, et al. The effects of acute and chronic exercise on PGC-1alpha, irisin and browning of subcutaneous adipose tissue in humans. FEBS J 2014;281(3):739–49.

58. Ellefsen S, Vikmoen O, Slettalokken G, et al. Irisin and FNDC5: effects of 12-week strength training, and relations to muscle phenotype and body mass composition in untrained women. Eur J Appl Physiol 2014;114(9):1875–88.

59. Vosselman MJ, Hoeks J, Brans B, et al. Low brown adipose tissue activity in endurance-trained compared with lean sedentary men. Int J Obes (Lond) 2015;39(12):1696–702.

60. Qiu S, Cai X, Sun Z, et al. Chronic exercise training and circulating Irisin in adults: a meta-analysis. Sports Med 2015;45(11):1577–88.

61. Raschke S, Elsen M, Gassenhuber H, et al. Evidence against a beneficial effect of irisin in humans. PLoS One 2013;8(9):e73680.

62. Roca-Rivada A, Castelao C, Senin LL, et al. FNDC5/irisin is not only a myokine but also an adipokine. PLoS One 2013;8(4):e60563.

63. Palacios-Gonzalez B, Vadillo-Ortega F, Polo-Oteyza E, et al. Irisin levels before and after physical activity among school-age children with different BMI: a direct relation with leptin. Obesity (Silver Spring) 2015;23(4):729–32.

64. Pardo M, Crujeiras AB, Amil M, et al. Association of irisin with fat mass, resting energy expenditure, and daily activity in conditions of extreme body mass index. Int J Endocrinol 2014;2014:857270.

65. Viitasalo A, Agren J, Venalainen T, et al. Association of plasma fatty acid composition with plasma irisin levels in normal weight and overweight/obese children. Pediatr Obes 2015. [Epub ahead of print].

66. Steensberg A, van Hall G, Osada T, et al. Klarlund Pedersen B. Production of interleukin-6 in contracting human skeletal muscles can account for the exercise-induced increase in plasma interleukin-6. J Physiol 2000;529(Pt 1): 237–42.

67. Wolsk E, Mygind H, Grondahl TS, et al. IL-6 selectively stimulates fat metabolism in human skeletal muscle. Am J Physiol Endocrinol Metab 2010;299(5):E832–40.

68. Knudsen JG, Murholm M, Carey AL, et al. Role of IL-6 in exercise training- and cold-induced UCP1 expression in subcutaneous white adipose tissue. PLoS One 2014;9(1):e84910.

69. Rao RR, Long JZ, White JP, et al. Meteorin-like is a hormone that regulates immune-adipose interactions to increase beige fat thermogenesis. Cell 2014; 157(6):1279–91.

70. Carriere A, Jeanson Y, Berger-Muller S, et al. Browning of white adipose cells by intermediate metabolites: an adaptive mechanism to alleviate redox pressure. Diabetes 2014;63(10):3253–65.

71. Roberts LD, Bostrom P, O'Sullivan JF, et al. beta-Aminoisobutyric acid induces browning of white fat and hepatic beta-oxidation and is inversely correlated with cardiometabolic risk factors. Cell Metab 2014;19(1):96–108.

72. Sakamoto T, Takahashi N, Goto T, et al. Dietary factors evoke thermogenesis in adipose tissues. Obes Res Clin Pract 2014;8(6):e533–9.

73. Lettieri Barbato D, Tatulli G, Vegliante R, et al. Dietary fat overload reprograms brown fat mitochondria. Front Physiol 2015;6:272.

74. Fromme T, Klingenspor M. Uncoupling protein 1 expression and high-fat diets. Am J Physiol Regul Integr Comp Physiol 2011;300(1):R1–8.

75. Vosselman MJ, Brans B, van der Lans AA, et al. Brown adipose tissue activity after a high-calorie meal in humans. Am J Clin Nutr 2013;98(1):57–64.

76. Sadurskis A, Dicker A, Cannon B, et al. Polyunsaturated fatty acids recruit brown adipose tissue: increased UCP content and NST capacity. Am J Physiol 1995;269(2 Pt 1):E351–60.

77. Acheson KJ, Blondel-Lubrano A, Oguey-Araymon S, et al. Protein choices targeting thermogenesis and metabolism. Am J Clin Nutr 2011;93(3):525–34.

78. Petzke KJ, Riese C, Klaus S. Short-term, increasing dietary protein and fat moderately affect energy expenditure, substrate oxidation and uncoupling protein gene expression in rats. J Nutr Biochem 2007;18(6):400–7.

79. Saito M, Yoneshiro T, Matsushita M. Food ingredients as anti-obesity agents. Trends Endocrinol Metab 2015;26(11):585–7.

80. Saito M, Yoneshiro T. Capsinoids and related food ingredients activating brown fat thermogenesis and reducing body fat in humans. Curr Opin Lipidol 2013;24(1):71–7.

81. Choo JJ. Green tea reduces body fat accretion caused by high-fat diet in rats through beta-adrenoceptor activation of thermogenesis in brown adipose tissue. J Nutr Biochem 2003;14(11):671–6.

82. Lone J, Choi JH, Kim SW, et al. Curcumin induces brown fat-like phenotype in 3T3-L1 and primary white adipocytes. J Nutr Biochem 2016;27:193–202.

83. Wang S, Wang X, Ye Z, et al. Curcumin promotes browning of white adipose tissue in a norepinephrine-dependent way. Biochem Biophys Res Commun 2015;466(2):247–53.

84. Sugita J, Yoneshiro T, Hatano T, et al. Grains of paradise (Aframomum melegueta) extract activates brown adipose tissue and increases whole-body energy expenditure in men. Br J Nutr 2013;110(4):733–8.

85. Bueter M, Lowenstein C, Olbers T, et al. Gastric bypass increases energy expenditure in rats. Gastroenterology 2010;138(5):1845–53.

86. Flancbaum L, Choban PS, Bradley LR, et al. Changes in measured resting energy expenditure after Roux-en-Y gastric bypass for clinically severe obesity. Surgery 1997;122(5):943–9.

87. Farla SL, Faria OP, Buffington C, et al. Energy expenditure before and after Roux-en-Y gastric bypass. Obes Surg 2012;22(9):1450–5.

88. Rabl C, Rao MN, Schwarz JM, et al. Thermogenic changes after gastric bypass, adjustable gastric banding or diet alone. Surgery 2014;156(4):806–12.

89. Stylopoulos N, Hoppin AG, Kaplan LM. Roux-en-Y gastric bypass enhances energy expenditure and extends lifespan in diet-induced obese rats. Obesity (Silver Spring) 2009;17(10):1839–47.

90. Vijgen GH, Bouvy ND, Teule GJ, et al. Increase in brown adipose tissue activity after weight loss in morbidly obese subjects. J Clin Endocrinol Metab 2012;97(7):E1229–33.

91. Kirwan JP, Malin SK, Kullman EL, et al. Early diabetes remission after gastric bypass surgery is explained by exclusion of the foregut. San Francisco (CA): American Diabetes Association; 2014.

92. Ahmad NN, Pfalzer A, Kaplan LM. Roux-en-Y gastric bypass normalizes the blunted postprandial bile acid excursion associated with obesity. Int J Obes (Lond) 2013;37(12):1553–9.

93. Changchien EM, Ahmed S, Betti F, et al. B-type natriuretic peptide increases after gastric bypass surgery and correlates with weight loss. Surg Endosc 2011;25(7):2338–43.

94. Neinast MD, Frank AP, Zechner JF, et al. Activation of natriuretic peptides and the sympathetic nervous system following Roux-en-Y gastric bypass is associated with gonadal adipose tissues browning. Mol Metab 2015;4(5):427–36.

95. Frayling TM, Timpson NJ, Weedon MN, et al. A common variant in the FTO gene is associated with body mass index and predisposes to childhood and adult obesity. Science 2007;316(5826):889–94.

96. Thorleifsson G, Walters GB, Gudbjartsson DF, et al. Genome-wide association yields new sequence variants at seven loci that associate with measures of obesity. Nat Genet 2009;41(1):18–24.

97. Willer CJ, Speliotes EK, Loos RJ, et al. Six new loci associated with body mass index highlight a neuronal influence on body weight regulation. Nat Genet 2009; 41(1):25–34.

98. Dina C, Meyre D, Gallina S, et al. Variation in FTO contributes to childhood obesity and severe adult obesity. Nat Genet 2007;39(6):724–6.

99. Fischer J, Koch L, Emmerling C, et al. Inactivation of the Fto gene protects from obesity. Nature 2009;458(7240):894–8.

100. Church C, Moir L, McMurray F, et al. Overexpression of Fto leads to increased food intake and results in obesity. Nat Genet 2010;42(12):1086–92.

101. Tews D, Fischer-Posovszky P, Fromme T, et al. FTO deficiency induces UCP-1 expression and mitochondrial uncoupling in adipocytes. Endocrinology 2013; 154(9):3141–51.

102. Claussnitzer M, Dankel SN, Kim KH, et al. FTO obesity variant circuitry and adipocyte browning in humans. N Engl J Med 2015;373(10):895–907.

103. Blaxter KL. Energy metabolism in animals and man. Cambridge (United Kingdom); New York: Cambridge University Press; 1989.

104. James WP, Trayhurn P. Thermogenesis and obesity. Br Med Bull 1981;37(1): 43–8.

105. Sims EA, Danforth E Jr. Expenditure and storage of energy in man. J Clin Invest 1987;79(4):1019–25.

106. Wang Z, O'Connor TP, Heshka S, et al. The reconstruction of Kleiber's law at the organ-tissue level. J Nutr 2001;131(11):2967–70.

107. Muzik O, Mangner TJ, Leonard WR, et al. 15O PET measurement of blood flow and oxygen consumption in cold-activated human brown fat. J Nucl Med 2013; 54(4):523–31.

108. Ozguven S, Ones T, Yilmaz Y, et al. The role of active brown adipose tissue in human metabolism. Eur J Nucl Med Mol Imaging 2016;43(2):355–61.

109. Chondronikola M, Volpi E, Borsheim E, et al. Brown adipose tissue improves whole-body glucose homeostasis and insulin sensitivity in humans. Diabetes 2014;63(12):4089–99.

110. Lee P, Smith S, Linderman J, et al. Temperature-acclimated brown adipose tissue modulates insulin sensitivity in humans. Diabetes 2014;63(11):3686–98.

111. Peirce V, Vidal-Puig A. Regulation of glucose homoeostasis by brown adipose tissue. Lancet Diabetes Endocrinol 2013;1(4):353–60.

112. Sidossis L, Kajimura S. Brown and beige fat in humans: thermogenic adipocytes that control energy and glucose homeostasis. J Clin Invest 2015;125(2):478–86.

113. Hao Q, Yadav R, Basse AL, et al. Transcriptome profiling of brown adipose tissue during cold exposure reveals extensive regulation of glucose metabolism. Am J Physiol Endocrinol Metab 2015;308(5):E380–92.

114. Stanford KI, Middelbeek RJ, Townsend KL, et al. Brown adipose tissue regulates glucose homeostasis and insulin sensitivity. J Clin Invest 2013;123(1):215–23.

115. Kharitonenkov A, Shiyanova TL, Koester A, et al. FGF-21 as a novel metabolic regulator. J Clin Invest 2005;115(6):1627–35.
116. Wente W, Efanov AM, Brenner M, et al. Fibroblast growth factor-21 improves pancreatic beta-cell function and survival by activation of extracellular signal-regulated kinase 1/2 and Akt signaling pathways. Diabetes 2006;55(9):2470–8.
117. Yilmaz Y, Ones T, Purnak T, et al. Association between the presence of brown adipose tissue and non-alcoholic fatty liver disease in adult humans. Aliment Pharmacol Ther 2011;34(3):318–23.
118. Rosell M, Kaforou M, Frontini A, et al. Brown and white adipose tissues: intrinsic differences in gene expression and response to cold exposure in mice. Am J Physiol Endocrinol Metab 2014;306(8):E945–64.
119. Wang GX, Zhao XY, Meng ZX, et al. The brown fat-enriched secreted factor Nrg4 preserves metabolic homeostasis through attenuation of hepatic lipogenesis. Nat Med 2014;20(12):1436–43.
120. Dai YN, Zhu JZ, Fang ZY, et al. A case-control study: association between serum neuregulin 4 level and non-alcoholic fatty liver disease. Metabolism 2015;64(12):1667–73.

Genetics of Bariatric Surgery Outcomes

Olivier F. Noel, BS[a,b,c], Christopher D. Still, DO[d], Glenn S. Gerhard, MD[e],*

KEYWORDS

- Bariatric surgery • Genetics • Weight loss • Type 2 diabetes mellitus • NAFLD

KEY POINTS

- Outcomes after bariatric surgery can vary widely and seem to have a significant genetic component.
- Only a small number of candidate gene studies and genome-wide association studies (GWAS) have analyzed bariatric surgery outcomes.
- The role of bile acids in mediating the beneficial effects of bariatric surgery implicate genes regulated by the farnesoid X receptor (FXR) transcription factor.

INTRODUCTION

The lack of adequate medical therapies for morbid or extreme obesity (body mass index [BMI] >40 kg/m^2) and type 2 diabetes mellitus (T2D) has led to the use of bariatric surgery, in particular the Roux-en-Y gastric bypass (RYGB) and sleeve gastrectomy (SG) procedures. Several large observational studies have shown lasting (>5 years) weight loss and dramatic improvements in T2D after bariatric surgery,[1] which also seems to improve lipid parameters and decrease long-term cardiovascular events. Several clinical factors have been identified that can affect weight loss after RYGB[2] but few studies have addressed genetic influences on these outcomes.

The beneficial metabolic effects of bariatric surgery have been observed for more than 50 years[3] and have been confirmed by numerous subsequent studies in humans

Disclosure Statement: Dr C. Still receives grant and consulting support from Ethicon Endo-Surgery. This work was supported by R01 DK088231 from the National Institutes of Health and by Lewis Katz School of Medicine, Temple University, Department of Medical Genetics and Molecular Biochemistry.

a Lewis Katz School of Medicine, Temple University, 3500 North Broad Street, Philadelphia, PA 19140, USA; b Penn State College of Medicine, 500 University Drive, Hershey, PA 17033, USA; c DNAsimple, Philadelphia, PA, USA; d Department of Gastroenterology and Nutrition, Geisinger Clinic, 100 North Academy Avenue, Danville, PA 17822, USA; e Department of Medical Genetics and Molecular Biochemistry, Lewis Katz School of Medicine, Temple University, 960 Medical Education and Research Building (MERB), 3500 North Broad Street, Philadelphia, PA 19140, USA
* Corresponding author.
E-mail address: gsgerhard@Temple.edu

Endocrinol Metab Clin N Am 45 (2016) 623–632
http://dx.doi.org/10.1016/j.ecl.2016.04.011
0889-8529/16/$ – see front matter © 2016 Elsevier Inc. All rights reserved.
endo.theclinics.com

and animal models, but the molecular mechanisms underlying these effects are not yet well delineated. Much attention has also focused on incretins, in particular glucagon-like peptide 1 (GLP-1), although comprehensive reviews attributed only some or none of the antidiabetic effects to GLP-1.[4] The other main classes of hypotheses[5] are based on alterations in the flow and anatomic routing of ingested nutrients. The foregut hypothesis posits that bypass and exclusion from contact with ingested nutrients of the proximal small intestine (foregut), primarily the duodenum, changes the production of a mediator that produces direct anti-T2D effects. Procedures that cause malabsorption through intestinal bypass have dramatic effects on T2D. The lower intestinal or hindgut hypothesis is based on the premise that inappropriate delivery of ingested nutrients and/or digestive juices to more distal regions of the small intestine induces a putative molecular mediator that ameliorates T2D. Bile acids have been implicated as key molecules in this hypothesis.[3,4] A seeming confounder to this hypothesis is the SG, a restrictive and nonmalabsorptive operation that is increasingly used instead of RYGB, which is a partial gastrectomy in which the stomach becomes a vertical tube or sleeve. The SG also results in resolution of T2D, which seems to contradict the inappropriate delivery of nutrients and digestive components to the distal intestine hypothesis. Gastric transit is substantially increased in SG, however, expediting delivery of digesta, including bile acids through the duodenum into the distal intestine.[4]

Bile acids can bind to the G protein–coupled TGR5 cellular receptor to mediate signaling.[6] Bile acids also function as a ligand for a specific nuclear transcription factor, the FXR, which forms a heterodimeric complex with retinoid X receptor α that binds to an inverted repeat sequence in gene promoters.[7] Recently, FXR has been shown to be required for weight loss and improvements in glucose metabolism after SG in mice.[8] Further delineation of the molecular mechanisms underlying these beneficial effects could provide targets for the development of new nonsurgical treatments.

HERITABILITY OF WEIGHT LOSS OUTCOMES

Although RYGB surgery is among the most successful interventions for long-term weight loss in extreme obesity, the degree of weight loss after surgery is variable, with an estimated 20% of patients failing to achieve or maintain greater than 50% loss of their excess body weight.[9] Clinical factors affecting weight loss after RYGB include higher initial BMI and T2D.[2] Studies of twins and close relatives have provided strong evidence of a genetic component to dietary and surgical weight loss.[10] These data indicate that genetic factors may influence weight loss after bariatric surgery.

CANDIDATE GENES AND BARIATRIC WEIGHT LOSS

Several studies have analyzed the association of polymorphisms in candidate genes with weight loss after bariatric surgery. For example, patients with melanocortin-4 receptor (MC4R) mutations achieve superior weight loss outcomes from procedures, such as RYGB, that produce neurohormonal changes rather than gastric restriction alone, possibly through effects on appetite and satiety regulation.[11] Polymorphisms near the growth hormone secretagogue receptor gene, or ghrelin receptor, have been studied in association with weight loss outcomes 30 months after RYGB. Patients homozygous for the rs490683-CC genotype – located in the promoter region of the growth hormone secretagogue receptor gene – exhibited significantly more weight loss than those who carried the T allele.[12] An association between the variant rs9939609 located in the fat mass and obesity-associated protein (FTO) gene and short-term weight loss outcomes after biliopancreatic diversion surgery has been reported.[13] Two studies have analyzed the association of a small panels of variants, including rs660339 located in the mitochondrial uncoupling protein 2 gene, rs712221 located in the estrogen receptor 1 gene, and rs9939609 located in the FTO gene associated with significant decreases in BMI after RYGB.[14] A summative allelic burden score of variants in the insulin-induced gene 2, proprotein convertase subtilisin/kexin type 1, MC4R, and FTO loci were correlated with poorer weight loss outcome after RYGB.[15] A major drawback to such candidate gene approaches is that they are selected based on a priori knowledge of the underlying molecular mechanism, which in the case of bariatric surgery has not been well-defined; thus, the selected genes may not be relevant or play a significant role.

GENOME-WIDE ASSOCIATION STUDIES OF BARIATRIC WEIGHT LOSS

In contrast to analyzing 1 or a small number of selected candidates, genome-wide approaches survey variants across the entire genome. For example, several loci have been identified in GWAS meta-analyses of obesity and metabolic phenotypes, including an analysis of BMI in 339,224 individuals, in whom 97 BMI-associated loci were identified,[16] and another meta-analyses of waist and hip circumference and related traits analyzed in 224,459 individuals, in whom 49 loci were associated with waist-to-hip ratio adjusted for BMI and an additional 19 loci associated with related waist and hip circumference measures.[17] Few studies to date, however, have used a GWAS approach to identify variants associated with outcomes of bariatric surgery. The authors conducted the first study to apply GWAS to weight loss after RYGB, using an extreme-trait design followed by second-stage confirmation to identify single nucleotide polymorphisms (SNPs) associated with weight loss 2 years after RYGB surgery.[18] To minimize population stratification and potential confounders, a cohort of more than 1000 white patients who were treated at 1 institution in a uniform clinical program after undergoing a standardized RYGB bariatric procedure was analyzed. A total of 17 SNPs was associated with weight loss at 2 years after RYGB in or near several genes with potential biological relevance, including polycystic kidney and hepatic disease 1, 5-hydroxytryptamine receptor 1A, neuromedin B receptor, and insulinlike growth factor 1 (IGF1R).

The authors also conducted a GWAS of weight nadir occurring up to 3 years after RYGB. A genetic variant was identified on chromosome 9 with suggestive ($P < 10^{-7}$) evidence of association (**Fig. 1**) that resides in an intron of the COL5A1. The nearest gene to COL5A1 is the retinoid X receptor α. Bile acid binding to FXR leads to formation of a heterodimer with retinoid X receptor α.[19] This adds further support for a role for FXR in postbariatric weight loss.

A GWAS by another group of RYGB analyzed weight loss at nadir in 693 participants of European descent.[18] Weight nadir was defined as the lowest weight at least 10 months after surgery. A single genetic locus near *ST8SIA2* and *SLCO3A1* was identified that was significantly associated with weight loss after RYGB.

FARNESOID X RECEPTOR–REGULATED OBESITY GENES

The increasing evidence that bile acids operating through FXR may mediate several of the beneficial effects of bariatric surgery focuses attention on FXR-regulated genes. An analysis of genes with at least suggestive evidence of association in the authors' published and unpublished GWAS, genes from the other bariatric surgery GWAS,[18] and data from recent obesity GWAS of BMI[16] and waist and hip circumference and related traits,[17] as well as genes associated with mendelian forms of obesity and

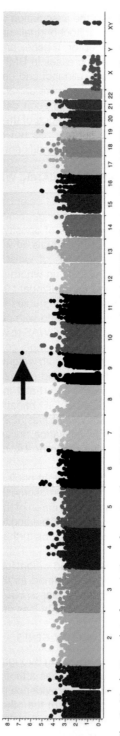

Fig. 1. Manhattan plot of association of greater than 650,000 genotypes on approximately 1500 patients with post-RYGB weight nadir data. Most significant SNP indicated by arrow.

other obesity-related genes,[20] was conducted to identify potential FXR-regulated obesity genes that may be influenced by changes in bile acids after bariatric surgery. Several genes, including APOBR, AS3MT, BDNF, GTF3A, HMGCR, IL27, MAP2K5, NT5C2, OLFM4, RPS3A, SEC16B, SH2B1, SULT1A2, TMEM184B, TMEM185A, IGF1R, MCHR1, and SIRT2, possess FXR-binding motifs. HMGCR,[21] BDNF,[22] MCHR1,[23] and SIRT2,[24] have all been implicated in bile acid metabolism or obesity, implicating them as candidates in the mechanisms of weight loss after bariatric surgery.

FARNESOID X RECEPTOR AND TYPE 2 DIABETES MELLITUS

The lack of a robust medical therapy for T2D has led to the increasing use of bariatric surgery. For example, in a single-center, nonblinded, randomized controlled trial of 60 patients (ages 30–60 years) with a BMI greater than 35 kg/m^2 with at least a 5-year history of T2D and a hemoglobin A_{1c} greater than 7% who were randomly assigned to receive conventional medical therapy or undergo RYGB, no patients in the medical therapy group achieved remission of T2D, defined as a fasting blood glucose less than 100 mg/dL and a hemoglobin A_{1c} less than 6.5% without use of medications, at 2 years, whereas 75% of the patients who underwent RYGB were in remission.[25] Based on the normalization of the hemoglobin A_{1c} and discontinuation of medications, glucose normalization occurred within hours to days of the surgery in most patients long before weight loss occurred.[26]

A mechanistic role for bile acids in glucose metabolism, in addition to their well-known roles in lipid absorption in the gut, seems part of a broader physiologic response to ingested nutrients.[19] This is consistent with the anabolic need to store fatty acids as triglycerides, which requires a glycerol-3-phosphate backbone[27] that is derived from glucose.[28,29] Bile acids thus seem to be involved in the regulation of glucose metabolism through modulation of FXR-regulated pathways. FXR−/− mice exhibited peripheral insulin resistance, reduced glucose disposal, and decreased adipose tissue and skeletal muscle insulin signaling, and, conversely, activation of FXR by the agonist GW4064 in insulin-resistant leptin-deficient (ob/ob) mice reduced hyperinsulinemia and improved glucose tolerance.[30] The role of FXR-regulated genes in the resolution of T2D after bariatric surgery has not yet been explored.

BARIATRIC LIPID OUTCOMES AND FARNESOID X RECEPTOR–REGULATED GENES

Dramatic changes in triglyceride (TRIG) and high-density lipoprotein (HDL) cholesterol levels can occur after RYGB surgery. TRIG levels decline and HDL levels increase in a majority of patients in the first year after surgery, with a substantial correlation between the degrees of change (**Fig. 2**). Similar results are seen in the second and third years after surgery.

An bioinformatic search for FXR motifs in a recent compilation of TRIG GWAS genes,[31] as well as the authors' own lipid GWAS loci,[32] identified motifs in METTL21C, APOC3, MAP3K12, METTL13, PLA2G6, PEPD, LPL, METTL6, MAP3K15, METTL7A, MAP3K14, and PINX1. LPL is the only 1 of 10 genes that were found associated with both TRIG and HDL by GWAS. Given the correlation in improvement in TRIG and HDL after bariatric surgery, LPL is a leading candidate as an FXR-mediated mechanism underlying the improvement in metabolic syndrome–related dyslipidemia characterized by high TRIG and low HDL.[33]

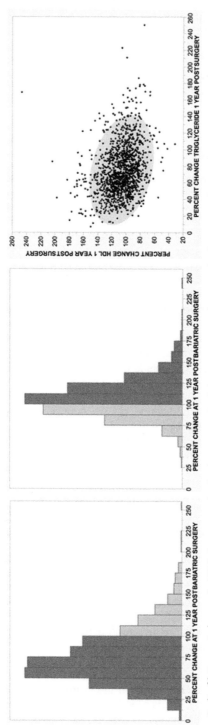

Fig. 2. (*Left*) Percent change in TRIG 1-year postbariatric surgery. Dark bars represent decreased values consistent with clinical improvement. (*Middle*) Percent change in HDL 1-year postbariatric surgery. Dark bars represent increased values consistent with clinical improvement. (*Right*) Plot of percentage 1-year change in TRIG versus HDL.

Table 1
Role of PNPLA3 I148M genetic variant on nonalcoholic fatty liver disease after bariatric surgery

	PNPLA3 NL	PNPLA3 I148M
Mean age (SD)	46.0 (9.5)	46.7 (8.5)
Female, % (n)	90% (19)	80% (12)
Caucasian, % (n)	95% (20)	100% (15)
Mean BMI, kg/m^2 (SD)	50.7 (11.3)	56.0 (12.8)
Liver pathology primary		
Normal, % (n)	43% (9)	13% (2)
Steatosis only, % (n)	33% (7)	47% (7)
Fibrosis, % (n)	24% (5)	40% (6)
Liver pathology revision		
Normal, % (n)	62% (13)	33% (5)
Steatosis only, % (n)	24% (5)	27% (4)
Fibrosis, % (n)	14% (3)	40% (6)
Mean interval, y (SD)	3.1 (1.9)	3.4 (2.2)

BARIATRIC SURGERY AND NONALCOHOLIC FATTY LIVER DISEASE

The metabolic liver disease nonalcoholic fatty liver disease (NAFLD) is an important but often clinically undiagnosed liver disorder. A primary treatment of NAFLD is weight loss through lifestyle modification.[34] Data also support a potential beneficial effect of bariatric surgery on NAFLD. A recent summary of 12 studies on NAFLD after RYGB reported a range of sample sizes from 7 to 116 individuals and postoperative follow-up periods ranging from 12 to 32 months.[35] The authors expanded this survey to include a total of 16 studies reporting on a total of 1024 patients who had undergone a primary bariatric surgery procedure and then a subsequent liver biopsy, most performed during a second surgical procedure.[36–51] Overall the data suggest that 50% to 75% of patients with NAFLD improve after a bariatric surgical intervention.

The PNPLA3 I148M genetic variant has been identified through GWAS as associated with NAFLD, which the authors confirmed in patients undergoing bariatric surgery.[52] The authors have also analyzed changes in liver histology between a primary bariatric surgery procedure and a subsequent revision surgery for 36 patients, also stratifying for the presence of the *PNPLA3* NAFLD risk G allele (**Table 1**). No statistically significant differences were present in the distribution of histologic phenotypes when stratifying by PNPLA3 genotype at the time of either biopsy, although limited sample size precludes detection of smaller differences. For patients with steatosis but no fibrosis at the primary surgery (see **Table 1**; 7 in both genotype groups), 4 of 7 without the *PNPLA3* NAFLD risk allele had normal histology on the subsequent revision surgery biopsy and none had fibrosis, whereas of the 7 who carried a risk allele, only 1 had normal histology but 4 of 7 had fibrosis (exact trend test, $P = .047$). These data suggest that carriers of the I148M allele may be resistant to the ameliorative effects of bariatric surgery.

SUMMARY

Bariatric surgery has pleiotropic effects on several medically important conditions. Given the wide variation among patient outcomes, the number of studies investigating the potential role for genetic predisposition has been small. Much more work is needed to further delineate the role of genetics after bariatric surgery.

REFERENCES

1. Courcoulas AP, Yanovski SZ, Bonds D, et al. Long-term outcomes of bariatric surgery: a National Institutes of Health symposium. JAMA Surg 2014;149(12): 1323–9.
2. Still CD, Wood GC, Chu X, et al. Clinical factors associated with weight loss outcomes after Roux-en-Y gastric bypass surgery. Obesity (Silver Spring) 2014; 22(3):888–94.
3. Allen RE, Hughes TD, Ng JL, et al. Mechanisms behind the immediate effects of Roux-en-Y gastric bypass surgery on type 2 diabetes. Theor Biol Med Model 2013;10:45.
4. Madsbad S, Dirksen C, Holst JJ. Mechanisms of changes in glucose metabolism and bodyweight after bariatric surgery. Lancet Diabetes Endocrinol 2014;2(2): 152–64.
5. Nguyen KT, Korner J. The sum of many parts: potential mechanisms for improvement in glucose homeostasis after bariatric surgery. Curr Diab Rep 2014;14(5):481.
6. Prawitt J, Caron S, Staels B. Bile acid metabolism and the pathogenesis of type 2 diabetes. Curr Diab Rep 2011;11(3):160–6.
7. Hoeke MO, Heegsma J, Hoekstra M, et al. Human FXR regulates SHP expression through direct binding to an LRH-1 binding site, independent of an IR-1 and LRH-1. PLoS One 2014;9(2):e88011.
8. Ryan KK, Tremaroli V, Clemmensen C, et al. FXR is a molecular target for the effects of vertical sleeve gastrectomy. Nature 2014;509(7499):183–8.
9. Eldar S, Heneghan HM, Brethauer SA, et al. Bariatric surgery for treatment of obesity. Int J Obes (Lond) 2011;35(Suppl 3):S16–21.
10. Hatoum IJ, Greenawalt DM, Cotsapas C, et al. Heritability of the weight loss response to gastric bypass surgery. J Clin Endocrinol Metab 2011;96(10): E1630–3.
11. Elkhenini HF, New JP, Syed AA. Five-year outcome of bariatric surgery in a patient with melanocortin-4 receptor mutation. Clin Obes 2014;4(2):121–4.
12. Matzko ME, Argyropoulos G, Wood GC, et al. Association of ghrelin receptor promoter polymorphisms with weight loss following Roux-en-Y gastric bypass surgery. Obes Surg 2012;22(5):783–90.
13. de Luis DA, Aller R, Conde R, et al. Effects of RS9939609 gene variant in FTO gene on weight loss and cardiovascular risk factors after biliopancreatic diversion surgery. J Gastrointest Surg 2012;16(6):1194–8.
14. Liou TH, Chen HH, Wang W, et al. ESR1, FTO, and UCP2 genes interact with bariatric surgery affecting weight loss and glycemic control in severely obese patients. Obes Surg 2011;21(11):1758–65.
15. Still CD, Wood GC, Chu X, et al. High allelic burden of four obesity SNPs is associated with poorer weight loss outcomes following gastric bypass surgery. Obesity (Silver Spring) 2011;19(8):1676–83.
16. Locke AE, Kahali B, Berndt SI, et al. Genetic studies of body mass index yield new insights for obesity biology. Nature 2015;518(7538):197–206.
17. Shungin D, Winkler TW, Croteau-Chonka DC, et al. New genetic loci link adipose and insulin biology to body fat distribution. Nature 2015;518(7538):187–96.

18. Hatoum IJ, Greenawalt DM, Cotsapas C, et al. Weight loss after gastric bypass is associated with a variant at 15q26.1. Am J Hum Genet 2013;92(5):827–34.

19. Kuipers F, Bloks VW, Groen AK. Beyond intestinal soap–bile acids in metabolic control. Nat Rev Endocrinol 2014;10(8):488–98.

20. van der Klaauw AA, Farooqi IS. The hunger genes: pathways to obesity. Cell 2015;161(1):119–32.

21. Duckworth PF, Vlahcevic ZR, Studer EJ, et al. Effect of hydrophobic bile acids on 3-hydroxy-3-methylglutaryl-coenzyme A reductase activity and mRNA levels in the rat. J Biol Chem 1991;266(15):9413–8.

22. Vivacqua G, Renzi A, Carpino G, et al. Expression of brain derived neurotrophic factor and of its receptors: TrKB and p75NT in normal and bile duct ligated rat liver. Ital J Anat Embryol 2014;119(2):111–29.

23. Verlaet M, Adamantidis A, Coumans B, et al. Human immune cells express ppMCH mRNA and functional MCHR1 receptor. FEBS Lett 2002;527(1–3): 205–10.

24. Krishnan J, Danzer C, Simka T, et al. Dietary obesity-associated Hif1alpha activation in adipocytes restricts fatty acid oxidation and energy expenditure via suppression of the Sirt2-NAD+ system. Genes Dev 2012;26(3):259–70.

25. Mingrone G, Panunzi S, De Gaetano A, et al. Bariatric surgery versus conventional medical therapy for type 2 diabetes. N Engl J Med 2012;366(17):1577–85.

26. Buchwald H, Estok R, Fahrbach K, et al. Weight and type 2 diabetes after bariatric surgery: systematic review and meta-analysis. Am J Med 2009;122(3): 248–56.e5.

27. Frayn KN, Humphreys SM. Metabolic characteristics of human subcutaneous abdominal adipose tissue after overnight fast. Am J Physiol Endocrinol Metab 2012;302(4):E468–75.

28. Fisette A, Poursharifi P, Oikonomopoulou K, et al. Paradoxical glucose-sensitizing yet proinflammatory effects of acute ASP administration in mice. Mediators Inflamm 2013;2013:713284.

29. Germinario R, Sniderman AD, Manuel S, et al. Coordinate regulation of triacylglycerol synthesis and glucose transport by acylation-stimulating protein. Metabolism 1993;42(5):574–80.

30. Cariou B, van Harmelen K, Duran-Sandoval D, et al. The farnesoid X receptor modulates adiposity and peripheral insulin sensitivity in mice. J Biol Chem 2006;281(16):11039–49.

31. Lange LA, Willer CJ, Rich SS. Recent developments in genome and exome-wide analyses of plasma lipids. Curr Opin Lipidol 2015;26(2):96–102.

32. Parihar A, Wood GC, Chu X, et al. Extension of GWAS results for lipid-related phenotypes to extreme obesity using electronic health record (EHR) data and the Metabochip. Front Genet 2014;5:222.

33. Lim S, Eckel RH. Pharmacological treatment and therapeutic perspectives of metabolic syndrome. Rev Endocr Metab Disord 2014;15(4):329–41.

34. Del Ben M, Polimeni L, Baratta F, et al. Modern approach to the clinical management of non-alcoholic fatty liver disease. World J Gastroenterol 2014;20(26): 8341–50.

35. Hafeez S, Ahmed MH. Bariatric surgery as potential treatment for nonalcoholic fatty liver disease: a future treatment by choice or by chance? J Obes 2013; 2013:839275.

36. Mattar SG, Velcu LM, Rabinovitz M, et al. Surgically-induced weight loss significantly improves nonalcoholic fatty liver disease and the metabolic syndrome. Ann Surg 2005;242(4):610–7 [discussion: 618–20].

37. Mottin CC, Moretto M, Padoin AV, et al. Histological behavior of hepatic steatosis in morbidly obese patients after weight loss induced by bariatric surgery. Obes Surg 2005;15(6):788–93.
38. Klein S, Mittendorfer B, Eagon JC, et al. Gastric bypass surgery improves metabolic and hepatic abnormalities associated with nonalcoholic fatty liver disease. Gastroenterology 2006;130(6):1564–72.
39. Barker KB, Palekar NA, Bowers SP, et al. Non-alcoholic steatohepatitis: effect of Roux-en-Y gastric bypass surgery. Am J Gastroenterol 2006;101(2):368–73.
40. Csendes A, Smok G, Burgos AM. Histological findings in the liver before and after gastric bypass. Obes Surg 2006;16(5):607–11.
41. de Almeida SR, Rocha PR, Sanches MD, et al. Roux-en-Y gastric bypass improves the nonalcoholic steatohepatitis (NASH) of morbid obesity. Obes Surg 2006;16(3):270–8.
42. Furuya CK Jr, de Oliveira CP, de Mello ES, et al. Effects of bariatric surgery on nonalcoholic fatty liver disease: preliminary findings after 2 years. J Gastroenterol Hepatol 2007;22(4):510–4.
43. Liu X, Lazenby AJ, Clements RH, et al. Resolution of nonalcoholic steatohepatits after gastric bypass surgery. Obes Surg 2007;17(4):486–92.
44. Weiner RA. Surgical treatment of non-alcoholic steatohepatitis and non-alcoholic fatty liver disease. Dig Dis 2010;28(1):274–9.
45. Moretto M, Kupski C, da Silva VD, et al. Effect of bariatric surgery on liver fibrosis. Obes Surg 2012;22(7):1044–9.
46. Ranlov I, Hardt F. Regression of liver steatosis following gastroplasty or gastric bypass for morbid obesity. Digestion 1990;47(4):208–14.
47. Stratopoulos C, Papakonstantinou A, Terzis I, et al. Changes in liver histology accompanying massive weight loss after gastroplasty for morbid obesity. Obes Surg 2005;15(8):1154–60.
48. Dixon JB, Bhathal PS, Hughes NR, et al. Nonalcoholic fatty liver disease: Improvement in liver histological analysis with weight loss. Hepatology 2004; 39(6):1647–54.
49. Dixon JB, Bhathal PS, O'Brien PE. Weight loss and non-alcoholic fatty liver disease: falls in gamma-glutamyl transferase concentrations are associated with histologic improvement. Obes Surg 2006;16(10):1278–86.
50. Mathurin P, Hollebecque A, Arnalsteen L, et al. Prospective study of the long-term effects of bariatric surgery on liver injury in patients without advanced disease. Gastroenterology 2009;137(2):532–40.
51. Kral JG, Thung SN, Biron S, et al. Effects of surgical treatment of the metabolic syndrome on liver fibrosis and cirrhosis. Surgery 2004;135(1):48–58.
52. DiStefano JK, Kingsley C, Craig Wood G, et al. Genome-wide analysis of hepatic lipid content in extreme obesity. Acta Diabetol 2015;52(2):373–82.

Leptin and Hormones

Energy Homeostasis

Georgios A. Triantafyllou, MD, Stavroula A. Paschou, MD, PhD,
Christos S. Mantzoros, MD, DSc, PhD h.c. mult.*

KEYWORDS

- Leptin • Energy homeostasis • Metabolism • Hormonal interactions • Obesity

KEY POINTS

- Leptin is a 167 amino acid adipokine; its interaction with the leptin receptor activates mainly the Janus kinase (JAK)–signal transducer and activator of transcription 3 (STAT3) signal transduction pathway.
- Leptin's primary action site is the central nervous system, especially the hypothalamus.
- Energy deprivation conditions, such as hypothalamic amenorrhea (HA) and lipodystrophy, are characterized by low leptin levels.
- Obesity is usually characterized by hyperleptinemia, but the hypothalamus is resistant or tolerant to the effects of increased leptin, except for the rare condition of congenital leptin deficiency due to leptin gene mutation.
- Leptin replacement treatment improves, and even normalizes, most of the endocrine and metabolic abnormalities in patients who suffer from conditions characterized by low leptin levels, such as lipodystrophy, HA, and congenital leptin deficiency.

INTRODUCTION

Leptin is an adipokine and its name derives from the Greek word λεπτός (*leptos*), which means thin. Since its initial discovery in 1994, important advances have been made, and human recombinant leptin is currently available and approved for pharmacologic use.[1–4] This article reviews the role of leptin in energy homeostasis. Specifically, the structure, production, and signaling of leptin are described first, followed by its action at both central and peripheral levels. Then, the role of leptin in conditions of energy deprivation or excess is discussed, along with leptin's existing and potential future therapeutic applications.

Disclosure Statement: The authors have nothing to disclose.
Division of Endocrinology, Diabetes and Metabolism, Department of Internal Medicine, Beth Israel Deaconess Medical Center, Harvard Medical School, 330 Brookline Avenue, ST 820, Boston, MA 02215, USA
* Corresponding author.
E-mail address: cmantzor@bidmc.harvard.edu

STRUCTURE, PRODUCTION, AND SIGNALING OF LEPTIN

Leptin is a 167 amino acid protein folded in a 4-helix bundle structure, which is produced by the expression of the *lep* gene.[5,6] It is expressed mainly in the white adipose tissue.[7] This is an approximately 20-kb gene located on chromosome 7, containing 3 exons separated by 2 introns.[8,9] In humans, leptin is secreted in a pulsatile fashion, with the highest levels present in the blood during evening hours, a pattern opposite to that of corticotropin and cortisol.[10] The total concentration of leptin is directly proportional to total body fat mass.[11] Its actions (discussed later) are mediated through binding to the leptin receptor, a single transmembrane-spanning protein,[12] member of the class I cytokine receptor family.[13] Several isoforms of that receptor exist, which are produced after alternate mRNA splicing.[14,15] One of them, the lep-Re isoform (soluble leptin receptor), represents the major leptin binding protein in the plasma.[16,17] The long leptin receptor isoform mediates signal transduction and is strongly expressed in the hypothalamus.[18]

The leptin-leptin receptor interaction activates mainly the JAK-STAT3 signal transduction pathway, which is the most important regulator of energy homeostasis.[19–21] Secondarily, the following pathways can be also activated: (1) phosphatidylinositol 3-kinase, which is important for regulation of both food intake and glucose homeostasis[22]; (2) mitogen-activated protein kinases/extracellular signal-regulated kinases pathway, which plays a role in fatty acid synthesis regulation[23]; (3) 5'-adenosine monophosphate–activated protein kinase, a potential coregulator pathway of pancreatic β-cell functions and insulin secretion[24]; and (4) mammalian target of rapamycin, a pathway that seems to promote intestinal cell proliferation.[25]

Signaling of leptin in peripheral blood mononuclear cells seems to reflect its signaling in other metabolically important tissues, such as muscle and adipose tissue.[26,27] A recent study conducted by the authors' group in obese women showed that 10% to 15% weight loss resulted in a decrease in leptin levels, in parallel with a decrease in baseline STAT3 phosphorylation of their peripheral blood mononuclear cells. Ex vivo treatment of those PMBCs with supraphysiologic leptin doses significantly increased extracellular signal–regulated kinase, STAT3, and protein kinase B phosphorylation. The phosphorylation levels of those proteins were higher after administration of supraphysiologic doses compared with either physiologic doses or no treatment.[28] Further studies are needed to elucidate the molecular pathways triggered by leptin as well as the potential therapeutic benefits that could derive from their manipulation.

CENTRAL ACTION OF LEPTIN

After its secretion from adipocytes, leptin circulates in the blood bound to lep-Re, acting as a marker of total body energy stored in fat and secondarily as marker of acute changes in energy intake.[29–31] It gets transferred through the blood-brain barrier via the short leptin receptor isoform to the hypothalamus, where it mediates most of its actions.[32–35] More specifically, it acts on the supraoptic nucleus, paraventricular nucleus, periventricular nucleus, arcuate nucleus, and lateral hypothalamus.[34,35] There, it interacts with a complex circuit, activating neurons that synthesize anorexigenic peptides, namely pro-opiomelanocortin (POMC)[36] and cocaine- and-amphetamine-regulated transcript (CART).[37] At the same time it suppresses the activity of orexigenic neurons, which express agouti-related peptide (AgRP) and neuropeptide Y (NPY).[38–40] Leptin's action at the hypothalamus is also responsible for counterbalancing the effect of ghrelin, which is a major orexigenic hormone.[41,42] In addition to the hypothalamus, leptin acts on the mesolimbic dopamine system, which is part of the brain reward system.[43] In a study involving leptin-sensitive hypoleptinemic patients, short-term metreleptin administration has been shown to increase food-derived reward, whereas long-term treatment decreased attention to food and the hedonic response to it after feeding.[44] Through its action on the neurons of the nucleus of the solitary tract, leptin also promotes satiety; possibly exerting a synergistic effect with incretins, such as glucagon-like peptide 1 (GLP-1) and cholecystokinin. The attenuation of leptin signaling after weight loss may blunt its effect on feeding inhibition in humans, thus possibly promoting weight regain.[45,46]

Leptin also regulates the hypothalamus-pituitary-endocrine organs axes via multiple ways.[10,47] Knowledge in this area is mostly derived from the effects of low levels of leptin on these axes and also from the changes observed after pharmacologic leptin administration.[10] Low leptin levels have been associated with hypogonadotropic hypogonadism, suppression of thyroid hormones, and growth hormone (GH) secretion. Leptin administration in replacement doses has resulted in restoration of thyroid hormones, luteinizing hormone (LH), and sex steroid levels in mice as well as in restoration of LH pulsatility and sex steroid levels in humans.[48–50] Regarding thyroid hormone regulation, leptin mainly up-regulates the pro–thyrotropin-releasing hormone (TRH) gene expression and induces the conversion of proTRH to TRH.[51,52] Leptin transmits the signal of adequate body energy stores to the gonadotropic axis and regulates the onset of puberty as well as the maintenance of the pulsatile rhythm of LH in reproductive life.[53] Gonadotropin-releasing hormone (GnRH) neurons do not express the leptin receptor, suggesting that these actions are indirect via NPY, POMC, and kisspeptin.[54–56] Leptin regulation of GH and hypothalamic-pituitary-adrenal axis is still unclear and seems to differ between species. In mice, leptin deficiency leads to an increase in corticotropin and corticosterone levels as well as to GH suppression. On the contrary, most studies in humans show that leptin effects insulinlike growth factor (IGF)-1 binding capacity rather than GH axis.[48,50,56,57]

PERIPHERAL ACTION OF LEPTIN
Adipose Tissue, Muscle, Liver, and Gastrointestinal Tract

Apart from its role in the central nervous system, leptin also acts on peripheral organs, such as adipose tissue, muscle, and liver. Through its action on adipocytes, insulin sensitivity is improved, lipolysis is reduced, and possibly browning of the adipose tissue occurs.[58] It has been found, in mice, that leptin administration increases basal oxygen consumption in fat tissue.[59] Its secretion for the mediation of the aforementioned actions is thought to be affected by peptide YY binding on receptors of adipocytes.[60] Furthermore, it seems that leptin limits total fat mass and lipid accumulation in nonadipose tissues, in a tissue-specific manner.[61] In skeletal muscle, leptin has been found to increase glucose uptake and oxidation, glycogen synthesis, and lactate formation.[62] This increase in insulin sensitivity seems to be mediated through leptin-induced expression of insulinlike growth factor binding protein 2.[63] Despite that insulinlike effect, leptin also opposes the accumulation of triacylglycerol in muscle, a process that is promoted by insulin.[64] In addition, leptin acts on the liver to reduce hepatic gluconeogenesis.[65] Two other liver enzymes, which are regulated, at least in part, by leptin are the 3-hydroxy-3-methylglutaryl–coenzyme A reductase and cholesterol 7 alpha-hydroxylase. These are the rate-limiting enzymes of cholesterol and bile acid synthesis, respectively.[66,67] Intracerebroventricular or continuous intravenous infusion of leptin was effective in decreasing the activity of those enzymes in Sprague-Dawley rats.[68] In humans, however, the correlation of leptin levels with lipid levels has been attributed to an underlying association of both lipid and leptin levels with body mass index.[69]

Besides adipose tissue, leptin is also secreted by the chief cells of the stomach.[70] In the lumen of the small intestine, by acting at specific apical receptors of the entero-cytes, leptin modulates the absorption of nutrients. Specifically, it decreases glucose, galactose, and amino acid absorption, whereas it increases the absorption of fructose and butyrate.[71]

Leptin and Other Peripheral Hormones

Recently, the potential interplay between leptin and other peripheral hormones has been considered. Studies examining the interaction of insulin and leptin have found evidence suggestive of those hormones being counter-regulated, because an in-crease in the levels of the one happens concomitantly with a decrease in the levels of the other.[72,73] This could be due to common actions shared by the 2 hormones. Apart from improving muscle insulin sensitivity (as discussed previously), leptin administration in leptin-deficient individuals has been shown to improve their lipid pro-file. Moreover, hepatic insulin sensitivity is improved in those patients after leptin administration, whereas lipolysis is decreased.[74]

Leptin also interacts with gastrointestinal hormones, such as GLP-1. In mouse models, leptin administration has been shown to increase the insulinotropic effect of exenatide, providing a new insight for a potential combination treatment of patients with type 2 diabetes mellitus and increased adiposity.[75] Some studies have found a decrease in leptin after GLP-1 analogs administration.[76,77] That negative feedback of GLP-1 on leptin could be suggestive of converging cellular mechanisms of action for the 2 hormones. Most interestingly, in a human study involving 58 subjects, liraglu-tide administration was shown to attenuate the decrease of leptin after weight loss.[78] Leptin was also found to prolongate the effects of peptide YY in appetite suppres-sion.[79] Another incretin, cholecystokinin, enhances the leptin-dependent weight reduction through its peripheral action.[80]

LEPTIN IN ENERGY DEPRIVATION
Starvation

The major physiologic role of leptin is the regulation of the neuroendocrine system during starvation.[81] In the fasted state, plasma leptin levels decline and the net result is an increase in appetite with a concomitant decrease in energy expenditure.[47] Pre-viously published findings from the authors' group suggest that leptin levels below approximately 3 ng/mL—albeit arbitrary and different from laboratory to labora-tory—signal an energy deprivation state.[53] This decrease in leptin levels happens rapidly, preceding any change in total fat mass and is thought to participate in the body's physiologic response to food deprivation.[82] This is supported by various studies, which have shown that the decrease in testosterone and thyroid-stimulating hormone levels, as well as the loss of LH pulsatility occurring after 72-hour fasting, are improved with leptin replenishment.[82–86] These changes have clin-ical implications in disease states, such as anorexia nervosa, HA, or lipodystrophy (discussed later).

Acquired Functional Decrease in Adipose Mass

Situations characterized by decreased energy intake in combination with increased energy expenditure may result in a decrease of adipose mass below a certain threshold. This can cause HA in women. HA refers to the cessation of menstrual cycles without any organic disorder and is caused by dysregulation of the hypothalamic-pituitary-gonadal axis[2] (**Table 1**). HA is seen in women with anorexia nervosa, athletes,

Table 1
The effects of hypoleptinemia on hypothalamic nuclei in states of energy deprivation

Preoptic Area	Paraventricular Nucleus	Arcuate Nucleus	Ventromedial Hypothalamic Nucleus	Lateral Hypothalamic Area
GNRH−	TRH−	AgRP/NPY+	BDNF−	Orexin+
	CRH+/−	POMC/CART−		MCH+

Note: States of energy excess, such as common obesity, are associated with hyperleptinemia, but the hypothalamus is resistant or tolerant to leptin.

Abbreviations: +, promotes secretion; −, inhibits secretion; BDNF, brain-derived neurotrophic factor; CRH, corticotropin-releasing hormone; MCH, melanin-concentrating hormone.

ballet dancers, gymnasts, and even in some normal weight women (with decreased adipose tissue) and is associated with reduced food intake, intense exercise, and stress. In athletes, HA is often accompanied by eating disorders and osteoporosis.[87] These 3 conditions comprise the athlete's triad. Initially, observational studies showed hypoleptinemia in women with HA.[86,88,89] Subsequently, phase II proof-of-concept trials showed that leptin replacement restored both the normality of menstrual cycles and the levels of estrogen, thyroid hormones, and IGF-1; at the same time it increased the levels of bone formation markers without any changes in bone resorption. Phase III randomized placebo control trials are expected to elucidate the potential therapeutic role of leptin in this condition.[26,85,86,90]

Partial or Total Decrease in Adipose Mass in Lipodystrophies

A not only generalized but also localized decrease in adipose mass is associated with hypoleptinemia.[91,92] Such conditions can be both congenital and acquired and are known by the term, *lipodystrophy*.[93] Congenital syndromes of lipodystrophy are rare, but several nonrandomized and case-controlled series have shown that leptin replacement treatment improved metabolic parameters, such as insulin sensitivity, lipid profile, glucose control, and hepatic steatosis.[93–98] Acquired lipodystrophy has become more common now, because it is a usually encountered comorbidity in HIV patients and is related to their anti-HIV treatment (up to 70% prevalence).[99] The authors' group has previously shown that these patients present with low leptin levels,[100] whereas leptin replacement therapy improved insulin sensitivity and lipid profile as well as reduced central fat mass.[100–103] These findings were confirmed by other investigators,[74] and it seems that leptin—alone or in combination with other insulin sensitizers—could soon find a place in the therapeutic armamentarium for the growing population of patients with lipodystrophy, even if concerns exist regarding the formation of neutralizing antibodies.

LEPTIN IN ENERGY EXCESS

The initial discovery of leptin showed that its deficiency through a mutation of the *lep* gene resulted in profound obesity and type 2 diabetes mellitus. This generated great enthusiasm about leptin's potential therapeutic applications in obesity.[1] Patients with inherited total leptin deficiency respond to leptin treatment, showing a decrease in their appetite and subsequent fat loss.[56,104–106] This condition is rare, but it should be considered in the differential diagnosis of young patients with obesity,[107] because they can be helped by the administration of leptin.

After the initially failed attempt to treat common obesity with leptin, however, the concept of leptin resistance came into play, indicating a complex role of leptin in human metabolism.[108–110] Obesity is usually characterized by hyperleptinemia both in humans and rodents. The hypothalamus, however, is resistant or tolerant to the effects of these increased levels of leptin. Only in 10% of the obese population are levels of leptin relatively lower (relative hypoleptinemia). Recent investigations are beginning to clarify the mechanisms leading to impaired response to leptin, desensitization of leptin receptor, and down-regulation of its intracellular signaling.[71,86]

A few clinical studies investigated the effect of leptin therapy on weight loss in obese individuals. At first, very high doses of leptin failed to induce any significant changes in body weight.[108] More recently, it was shown that the combination of leptin with pramlintide, an amylin analog, resulted in greater weight loss than each medication alone.[111,112] This could be attributed to the activation of overlapping signaling pathways from leptin and amylin in an additive manner.[113] The concept of leptin administration sounds even more interesting and promising in the case of weight maintenance. Weight loss leads to reduced leptin levels, which in turn act on the neuroendocrine system to increase energy intake while decreasing energy expenditure.[111]

LEPTIN THERAPEUTIC APPLICATIONS—FUTURE CONSIDERATIONS

As described previously, leptin replacement treatment has improved and even normalized most of the endocrine and metabolic parameters in patients who suffer from conditions with low leptin levels, such as lipodystrophy, HA, and congenital leptin deficiency.[90,97,112,114,115] The form currently available for therapy in humans is the recombinant methionyl human leptin (metreleptin [Myalept], Amylin Pharmaceuticals, San Diego, CA). Due to the formation of neutralizing antibodies in some cases, it has been Food and Drug Administration approved under risk evaluation and mitigation strategies only for patients with non-HIV generalized lipodystrophy and for compassionate use in subjects with congenital leptin deficiency.[116] Due to its beneficial effects, therapy with metreleptin has also been evaluated in obesity, type 2 diabetes mellitus, type 1 diabetes mellitus, and other syndromes. Recent data suggest that even patients with diseases like depression and dementia could possibly benefit from novel leptin-based therapeutic strategies in the future.[117]

REFERENCES

1. Blüher M, Mantzoros CS. From leptin to other adipokines in health and disease: facts and expectations at the beginning of the 21st century. Metabolism 2015; 64(1):131–45.

2. Chou SH, Mantzoros C. 20 years of leptin: role of leptin in human reproductive disorders. J Endocrinol 2014;223(1):T49–62.

3. Dalamaga M, Chou SH, Shields K, et al. Leptin at the intersection of neuroendocrinology and metabolism: current evidence and therapeutic perspectives. Cell Metab 2013;18(1):29–42.

4. Fiorenza CG, Chou SH, Mantzoros CS. Lipodystrophy: pathophysiology and advances in treatment. Nat Rev Endocrinol 2011;7(3):137–50.

5. Zhang Y, Proenca R, Maffei M, et al. Positional cloning of the mouse obese gene and its human homologue. Nature 1994;372(6505):425–32.

6. Kline AD, Becker GW, Churgay LM, et al. Leptin is a four-helix bundle: secondary structure by NMR. FEBS Lett 1997;407(2):239–42.

7. Masuzaki H, Ogawa Y, Isse N, et al. Human obese gene expression. Adipocyte-specific expression and regional differences in the adipose tissue. Diabetes 1995;44(7):855–8.

8. Geffroy S, De Vos P, Staels B, et al. Localization of the human OB gene (OBS) to chromosome 7q32 by fluorescence in situ hybridization. Genomics 1995;28(3): 603–4.

9. Isse N, Ogawa Y, Tamura N, et al. Structural organization and chromosomal assignment of the human obese gene. J Biol Chem 1995;270(46):27728–33.

10. Licinio J, Mantzoros C, Negrao AB, et al. Human leptin levels are pulsatile and inversely related to pituitary-adrenal function. Nat Med 1997;3(5):575–9.

11. Klein S, Coppack SW, Mohamed-Ali V, et al. Adipose tissue leptin production and plasma leptin kinetics in humans. Diabetes 1996;45(7):984–7.

12. Baumann H, Morella KK, White DW, et al. The full-length leptin receptor has signaling capabilities of interleukin 6-type cytokine receptors. Proc Natl Acad Sci U S A 1996;93(16):8374–8.

13. Haniu M, Arakawa T, Bures EJ, et al. Human leptin receptor. Determination of disulfide structure and N-glycosylation sites of the extracellular domain. J Biol Chem 1998;273(44):28691–9.

14. Fei H, Okano HJ, Li C, et al. Anatomic localization of alternatively spliced leptin receptors (Ob-R) in mouse brain and other tissues. Proc Natl Acad Sci U S A 1997;94(13):7001–5.

15. Sun Q, Cornelis MC, Kraft P, et al. Genome-wide association study identifies polymorphisms in LEPR as determinants of plasma soluble leptin receptor levels. Hum Mol Genet 2010;19(9):1846–55.

16. Sun Q, van Dam RM, Meigs JB, et al. Leptin and soluble leptin receptor levels in plasma and risk of type 2 diabetes in U.S. women: a prospective study. Diabetes 2010;59(3):611–8.

17. Yang G, Ge H, Boucher A, et al. Modulation of direct leptin signaling by soluble leptin receptor. Mol Endocrinol 2004;18(6):1354–62.

18. Vaisse C, Halaas JL, Horvath CM, et al. Leptin activation of Stat3 in the hypothalamus of wild-type and ob/ob mice but not db/db mice. Nat Genet 1996;14(1): 95–7.

19. Bates SH, Stearns WH, Dundon TA, et al. STAT3 signalling is required for leptin regulation of energy balance but not reproduction. Nature 2003;421(6925): 856–9.

20. Moon HS, Huh JY, Dincer F, et al. Identification and saturable nature of signaling pathways induced by metreleptin in humans: comparative evaluation of in vivo, ex vivo, and in vitro administration. Diabetes 2015;64(3):828–39.

21. Chan JL, Moschos SJ, Bullen J, et al. Recombinant methionyl human leptin administration activates signal transducer and activator of transcription 3 signaling in peripheral blood mononuclear cells in vivo and regulates soluble tumor necrosis factor-alpha receptor levels in humans with relative leptin deficiency. J Clin Endocrinol Metab 2005;90(3):1625–31.

22. Niswender KD, Morton GJ, Stearns WH, et al. Intracellular signalling. Key enzyme in leptin-induced anorexia. Nature 2001;413(6858):794–5.

23. Mauvoisin D, Prevost M, Ducheix S, et al. Key role of the ERK1/2 MAPK pathway in the transcriptional regulation of the Stearoyl-CoA Desaturase (SCD1) gene expression in response to leptin. Mol Cell Endocrinol 2010;319(1–2):116–28.

24. Chen PC, Kryukova YN, Shyng SL. Leptin regulates KATP channel trafficking in pancreatic beta-cells by a signaling mechanism involving AMP-activated

protein kinase (AMPK) and cAMP-dependent protein kinase (PKA). J Biol Chem 2013;288(47):34098–109.

25. Fazolini NP, Cruz AL, Werneck MB, et al. Leptin activation of mTOR pathway in intestinal epithelial cell triggers lipid droplet formation, cytokine production and increased cell proliferation. Cell Cycle 2015;14(16):2667–76.

26. Matarese G, La Rocca C, Moon HS, et al. Selective capacity of metreleptin administration to reconstitute CD4+ T-cell number in females with acquired hypoleptinemia. Proc Natl Acad Sci U S A 2013;110(9):E818–27.

27. Procaccini C, Pucino V, Mantzoros CS, et al. Leptin in autoimmune diseases. Metabolism 2015;64(1):92–104.

28. Sahin-Efe A, Polyzos SA, Dincer F, et al. Intracellular leptin signaling following effective weight loss. Metabolism 2015;64(8):888–95.

29. Considine RV, Sinha MK, Heiman ML, et al. Serum immunoreactive-leptin concentrations in normal-weight and obese humans. N Engl J Med 1996;334(5):292–5.

30. Hamnvik OP, Liu X, Petrou M, et al. Soluble leptin receptor and leptin are associated with baseline adiposity and metabolic risk factors, and predict adiposity, metabolic syndrome, and glucose levels at 2-year follow-up: the Cyprus Metabolism Prospective Cohort Study. Metabolism 2011;60(7):987–93.

31. Yannakoulia M, Yiannakouris N, Blüher S, et al. Body fat mass and macronutrient intake in relation to circulating soluble leptin receptor, free leptin index, adiponectin, and resistin concentrations in healthy humans. J Clin Endocrinol Metab 2003;88(4):1730–6.

32. Bjorbaek C, Elmquist JK, Michl P, et al. Expression of leptin receptor isoforms in rat brain microvessels. Endocrinology 1998;139(8):3485–91.

33. Tartaglia LA, Dembski M, Weng X, et al. Identification and expression cloning of a leptin receptor, OB-R. Cell 1995;83(7):1263–71.

34. Hakansson ML, Brown H, Ghilardi N, et al. Leptin receptor immunoreactivity in chemically defined target neurons of the hypothalamus. J Neurosci 1998;18(1):559–72.

35. Woods AJ, Stock MJ. Leptin activation in hypothalamus. Nature 1996;381(6585):745.

36. Seeley RJ, Yagaloff KA, Fisher SL, et al. Melanocortin receptors in leptin effects. Nature 1997;390(6658):349.

37. Kristensen P, Judge ME, Thim L, et al. Hypothalamic CART is a new anorectic peptide regulated by leptin. Nature 1998;393(6680):72–6.

38. Mizuno TM, Mobbs CV. Hypothalamic agouti-related protein messenger ribonucleic acid is inhibited by leptin and stimulated by fasting. Endocrinology 1999;140(2):814–7.

39. Erickson JC, Hollopeter G, Palmiter RD. Attenuation of the obesity syndrome of ob/ob mice by the loss of neuropeptide Y. Science 1996;274(5293):1704–7.

40. Mantzoros CS, Qu D, Frederich RC, et al. Activation of beta(3) adrenergic receptors suppresses leptin expression and mediates a leptin-independent inhibition of food intake in mice. Diabetes 1996;45(7):909–14.

41. Nakazato M, Murakami N, Date Y, et al. A role for ghrelin in the central regulation of feeding. Nature 2001;409(6817):194–8.

42. Ueno N, Dube MG, Inui A, et al. Leptin modulates orexigenic effects of ghrelin and attenuates adiponectin and insulin levels and selectively the dark-phase feeding as revealed by central leptin gene therapy. Endocrinology 2004;145(9):4176–84.

43. Fulton S, Pissios P, Manchon RP, et al. Leptin regulation of the mesoaccumbens dopamine pathway. Neuron 2006;51(6):811–22.

44. Farr OM, Fiorenza C, Papageorgiou P, et al. Leptin therapy alters appetite and neural responses to food stimuli in brain areas of leptin-sensitive subjects without altering brain structure. J Clin Endocrinol Metab 2014;99(12):E2529–38.

45. Kissileff HR, Thornton JC, Torres MI, et al. Leptin reverses declines in satiation in weight-reduced obese humans. Am J Clin Nutr 2012;95(2):309–17.

46. Garfield AS, Patterson C, Skora S, et al. Neurochemical characterization of body weight-regulating leptin receptor neurons in the nucleus of the solitary tract. Endocrinology 2012;153(10):4600–7.

47. Chan JL, Matarese G, Shetty GK, et al. Differential regulation of metabolic, neuroendocrine, and immune function by leptin in humans. Proc Natl Acad Sci U S A 2006;103(22):8481–6.

48. Chan JL, Heist K, DePaoli AM, et al. The role of falling leptin levels in the neuro-endocrine and metabolic adaptation to short-term starvation in healthy men. J Clin Invest 2003;111(9):1409–21.

49. Ahima RS, Prabakaran D, Mantzoros C, et al. Role of leptin in the neuroendo-crine response to fasting. Nature 1996;382(6588):250–2.

50. Park HK, Ahima RS. Physiology of leptin: energy homeostasis, neuroendocrine function and metabolism. Metabolism 2015;64(1):24–34.

51. Legradi G, Emerson CH, Ahima RS, et al. Leptin prevents fasting-induced sup-pression of prothyrotropin-releasing hormone messenger ribonucleic acid in neurons of the hypothalamic paraventricular nucleus. Endocrinology 1997; 138(6):2569–76.

52. Sanchez VC, Goldstein J, Stuart RC, et al. Regulation of hypothalamic prohor-mone convertases 1 and 2 and effects on processing of prothyrotropin-releasing hormone. J Clin Invest 2004;114(3):357–69.

53. Mantzoros CS, Flier JS, Rogol AD. A longitudinal assessment of hormonal and physical alterations during normal puberty in boys. V. Rising leptin levels may signal the onset of puberty. J Clin Endocrinol Metab 1997;82(4):1066–70.

54. Quennell JH, Mulligan AC, Tups A, et al. Leptin indirectly regulates gonadotropin-releasing hormone neuronal function. Endocrinology 2009; 150(6):2805–12.

55. Hausman GJ, Barb CR, Lents CA. Leptin and reproductive function. Biochimie 2012;94(10):2075–81.

56. Farooqi IS, Jebb SA, Langmack G, et al. Effects of recombinant leptin therapy in a child with congenital leptin deficiency. N Engl J Med 1999;341(12):879–84.

57. Hukshorn CJ, van Dielen FM, Buurman WA, et al. The effect of pegylated recom-binant human leptin (peg-ob) on weight loss and inflammatory status in obese subjects. Int J Obes Relat Metab Disord 2002;26(4):504–9.

58. Siegrist-Kaiser CA, Pauli V, Juge-Aubry CE, et al. Direct effects of leptin on brown and white adipose tissue. J Clin Invest 1997;100(11):2858–64.

59. Marti A, Novo FJ, Martinez-Anso E, et al. Leptin gene transfer into muscle in-creases lipolysis and oxygen consumption in white fat tissue in ob/ob mice. Bio-chem Biophys Res Commun 1998;246(3):859–62.

60. Serradeil-Le Gal C, Lafontan M, Raufaste D, et al. Characterization of NPY re-ceptors controlling lipolysis and leptin secretion in human adipocytes. FEBS Lett 2000;475(2):150–6.

61. Gallardo N, Bonzon-Kulichenko E, Fernandez-Agullo T, et al. Tissue-specific ef-fects of central leptin on the expression of genes involved in lipid metabolism in liver and white adipose tissue. Endocrinology 2007;148(12):5604–10.

62. Ceddia RB, William WN Jr, Curi R. Comparing effects of leptin and insulin on glucose metabolism in skeletal muscle: evidence for an effect of leptin on glucose uptake and decarboxylation. Int J Obes Relat Metab Disord 1999; 23(1):75–82.

63. Yau SW, Henry BA, Russo VC, et al. Leptin enhances insulin sensitivity by direct and sympathetic nervous system regulation of muscle IGFBP-2 expression: evidence from nonrodent models. Endocrinology 2014;155(6):2133–43.

64. Muoio DM, Dohm GL, Tapscott EB, et al. Leptin opposes insulin's effects on fatty acid partitioning in muscles isolated from obese ob/ob mice. Am J Physiol 1999; 276(5 Pt 1):E913–21.

65. Perry RJ, Zhang XM, Zhang D, et al. Leptin reverses diabetes by suppression of the hypothalamic-pituitary-adrenal axis. Nat Med 2014;20(7):759–63.

66. Marcuzzi A, Piscianz E, Loganes C, et al. Innovative Target Therapies Are Able to Block the Inflammation Associated with Dysfunction of the Cholesterol Biosynthesis Pathway. Int J Mol Sci 2015;17(1). pii: E47.

67. Schwarz M, Lund EG, Russell DW. Two 7 alpha-hydroxylase enzymes in bile acid biosynthesis. Curr Opin Lipidol 1998;9(2):113–8.

68. Vanpatten S, Karkanias GB, Rossetti L, et al. Intracerebroventricular leptin regulates hepatic cholesterol metabolism. Biochem J 2004;379(Pt 2):229–33.

69. Gannage-Yared MH, Khalife S, Semaan M, et al. Serum adiponectin and leptin levels in relation to the metabolic syndrome, androgenic profile and somatotropic axis in healthy non-diabetic elderly men. Eur J Endocrinol 2006;155(1): 167–76.

70. Bado A, Levasseur S, Attoub S, et al. The stomach is a source of leptin. Nature 1998;394(6695):790–3.

71. Sáinz N, Barrenetxe J, Moreno-Aliaga MJ, et al. Leptin resistance and diet-induced obesity: central and peripheral actions of leptin. Metabolism 2015; 64(1):35–46.

72. Fehmann HC, Berghofer P, Brandhorst D, et al. Leptin inhibition of insulin secretion from isolated human islets. Acta Diabetol 1997;34(4):249–52.

73. Poitout V, Rouault C, Guerre-Millo M, et al. Inhibition of insulin secretion by leptin in normal rodent islets of Langerhans. Endocrinology 1998;139(3):822–6.

74. Mulligan K, Khatami H, Schwarz JM, et al. The effects of recombinant human leptin on visceral fat, dyslipidemia, and insulin resistance in patients with human immunodeficiency virus-associated lipoatrophy and hypoleptinemia. J Clin Endocrinol Metab 2009;94(4):1137–44.

75. Sakai T, Kusakabe T, Ebihara K, et al. Leptin restores the insulinotropic effect of exenatide in a mouse model of type 2 diabetes with increased adiposity induced by streptozotocin and high-fat diet. Am J Physiol Endocrinol Metab 2014;307(8):E712–9.

76. Patel V, Joharapurkar A, Dhanesha N, et al. Co-agonist of glucagon and GLP-1 reduces cholesterol and improves insulin sensitivity independent of its effect on appetite and body weight in diet-induced obese C57 mice. Can J Physiol Pharmacol 2013;91(12):1009–15.

77. Clemmensen C, Chabenne J, Finan B, et al. GLP-1/glucagon coagonism restores leptin responsiveness in obese mice chronically maintained on an obesogenic diet. Diabetes 2014;63(4):1422–7.

78. Iepsen EW, Lundgren J, Dirksen C, et al. Treatment with a GLP-1 receptor agonist diminishes the decrease in free plasma leptin during maintenance of weight loss. Int J Obes (Lond) 2015;39(5):834–41.

79. Unniappan S, Kieffer TJ. Leptin extends the anorectic effects of chronic PYY(3-36) administration in ad libitum-fed rats. Am J Physiol Regul Integr Comp Physiol 2008;295(1):R51–8.

80. Matson CA, Reid DF, Cannon TA, et al. Cholecystokinin and leptin act synergistically to reduce body weight. Am J Physiol Regul Integr Comp Physiol 2000;278(4):R882–90.

81. Chan JL, Mantzoros CS. Role of leptin in energy-deprivation states: normal human physiology and clinical implications for hypothalamic amenorrhoea and anorexia nervosa. Lancet 2005;366(9479):74–85.

82. Boden G, Chen X, Mozzoli M, et al. Effect of fasting on serum leptin in normal human subjects. J Clin Endocrinol Metab 1996;81(9):3419–23.

83. Mantzoros CS, Ozata M, Negrao AB, et al. Synchronicity of frequently sampled thyrotropin (TSH) and leptin concentrations in healthy adults and leptin-deficient subjects: evidence for possible partial TSH regulation by leptin in humans. J Clin Endocrinol Metab 2001;86(7):3284–91.

84. Licinio J, Negrão AB, Mantzoros C, et al. Synchronicity of frequently sampled, 24-h concentrations of circulating leptin, luteinizing hormone, and estradiol in healthy women. Proc Natl Acad Sci U S A 1998;95(5):2541–6.

85. Chan JL, Williams CJ, Raciti P, et al. Leptin does not mediate short-term fasting-induced changes in growth hormone pulsatility but increases IGF-I in leptin deficiency states. J Clin Endocrinol Metab 2008;93(7):2819–27.

86. Kelesidis T, Kelesidis I, Chou S, et al. Narrative review: the role of leptin in human physiology: emerging clinical applications. Ann Intern Med 2010;152(2):93–100.

87. Foo JP, Polyzos SA, Anastasilakis AD, et al. The effect of leptin replacement on parathyroid hormone, RANKL-osteoprotegerin axis, and Wnt inhibitors in young women with hypothalamic amenorrhea. J Clin Endocrinol Metab 2014;99(11):E2252–8.

88. Audi L, Mantzoros CS, Vidal-Puig A, et al. Leptin in relation to resumption of menses in women with anorexia nervosa. Mol Psychiatry 1998;3(6):544–7.

89. Mantzoros C, Flier JS, Lesem MD, et al. Cerebrospinal fluid leptin in anorexia nervosa: correlation with nutritional status and potential role in resistance to weight gain. J Clin Endocrinol Metab 1997;82(6):1845–51.

90. Welt CK, Chan JL, Bullen J, et al. Recombinant human leptin in women with hypothalamic amenorrhea. N Engl J Med 2004;351(10):987–97.

91. Pardini VC, Victoria IM, Rocha SM, et al. Leptin levels, beta-cell function, and insulin sensitivity in families with congenital and acquired generalized lipoatropic diabetes. J Clin Endocrinol Metab 1998;83(2):503–8.

92. Nagy GS, Tsiodras S, Martin LD, et al. Human immunodeficiency virus type 1-related lipoatrophy and lipohypertrophy are associated with serum concentrations of leptin. Clin Infect Dis 2003;36(6):795–802.

93. Mantzoros CS. Leptin in relation to the lipodystrophy-associated metabolic syndrome. Diabetes Metab J 2012;36(3):181–9.

94. Crowell JA, Davis CR, Joung KE, et al. Metabolic pathways link childhood adversity to elevated blood pressure in midlife adults. Obes Res Clin Pract 2015. http://dx.doi.org/10.1016/j.orcp.2015.10.009.

95. Javor ED, Cochran EK, Musso C, et al. Long-term efficacy of leptin replacement in patients with generalized lipodystrophy. Diabetes 2005;54(7):1994–2002.

96. Javor ED, Ghany MG, Cochran EK, et al. Leptin reverses nonalcoholic steatohepatitis in patients with severe lipodystrophy. Hepatology 2005;41(4):753–60.

97. Oral EA, Simha V, Ruiz E, et al. Leptin-replacement therapy for lipodystrophy. N Engl J Med 2002;346(8):570–8.

98. Petersen KF, Oral EA, Dufour S, et al. Leptin reverses insulin resistance and hepatic steatosis in patients with severe lipodystrophy. J Clin Invest 2002;109(10): 1345–50.

99. Jacobson DL, Knox T, Spiegelman D, et al. Prevalence of, evolution of, and risk factors for fat atrophy and fat deposition in a cohort of HIV-infected men and women. Clin Infect Dis 2005;40(12):1837–45.

100. Brennan AM, Lee JH, Tsiodras S, et al. r-metHuLeptin improves highly active antiretroviral therapy-induced lipoatrophy and the metabolic syndrome, but not through altering circulating IGF and IGF-binding protein levels: observational and interventional studies in humans. Eur J Endocrinol 2009;160(2):173–6.

101. Paruthi J, Gill N, Mantzoros CS. Adipokines in the HIV/HAART-associated lipodystrophy syndrome. Metabolism 2013;62(9):1199–205.

102. Moon HS, Dalamaga M, Kim SY, et al. Leptin's role in lipodystrophic and nonlipodystrophic insulin-resistant and diabetic individuals. Endocr Rev 2013;34(3): 377–412.

103. Lee JH, Chan JL, Sourlas E, et al. Recombinant methionyl human leptin therapy in replacement doses improves insulin resistance and metabolic profile in patients with lipoatrophy and metabolic syndrome induced by the highly active antiretroviral therapy. J Clin Endocrinol Metab 2006;91(7):2605–11.

104. Strobel A, Issad T, Camoin L, et al. A leptin missense mutation associated with hypogonadism and morbid obesity. Nat Genet 1998;18(3):213–5.

105. Ozata M, Ozdemir IC, Licinio J. Human leptin deficiency caused by a missense mutation: multiple endocrine defects, decreased sympathetic tone, and immune system dysfunction indicate new targets for leptin action, greater central than peripheral resistance to the effects of leptin, and spontaneous correction of leptin-mediated defects. J Clin Endocrinol Metab 1999;84(10):3686–95.

106. Wabitsch M, Funcke JB, Lennerz B, et al. Biologically inactive leptin and early-onset extreme obesity. N Engl J Med 2015;372(1):48–54.

107. Boeke CE, Mantzoros CS, Hughes MD, et al. Differential associations of leptin with adiposity across early childhood. Obesity (Silver Spring) 2013;21(7): 1430–7.

108. Heymsfield SB, Greenberg AS, Fujioka K, et al. Recombinant leptin for weight loss in obese and lean adults: a randomized, controlled, dose-escalation trial. JAMA 1999;282(16):1568–75.

109. Moon HS, Chamberland JP, Diakopoulos KN, et al. Leptin and amylin act in an additive manner to activate overlapping signaling pathways in peripheral tissues: in vitro and ex vivo studies in humans. Diabetes Care 2011;34(1):132–8.

110. Ravussin E, Smith SR, Mitchell JA, et al. Enhanced weight loss with pramlintide/ metreleptin: an integrated neurohormonal approach to obesity pharmacotherapy. Obesity (Silver Spring) 2009;17(9):1736–43.

111. Rosenbaum M, Goldsmith R, Bloomfield D, et al. Low-dose leptin reverses skeletal muscle, autonomic, and neuroendocrine adaptations to maintenance of reduced weight. J Clin Invest 2005;115(12):3579–86.

112. Chou SH, Chamberland JP, Liu X, et al. Leptin is an effective treatment for hypothalamic amenorrhea. Proc Natl Acad Sci U S A 2011;108(16):6585–90.

113. Moon HS, Chamberland JP, Mantzoros CS. Amylin and leptin activate overlapping signalling pathways in an additive manner in mouse GT1-7 hypothalamic, C_2C_{12} muscle and AML12 liver cell lines. Diabetologia 2012;55(1):215–25.

114. Magkos F, Brennan A, Sweeney L, et al. Leptin replacement improves postprandial glycemia and insulin sensitivity in human immunodeficiency virus-infected

lipoatrophic men treated with pioglitazone: a pilot study. Metabolism 2011;60(7): 1045–9.

115. Moon HS, Matarese G, Brennan AM, et al. Efficacy of metreleptin in obese patients with type 2 diabetes: cellular and molecular pathways underlying leptin tolerance. Diabetes 2011;60(6):1647–56.

116. Sinha G. Leptin therapy gains FDA approval. Nat Biotechnol 2014;32(4):300–2.

117. Paz-Filho G, Mastronardi CA, Licinio J. Leptin treatment: facts and expectations. Metabolism 2015;64(1):146–56.

Bariatric Surgery
Overview of Procedures and Outcomes

Dan E. Azagury, MD, John Magaña Morton, MD, MPH*

KEYWORDS

- Bariatric surgery • Outcomes • Weight loss • Comorbidities

KEY POINTS

- Bariatric surgery is currently the most effective and enduring weight loss therapy available.
- The safety of bariatric surgery has improved more than tenfold during the last decade with the advent of laparoscopy and accreditation.
- Bariatric surgical procedures are currently performed with very low mortality rates (less than 1 per 1400 cases in accredited centers).
- Gastric bypass surgery reduces diabetes-related mortality by 92% over 7 years.
- The long-lasting remission of type 2 diabetes after bariatric surgery has been demonstrated in observational studies with more than 10,000 subjects, as well as in multiple randomized controlled trials.

INTRODUCTION

Bariatric surgery has been demonstrated to be the single most effective weight loss therapy available.[1] These therapies are now very well standardized and the evidence demonstrating their efficacy is overwhelming. The overall effect on mortality alone has been studied in multiple large landmark trials. The Swedish Obese Subjects Study is a prospective controlled trial that included 2000 surgical and 2000 control subjects. The follow-up period ranged from 10 to 15 years, and the main results were published nearly 10 years ago. This study, although incorporating older procedures, demonstrated an overall reduction in mortality after bariatric surgery with an adjusted odds ratio of 0.71 compared with the control group. The average weight change in the control group was less than plus or minus 2% over the study period. In contrast, the average total weight loss 10 years after gastric bypass was 25%.[2]

Another long-term study published in the *New England Journal of Medicine* 9 years ago studied mortality among 7925 gastric bypass subjects and 7925 carefully matched severely obese subjects. Over the 7-year follow-up, mortality decreased 40% in the

The authors have nothing to disclose.

Section of Bariatric and Minimally Invasive Surgery, Stanford University School of Medicine, Stanford University, 300 Pasteur Drive, H3680A, Stanford, CA 94305-5655, USA

* Corresponding author.

E-mail address: morton@stanford.edu

surgical group, and diabetes-related deaths were reduced by 92%.[3] A smaller study of 1000 surgical subjects and 5700 controls demonstrated similar benefits over 5 years with a reduction in the risk of death of 89%.[4] A more recent study analyzed the effect of surgery on 6100 type 2 diabetic subjects undergoing gastric bypass surgery and 6100 matched controls. Over 3.5 years, the overall mortality risk decreased by 58% and the risk of myocardial infarction was cut in half.[5] These findings were also confirmed among the US veterans population in 2500 subjects (74% men) who underwent bariatric surgery were matched to 7462 control subjects. Over the 14-year follow-up, overall mortality decreased after 1 to 5 years (hazard ratio [HR], 0.45) and 5 to 14 years (HR, 0.47).[6]

These studies predate the era of laparoscopy. Laparoscopy has led to a significant decrease in perioperative mortality and the benefits of bariatric surgery on life expectancy are, therefore, likely to be even more positive today. The most recent data demonstrated a 30-day mortality of 0.07% in accredited centers, representing less than 1 in 1400 surgeries.[7]

CURRENT SURGICAL BARIATRIC PROCEDURES

The type of bariatric procedures performed in the United States has evolved over the past 5 years (**Table 1**).[8] The laparoscopic gastric banding (LGB) was a very popular procedure during the last decade and is now in steep decline. The laparoscopic sleeve gastrectomy (LSG) now constitutes more than half of all procedures performed. Even if it is no longer the most common procedure performed, the laparoscopic Roux-en-Y gastric bypass (LRYGB) remains the gold standard of bariatric procedures.

To qualify for bariatric surgery, the current National Institutes of Health guidelines require a body mass index (BMI) equal to or greater than 40 kg/m^2 or a BMI equal to or greater than 35 kg/m^2 with high-risk comorbid conditions such as life-threatening cardiopulmonary problems, severe diabetes mellitus, or obesity-induced physical problems interfering with lifestyle. Patients must have failed attempts at diet and exercise, be motivated and well informed, and free of significant psychological disease. In addition, the expected benefits of the operation must outweigh the risks.[9] The LGB is approved by the Food and Drug Administration (FDA) for patients with a BMI of 30 to 40 with 1 or more obesity-related medical conditions, such as high blood pressure, heart disease, diabetes, or sleep apnea.[10]

LAPAROSCOPIC ROUX-EN-Y GASTRIC BYPASS

RYGB was first described by Mason and Ito[11] in the mid-1960s and is now performed laparoscopically. A small proximal gastric pouch is created (approximately 15–20 cc).

Table 1
Estimate of bariatric surgery procedures in the United States

Year	2011	2012	2013	2014
Total	158,000	173,000	179,000	193,000
Roux-en-Y	36.7%	37.5%	34.2%	26.8%
Band	35.4%	20.2%	14%	9.5%
Sleeve	17.8%	33%	42.1%	51.7%
Biliopancreatic diversion with duodenal switch	0.9%	1%	1%	0.4%
Revisions	6%	6%	6%	11.5%
Other	3.2%	2.3%	2.7%	0.1%

Data from American Society for Metabolic and Bariatric Surgery.

The small bowel is then divided approximately 40 to 60 cm from the ligament of Treitz. The distal portion is then brought up and anastomosed to the neostomach (Roux limb). The proximal portion is then reconnected to the distal Roux limb, approximately 150 cm from the stomach, creating a functional nonabsorptive bypass because the bile is not in contact with ingested food in this proximal portion (**Fig 1**).

Weight Loss Results

LRYGB not only presents with the best weight loss results among the most common procedures but maintenance over time is well demonstrated.[12] Average percent excess body weight lost (%EBWL) at 1 year is approximately 68%[13] (ranges quoted 48%–77%). In a review of 10-year outcomes after gastric bypass, weighted mean excess weight loss at greater than or equal to 10 years was 61.4% plus or minus 13.5.[14] In terms of total weight lost, a study of more than 1700 RYGB subjects demonstrated median weight loss of 41 kg at 3 years postoperative, corresponding to a percentage of baseline weight of 31.5%.[15] On average, LRYGB subjects lost greater than 15 BMI points at 1 year.[16]

Resolution of Comorbidities

Improvement in hypertension after gastric bypass has been reported in approximately 87% of patients with complete remission in 61% to 81%.[13,17] A systematic review with follow-up at more than 2 years showed a remission rate of 38%.[18] In a recent study of

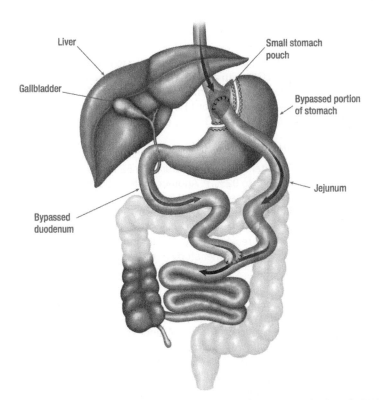

Fig. 1. Roux-en-Y gastric bypass. (*Courtesy of* Ethicon Endo-Surgery, Cincinnati, OH.)

more than 1000 subjects, remission was maintained at 6 years in 42% of subjects.[19] Similarly, improvement in hyperlipidemia was seen in 94% of subjects, with resolution in 63% to 91%; 60% at more than 2 years, and maintained remission of 71% at 6 years.[13,17–19] Obstructive sleep apnea improved in 95% of subjects after RYGB and resolved in 80%.[13]

Morbidity and Mortality

Short-term mortality rates after bariatric surgery has been constantly decreasing. For RYGB, the short-term mortality rate has been reduced by one-third between 2007 and 2012, according to a large French study of more than 133,000 subjects.[20] Currently, 30-day mortality is reported to be between 0.07% and 0.38%,[7,16,17,21,22] with reports from US accredited centers ranging between 0.07% and 0.14%.[7,16] Chang and colleagues[17] reported an overall complication rate between 12% and 21%, and reoperations rates of 2.56% to 5.34%.

LAPAROSCOPIC SLEEVE GASTRECTOMY

The LSG was originally described 15 years ago as the first step preceding biliopancreatic diversion with duodenal switch (BPD/DS) in superobese patients (BMI >50 kg/m2). The BPD/DS was scheduled approximately 1 year later but the significant weight loss observed during the interval led to the adoption of this procedure as stand-alone.[23] It is performed laparoscopically and a gastric conduit of approximately 100 cc is created along the lesser curve of the stomach. The remnant stomach, including the fundus, is then resected (**Fig 2**).

Weight Loss Results

Average weight loss 1 year after LSG has been reported to be comparable, and sometimes superior, to that of LRYGB, with a %EBWL of 69% at 1 year in a blinded randomized controlled trial.[24] However, long-term maintenance of weight loss has not yet been demonstrated to be as good as for LRYGB. A recent study showed a 76.8%, 69.7%, and 56.1% %EBWL at 1-year, 3-year, and 5-year follow-up, respectively.[25]

Resolution of Comorbidities

Remission of hypertension after LSG was greater than 82% in a recent systematic review with reported ranges 68% to 92%.[17] Another systematic review with follow-up of more than 2 years showed a remission rate of 38%.[18] In a more recent study, resolution of hypertension was maintained at 5 years post-LSG in 61%.[26] Hypertriglyceridemia completely resolved at 1 year in 72% of patients[25] and overall dyslipidemia resolution rate was 82% in a recent review.[17] Obstructive sleep apnea resolution was 90% in that same review and another study demonstrated a maintained resolution rate of 73% 5 years post-LSG.[26]

Morbidity and Mortality

Similarly to RYGB, the mortality rate of LSG has been improving since its inception, with a similar 3-fold decrease between 2007 and 2012 in a large French study (0.36% to 0.11%).[20] In a recent meta-analysis, 30-day mortality after LSG was reported to be 0.29% (retrospective studies) and reoperation rates were 2.96% (retrospective studies) to 9.05% (randomized controlled trials).[17] In the American College of Surgeons Bariatric Surgery Center Network report (944 LSG subjects), 30-day mortality was 0.11%, with a 30-day morbidity was 5.6%.[16]

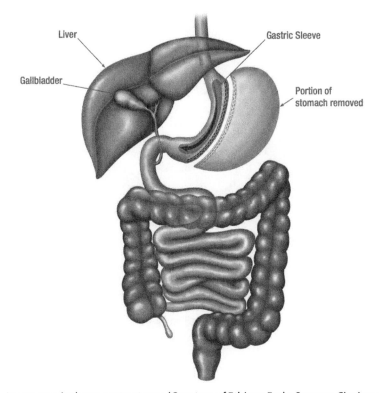

Fig. 2. Laparoscopic sleeve gastrectomy. (*Courtesy of* Ethicon Endo-Surgery, Cincinnati, OH.)

LAPAROSCOPIC ADJUSTABLE GASTRIC BANDING

Laparoscopic adjustable gastric banding (LAGB) is an inert inflatable band placed around the proximal portion of the stomach. It is inflated using a subcutaneous port, offering the opportunity of adjusting of the degree of restriction (**Fig 3**). LAGB has gained fast and wide popularity in Europe and Australia in the mid and late 1990s, as well as in the United States a decade later, after its FDA approval in 2001. It has demonstrated very low perioperative mortality and morbidity but the advent of the LSG has made the LAGB much less attractive with less than 10% of procedures currently used in the United States versus more than one-third only 5 years ago (see **Table 1**).

Weight Loss Results

One of the reasons for the decreasing number of LAGB procedures performed is the significant variability in weight-loss results. Variability in weight loss is significantly greater than the other bariatric procedures and requires close follow-up for iterative adjustments. At 1 year, %EBWL loss ranges from 29% to 49% with an average of 42%.[13] In the American College of Surgeons Bariatric Surgery Center Network report (>12,000 LAGB patients) the average BMI lost at 1 year was 7 kg/m^2.[16] Over time, %EBWL has been reported to be between 44% and 59% at follow-up of more than 5 years and 42% at more than 12 years.[27–29]

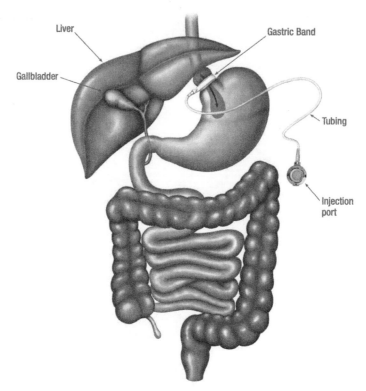

Fig. 3. Laparoscopic adjustable gastric banding. (*Courtesy of* Ethicon Endo-Surgery, Cincinnati, OH.)

Resolution of Comorbidities

One year after LAGB, hyperlipidemia improved in 59% of subjects, hypercholesterolemia in 78%, and hypertriglyceridemia in 77%. Hypertension resolved in 43% and improved in 71%. Obstructive apnea syndrome improved in 95% and resolved in 68% of LAGB subjects.[13] At 2 years or more, remission of hypertension was 17.4% and 22.7% for hyperlipidemia.[18] Obstructive sleep apnea remission ranged between 71% (observational studies) and 94% (randomized controlled trials).[17]

Morbidity and Mortality

The perioperative morbidity and mortality rates of the LAGB have been consistently very low with a 30-day mortality at or below 0.05%, including no deaths in more than 1200 cases in the Longitudinal Assessment of Bariatric Surgery (LABS) Consortium study.[16,30] Short-term (30-day) reoperation rates are also low (0.92%).[16] The Achilles heel of this procedure (and a significant cause for its decreasing use) has emerged over time. The removal (reoperation) rate is significant and ranges from 25% to greater than 50% in long-term studies.[27,28] Grounds for removal include inadequate weight loss, gastroesophageal reflux, dysphagia with or without slippage, and erosion.

DIABETES REMISSION AFTER BARIATRIC SURGERY

The impact of a bariatric procedure on diabetes was not expected and is truly remarkable. RYGB reduces 3-year diabetes-associated mortality by 58% in type 2 diabetes mellitus (T2DM). Similarly, cardiovascular-related mortality is reduced by 59% and the risk of myocardial infarction in half.[5]

Furthermore, bariatric surgery has provided patients with a potential for long-lasting and complete remission of T2DM and has offered the medical community a novel understanding of this complex disease.[31]

Even if LAGB has demonstrated very positive outcomes in T2DM patients, the mechanisms of action and timeline for resolution are different from those of RYGB or even LSG. In the case of RYGB or LSG, improvement or resolution of diabetes is witnessed within days of the procedure. In LAGB patients, resolution of diabetes is depends more on weight loss. Remission rates of T2DM after LAGB range from 28.6% to 73% of patients and improvement was seen in 80% of patients.[13,17,18]

The mechanisms behind the effect of LSG on T2DM are yet to be fully understood and its efficacy on the disease seems to lie between LAGB and RYGB.[32] Improvement or resolution of diabetes was greater than 60% within the first 30 days.[16] T2DM remission rates of 79% to 85% have been reported at 1 year[17,26] and 40% at 5 years.[33]

The substantial effect of Roux-en-Y gastric bypass on T2DM was described 20 years ago. Pories and colleagues[34] published an article entitled "Who would have thought it? An operation proves to be the most effective therapy for adult-onset diabetes mellitus." The study described a series of 146 T2DM subjects having undergone an RYGB with 83% of them showing remission of their diabetes.

Since this initial publication, multiple observational studies, analyzing more than 10,000 subjects have confirmed these findings. A retrospective cohort in the United Kingdom identified 569 surgical subjects with T2DM and matched them to 1881 diabetic subjects. Remission was defined as absence of medication and a hemoglobin A1c (HbA1c) level below 6.0%. In the bariatric surgery group, 94.5 diabetes mellitus remissions were found per 1000 person-years compared with 4.9 in control subjects. The remission rate in the RYGB group was 43 times that of the control group.[32]

Two recent reviews including more than 60,000 subjects reported remission rates between 66.7% and 70.9% at 2 years or more. At less than 2 years, the resolution rate was 81.6%.[18,35] The LABS consortium published their 3-year results (>2400 subjects) and the T2DM remission rate was 67.5%.[15] Very long-term remission rates remain high at 58% at 10 years.[12]

This overwhelming evidence paved the way for 2 prospective randomized controlled trials. The STAMPEDE trial published their 3-year results recently in the *New England Journal of Medicine*. In this trial, 150 obese subjects with uncontrolled T2DM were randomized to receive either intensive medical therapy alone or intensive medical therapy plus RYGB or LSG, with a goal of obtaining an HbA1c of 6.0% or less. This was achieved in 5% of the medical group subjects and 38% in the RYGB group. Of note, 35% of the subjects in the RYGB group achieved the primary endpoint without any medication and 65% of the subjects in this same group achieved an HbA1c lower than 7%. Subjects in the medical group were taking more than 5 diabetes medications versus an average of 1.4 in the RYGB group.[36] The 5-year results of another, similar, randomized controlled trial were published this year in *Lancet*. Sixty subjects were randomized to receive either medical treatment, RYGB, or biliopancreatic diversion. The primary endpoint was an HbA1c less than 6.5% without active pharmacologic treatment for 1 year. This endpoint was achieved and maintained at 5 years in 50% of the 38 surgical subjects (37% in the RYGB group) and in none of the 15 medically treated subjects. Five major complications of diabetes (including one fatal myocardial infarction) occurred in the medical group compared with one complication in the surgical group.[37]

Other endocrine effects of bariatric surgery have been demonstrated, including improvement in low testosterone syndrome with a doubling of testosterone at 1 year following gastric bypass surgery.[38] Finally, enhancement in women's fertility and birth events was also seen in a meta-analysis following bariatric surgery.[39]

REFERENCES

1. Shekelle PG, Morton SC, Maglione MA, et al. Pharmacological and surgical treatment of obesity. Evidence Report/Technology Assessment No. 103. (Prepared by the Southern California–RAND Evidence-Based Practice Center, Santa Monica, CA, under contract Number 290-02-0003.) AHRQ Publication No. 04-E028-2. Rockville (MD): Agency for Healthcare Research and Quality; 2004.
2. Sjöström L, Narbro K, Sjöström CD, et al. Effects of bariatric surgery on mortality in Swedish obese subjects. N Engl J Med 2007;357(8):741–52.
3. Adams TD, Gress RE, Smith SC, et al. Long-term mortality after gastric bypass surgery. N Engl J Med 2007;357(8):753–61.
4. Christou NV, Sampalis JS, Liberman M, et al. Surgery decreases long-term mortality, morbidity, and health care use in morbidly obese patients. Ann Surg 2004; 240(3):416–23 [discussion: 423–4].
5. Eliasson B, Liakopoulos V, Franzén S. Cardiovascular disease and mortality in patients with type 2 diabetes after bariatric surgery in Sweden: a nationwide, matched, observational cohort study. Lancet Diabetes Endocrinol 2015;3(11): 847–54.
6. Arterburn DE, Olsen MK, Smith VA, et al. Association between bariatric surgery and long-term survival. JAMA 2015;313(1):62.
7. Morton JM, Garg T, Nguyen N. Does hospital accreditation impact bariatric surgery safety? Ann Surg 2014;260(3):504–9.
8. ASMBS Estimates of Bariatric Procedures. Available at: https://asmbs.org/resources/estimate-of-bariatric-surgery-numbers. Accessed June 4, 2015.
9. NIH conference. Gastrointestinal surgery for severe obesity. Consensus Development Conference Panel. Ann Intern Med 1991;115:956–61.
10. FDA Approved Obesity Treatment Devices. Available at: http://www.fda.gov/MedicalDevices/ProductsandMedicalProcedures/ObesityDevices/ucm350134.htm. Accessed December 11, 2015.
11. Mason EE, Ito C. Gastric bypass. Ann Surg 1969;170(3):329–39.
12. Obeid NR, Malick W, Concors SJ, et al. Long-term outcomes after Roux-en-Y gastric bypass: 10- to 13-year data. Surg Obes Relat Dis 2016;12(1):11–20.
13. Buchwald H, Avidor PY, Braunwald ME, et al. Bariatric surgery review. JAMA 2004;292:14.
14. Hsieh T, Zurita L, Grover H, et al. 10-Year Outcomes of the Vertical Transected Gastric Bypass for Obesity: a Systematic Review. Obes Surg 2013;24(3):456–61.
15. Courcoulas AP. Weight change and health outcomes at 3 years after bariatric surgery among individuals with severe obesity. JAMA 2013;310(22):2416–25.
16. Hutter MM, Schirmer BD, Jones DB, et al. First Report from the American College of Surgeons Bariatric Surgery Center Network. Ann Surg 2011;254(3):410–22.
17. Chang S-H, Stoll CRT, Song J, et al. The effectiveness and risks of bariatric surgery. JAMA Surg 2014;149(3):275.
18. Puzziferri N, Roshek TB III, Mayo HG, et al. Long-term follow-up after bariatric surgery. JAMA 2014;312(9):934.

19. Adams TD, Davidson LE, Litwin SE, et al. Health benefits of gastric bypass surgery after 6 years. JAMA 2012;308(11):1122–31.
20. Lazzati A, Audureau E, Hemery F, et al. Reduction in early mortality outcomes after bariatric surgery in France between 2007 and 2012: a nationwide study of 133,000 obese patients. Surgery 2016;159(2):467–74.
21. Buchwald H, Estok R, Fahrbach K, et al. Trends in mortality in bariatric surgery: a systematic review and meta-analysis. Surgery 2007;142(4):621–35.
22. Carter J, Elliott S, Kaplan J, et al. Predictors of hospital stay following laparoscopic gastric bypass: analysis of 9,593 patients from the National Surgical Quality Improvement Program. Surg Obes Relat Dis 2015;11(2):288–94.
23. Marceau P, Biron S, Marceau S, et al. Biliopancreatic diversion-duodenal switch: independent contributions of sleeve resection and duodenal exclusion. Obes Surg 2014;24(11):1843–9.
24. Karamanakos SN, Vagenas K, Kalfarentzos F, et al. Weight loss, appetite suppression, and changes in fasting and postprandial ghrelin and peptide-YY levels after Roux-en-Y gastric bypass and sleeve gastrectomy: a prospective, double blind study. Ann Surg 2008;247(3):401–7.
25. Golomb I, Ben David M, Glass A, et al. Long-term Metabolic Effects of Laparoscopic Sleeve Gastrectomy. JAMA Surg 2015;150(11):1051–7.
26. Lemanu DP, Singh PP, Rahman H, et al. Five-year results after laparoscopic sleeve gastrectomy: a prospective study. Surg Obes Relat Dis 2015;11(3):518–24.
27. Nieuwenhove Y, Ceelen W, Stockman A, et al. Long-Term Results of a Prospective Study on Laparoscopic Adjustable Gastric Banding for Morbid Obesity. Obes Surg 2010;21(5):582–7.
28. Himpens J, Cadiere GB, Bazi M, et al. Long-term outcomes of laparoscopic adjustable gastric banding. Arch Surg 2011;146(7):802–7.
29. O'Brien PE, McPhail T, Chaston TB, et al. Systematic review of medium-term weight loss after bariatric operations. Obes Surg 2006;16(8):1032–40.
30. Longitudinal Assessment of Bariatric Surgery (LABS) Consortium, Flum DR, Belle SH, King WC, et al. Perioperative safety in the longitudinal assessment of bariatric surgery. N Engl J Med 2009;361(5):445–54.
31. Rubino F, Schauer PR, Kaplan LM, et al. Metabolic surgery to treat type 2 diabetes: clinical outcomes and mechanisms of action. Annu Rev Med 2010;61(1): 393–411.
32. Yska JP, van Roon EN, de Boer A, et al. Remission of type 2 diabetes mellitus in patients after different types of bariatric surgery. JAMA Surg 2015;150(12):1126–33.
33. Boza C, Daroch D, Barros D, et al. Long-term outcomes of laparoscopic sleeve gastrectomy as a primary bariatric procedure. Surg Obes Relat Dis 2014;10(6): 1129–33.
34. Pories WJ, Swanson MS, MacDonald KG, et al. Who would have thought it? An operation proves to be the most effective therapy for adult-onset diabetes mellitus. Ann Surg 1995;222(3):339–50 [discussion:350–2].
35. Buchwald H, Estok R, Fahrbach K, et al. Weight and Type 2 Diabetes after Bariatric Surgery: Systematic Review and Meta-analysis. Am J Med 2009;122(3): 248–56.e5.
36. Schauer PR, Bhatt DL, Kirwan JP, et al. Bariatric surgery versus intensive medical therapy for diabetes — 3-year outcomes. N Engl J Med 2014;370(21): 2002–13.
37. Mingrone G, Panunzi S, De Gaetano A, et al. Bariatric–metabolic surgery versus conventional medical treatment in obese patients with type 2 diabetes: 5 year

follow-up of an open-label, single-centre, randomised controlled trial. Lancet 2015;386(9997):964–73.

38. Woodard G, Ahmed S, Podelski V, et al. Effect of Roux-en-Y gastric bypass on testosterone and prostate-specific antigen. Br J Surg 2012;99(5):693–8.

39. Maggard MA, Yermilov I, Li Z, et al. Pregnancy and fertility following bariatric surgery: a systematic review. JAMA 2008;300(19):2286–96.

Medical Devices in the Treatment of Obesity

Julietta Chang, MD*, Stacy Brethauer, MD

KEYWORDS

- Obesity • Endoscopic therapy • Diabetes • Weight loss • Devices

KEY POINTS

- There is a need for obesity treatment options with a risk/benefit profile that is intermediate between medical and surgical therapy.
- Recently, the FDA has approved three medical devices for the treatment of obesity including intragastric balloons and vagal blockade devices.
- Intragastric balloon therapy is indicated in patients with a BMI of 30 to 40 for a 6-month period of therapy.
- Vagal blockade is a minimally invasive surgical procedure that provides intermittent neuromodulation of the infradiaphragmatic vagal trunks.
- The international experience with intragastric balloons suggests that this therapy is effective for patients with lower BMI or as a method to decrease weight before definitive surgical therapy.

INTRODUCTION

Obesity, defined as body mass index (BMI) equal to or greater than 30 kg/m^2, is a rising epidemic in the western patient population with incidence more than doubling in the past 25 years.[1] In 1998, the World Health Organization identified obesity as a chronic disease with multiple comorbid conditions, including detrimental effects on the cardiovascular system (eg, hypertension, hyperlipidemia, stroke, and cardiac disease), metabolic disorders including type 2 diabetes, and certain cancers including esophageal and colon adenocarcinoma.[2] The initial treatment of obesity includes medical therapies, such as behavioral therapy, pharmacotherapies, and dietary modification.[3] These approaches result in modest weight loss and high recidivism rates long-term. Numerous studies have clearly demonstrated the safety and efficacy of bariatric surgery. These operations result in greater and more durable weight loss than medical therapy and result in more durable remission of comorbid conditions and cardiovascular risk factors compared with medical management.[4–6] The most common surgical

The authors have nothing to disclose.
Digestive Diseases Institute, Cleveland Clinic Foundation, 9500 Euclid Avenue, Cleveland, OH 44195, USA
* Corresponding author.
E-mail address: juliettac@gmail.com

interventions performed today are laparoscopic Roux-en-Y gastric bypass (LRYGB), laparoscopic sleeve gastrectomy (LSG), and laparoscopic adjustable gastric banding. Although LRYGB has been the most popular bariatric surgery overall in the modern era, LSG has recently overtaken gastric bypass as the most commonly performed operation because of similar weight loss outcomes to LRYGB with fewer potential risks.[6,7] It is this current trend for less invasive approaches that has set the stage for endoscopic therapy and obesity treatment devices to enter the market.

There is clearly a need for therapy modalities that offer better and more durable weight loss than medical therapy while being less invasive than surgical interventions. Candidates for such therapy may include those with severe comorbid conditions precluding surgery or the supermorbid obese patients who may need a bridge to definitive surgical therapy. This concept of "downstaging" patients before undergoing definitive bariatric surgery[8] is a proven concept and has been shown to aid in ease of operation by decreasing liver size and visceral fat stores. In addition, there are many patients who simply do not want surgical treatment of their obesity. Although there are many reasons for this, the fact remains that only 1% of patients who would be eligible for bariatric surgery are receiving this type of therapy. Other options are needed, therefore, that can provide effective therapy with acceptable risk. There has been an increase in the number of obesity medications and medical devices that aim to provide meaningful weight loss with reproducible results and decreased morbidity compared with surgery. Current devices aim to aid in weight loss via different mechanisms including gastric distention with balloons, vagal blockade, malabsorption to mimic exclusion of the duodenum and jejunum, and gastrostomy tubes for the aspiration of gastric contents. This article reviews these new devices and current data regarding their efficacy.

SPACE-OCCUPYING DEVICES
Orbera BioEnterics Intragastric Balloon

Intragastric balloons for the treatment of obesity originate from the observation of patients with ingested gastric bezoars in the 1980s[2] resulting in early satiety and decreased food intake. Early versions of air-filled gastric balloons were plagued with high complications rates including mucosal erosions (26%), gastric ulcers (14%), and small bowel obstructions caused by migration (2%). Modern saline-filled intragastric balloons have been used outside the United States since 1997 with reported percent excess weight loss (%EWL) from 25% to 40%.[9]

One recent iteration of this concept is the Orbera BioEnterics Intragastric Balloon (Allergan BioEnterics Corporation, Irvine, TX) (**Fig. 1**). This Food and Drug Administration (FDA)-approved device is a silicone sphere placed endoscopically into the gastric lumen and filled with 400 to 700 mL of sterile saline. The device can be placed using moderate or deep sedation, thus eliminating the need for and cost of the operating suite. Ten milliliters of methylene blue can be mixed with the saline. In the event of balloon deflation, the dye is absorbed and excreted renally, causing urine to turn a distinctive green hue, alerting the patient to balloon deflation.[2] Although this potentially prevents migration of a deflated balloon into the intestine, balloon rupture is a rare event with the current technology. The balloons are left in situ for up to 6 months, and then removed endoscopically. Removal involves puncturing the balloon, aspirating the fluid, and removing the balloon using a grasping device through the endoscope. The balloons provide early satiety because of gastric distention. However, it has been proposed that gastric stretch secondary to the balloon causes release of cholecystokinin, which decreases gastric emptying and may also lead to early satiety.[10]

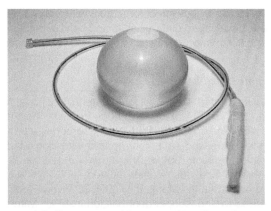

Fig. 1. Orbera intragastric balloon system. (*Courtesy of* Apollo Endosurgery, Inc, Austin, TX.)

One indication for Orbera is to place it in patients with high BMI or high-risk patients before bariatric surgery to reduce the risk of anesthesia, decrease liver size, and thus enhance intraoperative visualization. Another potential use is to predict how well a patient will respond to a purely restrictive bariatric procedure (eg, LSG); those that lose a significant amount of weight with the BioEnterics Intragastric Balloon would, in theory, respond better to surgical procedures that involve only gastric volume reduction instead of intestinal bypass.[2] The ability of the balloon to predict success after a particular surgical treatment, however, requires further investigation. One challenge in the United States for using the balloon to downstage patients with high BMI for surgery is that the current indication is for BMI of 30 to 40 mg/kg^2, making this an off-label use of the device. The approach, however, has been shown to be valid in international studies. Contraindications to BioEnterics Intragastric Balloon placement include contraindications to endoscopy, alterations of normal gastric anatomy including prior gastric surgery and hiatal hernias greater than 5 cm, potential bleeding lesions of the stomach and severe liver disease, ongoing alcohol or drug addiction, and pregnancy.[2]

The device has been studied extensively in Europe and has shown successful weight loss for a range of BMI. A multicenter European study enrolled overweight patients with a BMI of 27 to 30 mg/kg^2. They demonstrated a mean %EWL of 55.6% at time of removal, and maintained a mean %EWL of 29.1% at 3 years following removal.[11] In the largest reported series, more than 2500 obese patients with mean BMI of 44 underwent balloon placement with a reported mean %EWL of 33%.[12]

Early removal is most commonly caused by patient intolerance usually in the form of persistent nausea, and occurs in 2.43% to 4.2% of patients.[2] Perforation is the most feared complication and, in the largest series, less than 1% of patients developed gastric perforation. Prior gastric surgery was found to be a risk factor for perforation after balloon placement in that series and is now an absolute contraindication to placement of the Orbera balloon.[12]

Studies demonstrate that this device is relatively safe and effective; however, the main drawback to the Orbera device is the temporary nature of the therapy for the treatment of a chronic disease. In one study of 100 morbidly obese patients, only 28 of 100 patients were able to maintain %EWL greater than 10% at 2.5 years; the remainder regained most of their lost weight, underwent further bariatric procedures, or underwent a second balloon placement.[13] There may still be a role for use as an adjunct to medical management of obesity, as a staging procedure in preparation of bariatric surgery, or in those who are too sick to undergo bariatric surgery. The device does seem to have a legacy effect for up to a year with some persistent weight loss (perhaps caused by changed dietary habits and behavior); thus repeated therapy may become the most common paradigm for this device to maintain some effect long-term.

ReShape Duo Integrated Dual Balloon System

The ReShape Duo Integrated Dual Balloon System (ReShape Medical Inc, San Clemente, CA) **(Fig. 2)** is an FDA-approved endoscopically implanted device that is retrieved 6 months later. The double-balloon profile purportedly provides better intragastric filling and thus increased satiety compared with single-balloon systems. In addition, in the event of balloon rupture, there may be decreased risk of migration because the other separate balloon remains inflated.

The largest randomized trial thus far is the REDUCE Pivotal Trial, in which 326 patients were randomized to endoscopic dual-balloon insertion with diet and exercise versus sham endoscopy followed by diet and exercise.[9] The devices were removed at 24 weeks, and the patients were followed to 48 weeks. This found that there was significantly greater weight loss in the balloon therapy group at 24 weeks with mean %EWL of 25.1% versus 11.3% in the sham group. In addition, the balloon therapy group maintained significant beneficial changes in comorbid conditions, such as hemoglobin A_{1c}, high- and low-density lipoproteins, and systolic and diastolic blood pressure at 48 weeks, 24 weeks after device retrieval. The most common complication was gastric ulceration, which was observed in 35% of balloon patients even in the presence of mandatory proton pump inhibitor therapy. Most had no clinical significance but one bleeding ulcer at the gastroesophageal junction required transfusion. Symptoms of accommodation to the device including nausea and abdominal pain necessitated early retrieval in 9.1% of patients. Device deflation occurred in 6% of patients, and none were associated with device migration. There was a 99.4% success rate in device placement and 100% successful retrieval rate with short procedure

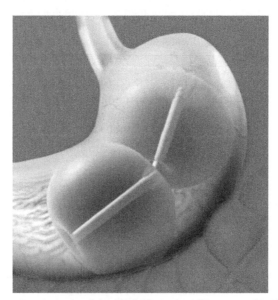

Fig. 2. The ReShape Duo integrated dual balloon system. (*Courtesy of* ReShape Medical Inc, San Clemente, CA.)

times. The trial demonstrated that ReShape dual-balloon therapy resulted in twice the weight loss as observed with diet and exercise alone, whereas a significant amount of weight loss and improvement in comorbid conditions persisted after device removal.[9]

VAGAL BLOCKADE
Maestro System

The Maestro System (EnteroMedics Inc, St Paul, MN) is a surgically placed device that reversibly blocks afferent and efferent signals from the anterior and posterior vagus nerve at the level of the gastroesophageal junction (**Fig. 3**). Implantation requires a laparoscopic procedure and dissection around the diaphragmatic hiatus to identify and circumferentially dissect both vagus nerve trunks. Although the device requires surgical placement, it has a much lower complication profile compared with other bariatric surgeries, such as LRYGB or LSG, and does not permanently alter the anatomy and thus falls under the category of devices in the treatment of obesity. Through vagal modulation, the device purports to increase satiety, perhaps by decreasing gastric emptying and inhibiting gastric relaxation during meals. However, mechanism of weight loss is still largely speculative.

The first iteration of the device required an externally worn device charger, and the duration of treatment relied on patient compliance. The EMPOWER trial[14] enrolled 294 patients to undergo implantation of the Maestro device. In the treatment group, the device was fully functional and operating while the external controller was placed directly over the implanted neuroregulator. In the control group, a fully functional

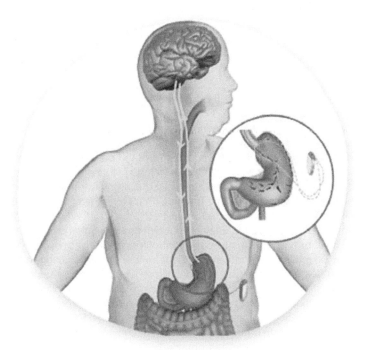

Fig. 3. The Maestro System contains electrodes placed on the infradiaphragmatic vagal trunks to provide neuromodulation of the afferent and efferent fibers. (*Courtesy of* EnteroMedics, Inc, St. Paul, MN.)

device was implanted but did not deliver impulses other than those associated with control checks. This study found no statistical difference in weight loss among the treatment and control groups, with %EWL of 17% versus 16%, respectively. However, the study found that there was improved %EWL with increased device usage, specifically greater than 12 hours a day. However, this difference was seen in control and treatment groups, raising the question as to whether the observed weight loss was caused by patient motivation and thus increased device compliance, versus low-dose vagal blockade from the control group caused by electrical input during device checks from the neuromodulator.

In the ReCharge study, the device used did not require an external battery, but did require charging every 1 to 2 days.[15] In addition, in the control group, a sham procedure was performed where a nonfunctioning neuroregulator was placed in the subcutaneous space and skin incisions for laparoscopic ports made, but the peritoneum was not violated. This eliminated the possibility of inadvertent therapy being delivered during impedance monitoring from the device. The predetermined efficacy objective was defined as a difference in %EWL of 10% or greater, which this study did not demonstrate. However, the treatment group did have significantly greater weight loss than the control as evidenced by a greater %EWL (24.4% vs 15.9% in the sham group).[15]

The main side effects reported are symptoms of delayed gastric emptying, such as belching, abdominal pain, heartburn, and dyspepsia.[15] In both trials, the presence of a large hiatal hernia requiring extensive dissection and inability to isolate both vagus nerves were causes of implantation failure. Compared with other endoscopic procedures, the device mandates intraperitoneal violation, and placement of the device requires advanced laparoscopic skills, both of which may limit patient selection and procedure availability for patients.

INVESTIGATIONAL DEVICES
Endobarrier

The duodenal-jejunal bypass sleeve (EndoBarrier; GI Dynamics, Inc, Lexington, MA) is a device that is endoscopically placed in the duodenal bulb by way of a self-expanding anchoring system. A 60-cm fluoropolymer sleeve extends distal to the anchoring system and prevents nutrient interaction with biliopancreatic fluid and the mucosa for the length of the device (**Fig. 4**).[8] Digestive juices from the pancreas and biliary system flow outside the sleeve to mix with chyme in the jejunum, further decreasing enzymatic digestion of ingested nutrients. There are also gut hormonal changes that induce satiety, specifically an increase in PYY (peptide YY) 3 to 36, similar to RYGB. Weight loss with this device has been reported to be 11.9% to 32% EWL.[8,16]

In addition, exclusion of duodenal-jejunal nutrient flow (as with the gastric bypass) is associated with improvements in glycemic control for patients with diabetes. Some of this effect may be related to modulations in gut hormones. Bypassing the duodenum has been shown to decrease glucagon release (foregut theory), whereas the presence of undigested chyme in the ileum stimulates release of incretins, such as glucagon-like peptide 1 (hindgut theory), both of which may contribute to improved glycemic control. The indications for placing the device have changed over time from a weight loss procedure to a treatment of diabetes based on this mechanism and the outcomes from international studies. This device has obtained CE Mark approval in the European Union but currently does not have FDA approval for use in the United States.

The EndoBarrier has been shown in trials to lead to a decrease in glycolated hemoglobin (HbA_{1c}) of up to 2.1%.[17] In one Dutch study of 17 obese patients, after

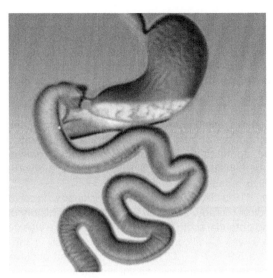

Fig. 4. EndoBarrier duodenal-jejunal liner. The 60-cm fluoropolymer tube is anchored in the proximal duodenum and excludes interaction between nutrients and the mucosa and biliopancreatic secretions for the length of the tube. (*Courtesy of* GI Dynamics, Inc, Lexington, MA.)

implantation of the sleeve, patients experienced a decreased in HbA_{1c} from 8.4% to 7.0%, with a mean weight loss of 12.7 kg. Furthermore, there were greater elevations in postprandial glucagon-like peptide 1 after device implantation.[18] The device has also been shown to improve HbA_{1c} in nonobese patients[16] with the implication that the device may be applicable in the management of type II diabetes in the absence of obesity. In the largest randomized control trial comparing the use of the EndoBarrier with medical therapy in the treatment of obesity and diabetes, the devices was implanted for 6 months and the patients were followed for 12 months. At 6 months, the EndoBarrier group had statistically significantly lower HbA_{1c}, %EWL, and cholesterol. At 12 months the EndoBarrier group maintained a lower %EWL compared with control. In addition, insulin requirement was significantly decreased in the EndoBarrier group.[16]

Adverse events reported with the EndoBarrier include abdominal pain, nausea, and emesis, which can usually be treated with conservative management; to more serious upper gastrointestinal bleeding, usually from the anchor; sleeve migration; sleeve occlusion; and reported esophageal and oropharyngeal trauma during deployment or extraction and duodenal perforation.[8,16] The early explantation rate of the EndoBarrier is 24% as demonstrated in a recent meta-analysis,[19] usually caused by patient intolerance or device migration. The FDA trial evaluating the safety and efficacy of the EndoBarrier system was halted early because of a higher than expected incidence of hepatic abscesses. This complication presumably resulted from translocation of bacteria related to the anchoring system but this is currently being evaluated by the company.

Most centers report placing the EndoBarrier under general anesthesia, although it has been reported to be successfully placed under conscious sedation similar to more common endoscopic procedures.[16] As experience with the device grows, it will likely be offered as a procedure under conscious sedation with increasing frequency.

AspireAssist

The AspireAssist device (Aspire Bariatrics, King of Prussia, PA) is an endoscopically placed gastrostomy tube that allows patients to aspirate gastric contents and ingested food. The device is placed using the standard pull technique as used with traditional percutaneous endoscopic gastrostomy tube placements. A 20F or 24F catheter tube is placed in the greater curvature of the stomach. The external portion is trimmed to 1 cm above skin level after 1 week and connected to the skin port, which contains a valve that prevents inadvertent leakage of gastric contents and unsupervised aspiration without the correct connector and reservoir. Patients are instructed to aspirate gastric contents 20 minutes after a meal containing greater than 200 kcal. Proton pump inhibitors and potassium chloride supplementation are used to minimize electrolyte losses.

In one pilot study,[20] 18 patients were randomly assigned to receive the device or undergo maximal medical therapy. They were screened for a history of eating disorders and depression, and potential subjects were excluded if there was evidence of psychiatric disease. There was significantly greater weight loss in the device group at 52 weeks (18.6% vs 5.9%; $P = .021$). Most weight loss occurred within the first 52 weeks and there was no further significant weight loss observed in the following 54 weeks. There were no major adverse events, and the most common adverse event was pain around the tube site. The use of the device did not induce any adverse eating behaviors; however, this remains a significant concern in the use of this device. In addition, the device was not associated with a compensatory increase in ingested calories. A Swedish study group also demonstrated successful weight loss with the device, with a mean %EWL of 40.8% in a group of 25 obese men and women. Two hospitalizations occurred in this group: one for pain control, and one for an intra-abdominal fluid collection that did not require intervention.[21] This device remains investigational and is not yet FDA approved. Further research needs to be performed to study adverse effects, especially behavioral, and to determine the durability of weight loss achieved using the AspireAssist device.

FUTURE CONSIDERATIONS/SUMMARY

Obesity continues to be a growing epidemic worldwide. Although bariatric surgery remains the most effective and durable treatment of obesity and its comorbidities, there is a need for less invasive yet efficacious weight loss therapies. Currently the FDA has approved two endoscopically placed intragastric balloon devices and a surgically placed vagal blockade device. Another device that holds promise, particularly for the treatment of type 2 diabetes, is the endoscopically placed duodenojejunal bypass liner. Other potential endoscopic therapies include endoscopic aspiration gastrostomy devices, and endoscopic suturing and stapling devices that simulate surgical procedures, such as the LSG or gastroplasty procedures. Although these devices provide variable weight loss during treatment, the transient nature of weight loss associated with these devices suggests that they are unlikely to be used as a standalone therapy. Medical devices will likely require repeated therapy to produce durable weight loss, or will become integrated into part of a multimodal approach to obesity.

REFERENCES

1. Flegal KM, Carroll MD, Kit BK, et al. Prevalence of obesity and trends in the distribution of body mass index among US adults, 1999-2010. JAMA 2012; 307(5):491–7.

2. Swidnicka-Siergiejko A, Wroblewski E, Dabrowki A. Endoscopic treatment of obesity. Can J Gastroenterol 2011;25(11):627–33.
3. Kumar N. Endoscopic therapy for weight loss: gastroplasty, duodenal sleeves, intragastric balloons, and aspiration. World J Gastrointest Endosc 2015;7(9):847–59.
4. Gloy VL, Briel M, Bhatt DL, et al. Bariatric surgery versus non-surgical treatment for obesity: a systematic review and meta-analysis of randomised controlled trials. BMJ 2013;347:f5934.
5. Buchwald H, Avidor Y, Braunwald E, et al. Bariatric surgery: a systematic review and meta-analysis. JAMA 2004;292(14):1724–37.
6. Schauer PR, Kashyap SR, Wolski K, et al. Bariatric surgery versus intensive medical therapy in obese patients with diabetes. N Engl J Med 2012;366(17): 1567–76.
7. Colquitt JL, Pickett K, Loveman E, et al. Surgery for weight loss in adults. Cochrane Database Syst Rev 2014;(8):CD003641.
8. Patel S, Hakim D, Mason J, et al. The duodenal-jejunal bypass sleeve (EndoBarrier Gastrointestinal Liner) for weight loss and treatment of type 2 diabetes. Surg Obes Relat Dis 2013;9:482–4.
9. Ponce J, Woodman G, Swain J, et al. The REDUCE pivotal trial: a prospective, randomized controlled pivotal trial of a dual intragastric balloon for the treatment of obesity. Surg Obes Relat Dis 2015;11:874–81.
10. Majumder S, Birk J. A review of the current status of endoluminal therapy as a primary approach to obesity management. Surg Endosc 2013;27(7):2305–11.
11. Genco A, López-Nava G, Wahlen C, et al. Multi-centre European experience with intragastric balloon in overweight populations: 13 years of experience. Obes Surg 2013;23(4):515–21.
12. Genco A, Bruni T, Doldi SB, et al. BioEnterics intragastric balloon: the Italian experience with 2,515 patients. Obes Surg 2005;15(8):1161–4.
13. Dastis NS, François E, Deviere J, et al. Intragastric balloon for weight loss: results in 100 individuals followed for at least 2.5 years. Endoscopy 2009;41(7):575–80.
14. Sarr M, Billington CJ, Brancatisano R, et al. The EMPOWER Study: randomized, prospective, double-blind, multicenter trial of vagal blockade to induce weight loss in morbid obesity. Obes Surg 2012;22(11):1771–82.
15. Ikramuddin S, Blackstone RP, Brancatisano A, et al. Effect of reversible intermittent intra-abdominal vagal nerve blockade on morbid obesity. JAMA 2014;213(9): 915–22.
16. Koehestanie P, Betzel B, Dogan K, et al. The feasibility of delivering a duodenal-jejunal bypass liner (EndoBarrier) endoscopically with patients under conscious sedation. Surg Endosc 2014;28(1):325–30.
17. De Moura EG, Martins BC, Lopes GS, et al. Metabolic improvements in obese type 2 diabetes subjects implanted for 1 year with an endoscopically deployed duodenal-jejunal bypass liner. Diabetes Technol Ther 2012;14:183–9.
18. de Jonge C, Rensen SS, Verdam FJ, et al. Endoscopic duodenal-jejunal bypass liner rapidly improves type 2 diabetes. Obes Surg 2013;23(9):1354–60.
19. Zechmeister-Koss I, Huić M, Fischer S, European Network for Health Technology Assessment (EUnetHTA). The duodenal-jejunal bypass liner for the treatment of type 2 diabetes mellitus and/or obesity: a systematic review. Obes Surg 2014; 24(2):310–23.
20. Sullivan S, Stein R, Jonnalagadda S, et al. Aspiration therapy leads to weight loss in obese subjects: a pilot study. Gastroenterology 2013;145(6):1245–52.
21. Forssell H, Norén E. A novel endoscopic weight loss therapy using gastric aspiration: results after 6 months. Endoscopy 2015;47(1):68–71.

Update on Adolescent Bariatric Surgery

Nirav K. Desai, MD[a],*, Mark L. Wulkan, MD[b], Thomas H. Inge, MD, PhD[c]

KEYWORDS

- Adolescent bariatric surgery • Adolescent obesity • Obesity

KEY POINTS

- Adolescent severe obesity is associated with significant health complications.
- Bariatric surgery has shown significant improvements in health outcomes and is well tolerated.
- Careful preoperative assessment and postoperative follow-up is necessary.

BACKGROUND

Obesity is one of the most significant health problems facing children and adolescents today. Current data suggest that the prevalence of obesity among children and adolescents has plateaued and the rate of increase of obesity has slowed. Despite this, severe obesity has become the fastest-growing subcategory of obesity among children and adolescents.[1,2] Obesity is associated with a range of adverse immediate and long-term effects, including type 2 diabetes (T2D), obstructive sleep apnea, hypertension, nonalcoholic fatty liver disease, and dyslipidemia.[3–5] It is also clear that adolescent obesity predicts adult obesity and its many known metabolic complications. There is evidence that the increased risk of development of adult comorbidities is reduced if weight loss is achieved.[6]

Body mass index (BMI) norms in children vary with age and sex. Overweight in children is defined as a BMI between the 85th and less than 95th percentile, and obesity is greater than or equal to 95th percentile for age and sex. Severe obesity is defined as BMI greater than or equal to 120% of the 95th percentile or BMI greater than or equal

Disclosure Statement: T.H. Inge has received bariatric research grant funding from Ethicon Endosurgery and has served as consultant for Sanofi Corporation. Dr N.K. Desai and Dr M.L. Wulkan have nothing to disclose.
^a Division of Gastroenterology, Hepatology and Nutrition, Boston Children's Hospital, 300 Longwood Avenue, Boston, MA 02115, USA; ^b Department of Surgery, Emory University School of Medicine, Children's Healthcare of Atlanta, 1405 Clifton Road NE, Atlanta, GA 30322, USA; ^c Department of Surgery, University of Cincinnati College of Medicine, Cincinnati Children's Hospital Medical Center, 3333 Burnet Avenue, MLC 2023, Cincinnati, OH 45229-3039, USA
* Corresponding author.
E-mail address: Nirav.desai@childrens.harvard.edu

Endocrinol Metab Clin N Am 45 (2016) 667–676
http://dx.doi.org/10.1016/j.ecl.2016.04.015
0889-8529/16/$ – see front matter © 2016 Elsevier Inc. All rights reserved.

to 35 kg/m^2, whichever is lower (roughly the 99th percentile for age and sex).[7–9] Currently about one-third of children and adolescents in the United States are overweight (**Table 1**). The prevalence of adolescent (12–19 years) obesity in the United States increased from 11% in 1988 to 20% in 2012.[1] Severe obesity is seen in 8% of adolescent girls and 7% of adolescent boys.[10] The severity of obesity in adolescence is a predictor of whether obesity will persist into adulthood.[11] In one study about 75% of adolescents with severe obesity remained severely obese as adults.[12]

ROLE OF BARIATRIC SURGERY

First-line treatment of obesity consists of structured diet and exercise programs. The American Academy of Pediatrics recommends a stepwise approach that begins with the primary care physician.[13] Use of medication and meal replacements is gaining interest; however, pharmacologic options are limited by the lack of safety and efficacy data in adolescents.[14] Behavioral treatment is the recommended starting point for treatment of pediatric obesity, although it is seldom effective for adolescents with severe obesity. In one example, after 3 years of behavioral treatment, the response was distinctly better for the 6 to 10 year olds with severe obesity and no weight improvement was seen for 14 to 16 year olds. Only 2% of the adolescents were able to achieve a clinically meaningful response (BMI Standard Deviation Score improvement of $\geq$0.5). These findings led authors to question the ethics of insisting on therapy that verges on futile, particularly given the potential for treatment failure to adversely affect already compromised self-esteem.[15]

Bariatric surgery, however, has proven to be more effective than nonsurgical obesity management for weight loss and the resolution of comorbid conditions, such as cardiovascular risk factors and diabetes.[16] The first gastric bypass, the precursor to the current Roux-en-y gastric bypass (RYGB), was performed by Mason and Ito[17] in 1967. Surgical weight loss techniques for adolescents were reported in the 1980s but did not gain momentum until the 2000s.[18] Data from the US National Inpatient Sample indicate that 2744 adolescent bariatric surgeries were performed in the United States from 1996 to 2003,[19] whereas more recent estimates show that approximately 1600 cases per year were done in 2009.[20] However, despite evidence showing health benefits of surgery, many remain reluctant to recommend surgery for adolescents with severe obesity. In 2010, nearly half of physicians surveyed said they would never refer an adolescent for bariatric surgery, and 65% suggested a minimal age of 18 years for a patient to undergo surgery.[21] The three most commonly performed adolescent bariatric procedures are RYGB, adjustable gastric band (AGB), and vertical sleeve gastrectomy (VSG). The US Food and Drug Administration has not approved the use of AGB in patients younger than 18 years of age.

Table 1
Definitions and prevalence of obesity 1999–2012

Category	BMI Percentile	% Prevalence Ages 12–19 y
Normal weight	<85th	—
Overweight	$\geq$85th	33
Obesity	$\geq$95th	18
Class II obesity	$\geq$120% of the 95th or BMI $\geq$35 kg/m^2	7
Class III obesity	$\geq$140% of the 95th or BMI $\geq$40 kg/m^2	2

Data from Skinner AC, Skelton JA. Prevalence and trends in obesity and severe obesity among children in the United States, 1999-2012. JAMA Pediatr 2014;168(6):561–6.

ELIGIBILITY CRITERIA

Surgical practice guidelines based on expert opinion have outlined criteria for selecting adolescent patients for bariatric surgery.[22–24] Patients with a BMI greater than or equal to 35 kg/m^2 with a severe comorbidity, such as moderate to severe obstructive sleep apnea, T2D, benign intracranial hypertension, or nonalcoholic steatohepatitis, can be considered. Patients with a BMI greater than or equal to 40 kg/m^2 and less severe comorbidities can be considered. Most guidelines suggest that patients should have attained Tanner stage IV or 95% of linear growth (based on bone age). However, these physiologic maturity criteria may be set aside in special cases of rapid weight gain because of defined medically recalcitrant causes (eg, hypothalamic obesity) if the mortality risk of comorbidities outweighs the theoretic risk of growth impairment following surgery. Patients and families must understand the importance of behavioral change, role of diet, and physical activity necessary for long-term success following surgery. Generally accepted contraindications for surgical weight loss procedures include a medically correctable cause of obesity; active substance abuse problem; and psychosocial, medical, unstable psychiatric, or cognitive conditions that prevent adherence to recommendations or impair decision-making ability. In addition, current or planned pregnancy (within 18 months of surgery) and inability to understand the risks and benefits of weight loss surgery are also contraindications.[22–24]

PREOPERATIVE EVALUATION

A multidisciplinary, team-based approach is recommended for evaluation of severely obese adolescents for bariatric surgery. The team should include an experienced bariatric surgeon, pediatric obesity specialist, nurse, dietitian, exercise specialist, and a psychologist/psychiatrist with pediatric expertise. Programs should have access to other pediatric subspecialists for management of other coexisting conditions as needed. Preoperative medical evaluation should identify and characterize the severity of comorbidities and presence of nutritional deficiencies, specifically to identify targets for preoperative optimization. All patients should undergo a psychosocial/behavioral evaluation. Obesity is a known risk factor for vitamin and micronutrient deficiencies. Low ferritin and vitamin A levels have been measured in 5% to 10% of severely obese adolescents, and vitamin D insufficiency in approximately half. Deficiencies in other micronutrients, such as vitamin B_{12}, B_1, and folic acid, were reported in less than 5%.[25] Thus screening everyone for nutrient deficiencies may not be cost effective. Assuming various mild deficiencies may exist and treating everyone with multivitamins preoperatively (one standard multivitamin with iron and 1000 IU vitamin D) may be more appropriate. *Helicobacter pylori* screening should be done in high-prevalence areas. It is also recommended patients undergo a cardiac evaluation and sleep apnea screening if indicated before bariatric surgery. Additional evaluations including upper endoscopy and endocrinology evaluation (diabetes, thyroid disease, polycystic ovary syndrome) should be done based on symptoms.[24]

WEIGHT LOSS PROCEDURES

All modern bariatric procedures are typically minimally invasive, with the aid of laparoscopy (**Fig. 1**).

Adjustable Gastric Band

The AGB is a purely restrictive procedure. It involves the laparoscopic placement of an adjustable silicone band around the stomach 1 to 2 cm below the gastroesophageal

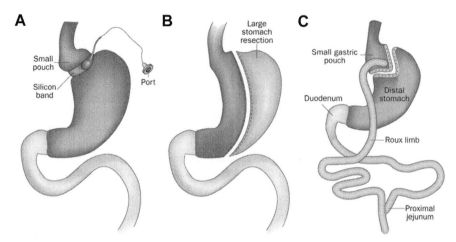

Fig. 1. Weight loss procedures. (*A*) Adjustable gastric band. (*B*) Vertical sleeve gastrectomy. (*C*) Roux-en-Y gastric bypass. (*From* Aron-Wisnewsky J, Doré J, Clement K. The importance of the gut microbiota after bariatric surgery. Nat Rev Gastroenterol Hepatol 2012;9:593; with permission.)

junction attached to a small reservoir that is implanted subcutaneously.[26] The band can be adjusted by altering the amount of fluid in the reservoir. The tighter the band, the slower the gastric pouch empties. Adult studies show that use of the band is decreasing, possibly because of the high rate of revisions, inadequate weight loss, and weight regain.[27]

Vertical Sleeve Gastrectomy

VSG involves the removal of most of the greater curvature of the stomach. The remaining tubular stomach is about 10% to 15% of its original size. This procedure was first performed as the initial stage of a two-stage weight loss procedure for adults who were extremely obese and believed to be poor surgical candidates for RYGB. Following initial weight loss after sleeve gastrectomy, a conversion to biliopancreatic diversion with duodenal switch or RYGB was prescribed as the next stage. However, because of the observation that significant short-term weight loss was achievable with VSG alone, the procedure has increasingly been described as a stand-alone operation that is associated with weight loss and comorbidity improvement.[28]

Roux-en-Y Gastric Bypass

In the RYGB, a small (approximately 30 mL) gastric pouch is created from the upper stomach. The small intestine is divided 30 to 50 cm distal to the duodenojejunal junction. This division creates a biliopancreatic limb (which transports secretions from the gastric body, liver, and pancreas) and also a Roux limb (also known as the alimentary limb). The proximal end of the Roux limb is anastomosed to the gastric pouch. The distal segment of the biliopancreatic limb is then connected to the alimentary limb, approximately 75 to 150 cm from the gastrojejunal anastomosis.[26]

OUTCOMES
Weight Loss/Maintenance

Data regarding long-term weight loss and weight regain for adolescents are limited. In a recent systematic review and meta-analysis of adolescent bariatric surgery, the average weighted mean BMI difference from baseline to 1 year was −13.5 kg/m² (95% confidence interval, −15.1 to −11.9 kg/m²). When examined by procedure type, weight loss was greatest for RYGB and smallest for AGB.[29] Inge and colleagues[30] found a 37% reduction in BMI at 1 year for patients undergoing RYGB regardless of starting BMI. More recently, data from the Teen-Longitudinal Assessment of Bariatric Surgery (Teen-LABS) have been published. In this study, 242 adolescents were enrolled (RYGB = 161, VSG = 67, AGB = 14) from five US centers. Three-year outcomes showed BMI reductions of 15.1 kg/m² (28%), 13.1 kg/m² (28%), and 3.8 kg/m² (8%) associated with RYGB, VSG, and AGB procedures, respectively (**Fig. 2**).[25] BMI data for 53 (of 72 eligible for 3-year follow-up; BMI of 48 kg/m²) pediatric patients who underwent VSG in Saudi Arabia showed a BMI decrease of 20 kg/m² over 3 years. This impressive 42% decline may in part be caused by a height increase of 5.8 cm on average for this cohort of preadolescents and adolescents.[31] Because adult studies have commonly shown a modest degree of weight regain from 3 to 10 years following essentially all operations,[32] longer term follow-up is needed to assess durability of adolescent weight loss outcomes.

Comorbidities Change

One of the most important objectives of performing weight loss surgery is to improve or reverse obesity-related comorbidities. Adult studies have shown better glycemic control in patients with T2D undergoing medical therapy in conjunction with bariatric surgery than medical therapy alone.[33] Other adult studies have shown resolution of T2D in 78% of patients, although variation in definitions of disease response makes extrapolation to individual patients difficult.[34] Adolescent studies have also shown resolution of T2D and improvements in obstructive sleep apnea, asthma, nonalcoholic fatty liver disease, and dyslipidemia.[31,35–38] Teen-LABS observed the reversal of diabetes (90% of patients), dyslipidemia (66%), hypertension (74%), and abnormal kidney function (86%).[25] These prospective data are consistent with other predominantly retrospective findings summarized in a recent systematic review.[39]

One study examining the psychological profile of 37 adolescents undergoing bariatric surgery demonstrated improvement in anxiety, depression, and self-concept at 4 months from baseline.[10] Studies in adults and adolescents have found the most substantial psychosocial improvements are seen in the first year after

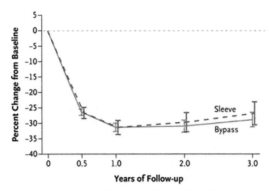

Fig. 2. Percent change in weight from baseline. (*From* Inge TH, Courcoulas AP, Jenkins TM, et al. Weight loss and health status 3 years after bariatric surgery in adolescents. N Engl J Med 2015;374(2):118; with permission.)

surgery, and tend to level off thereafter.[41,42] Adolescents report the greatest gains in physical comfort, and body esteem domains of quality of life.[42]

Complications

Few outcomes of bariatric surgery have been as inconsistently reported in the literature as complications of surgery. However, information about complications of surgery are enormously important for detailed and informative discussions of benefits and risks of treatment for care providers and families alike. Retrospective analyses of administrative databases have suggested that the frequency of complications of bariatric surgery may be lower in adolescents as compared with adults, but these findings have not been verified by prospective clinical research.[43]

A recent meta-analysis and systematic review found that approximately 11% of patients who undergo AGB experience band-related complications. Of those, 15% needed reintervention including cholecystectomy; however, most were band-related procedures, such as repositioning, removal, or port revision. Perioperative complications, such as wound infection, were noted 1% and intraoperative bleeding or conversion to laparotomy in less than 1%. Ten percent of patients experienced gastrointestinal issues, such as vomiting, nausea, acid reflux, diarrhea, and gallstones.[39]

The largest single-center series reporting detailed complication data for RYGB was derived from 77 consecutive cases in a children's hospital setting. The baseline BMI in this series was 59 kg/m^2. Intraoperative complications were seen in two (3%) and neither had postoperative consequences. Perioperative complications within 30 days were seen in 22% of patients, whereas 13% had a complication between 31 and 90 days. The most common types of postoperative complications included 17% with gastrojejunal anastomotic stricture, reoperation in 13%, leak in 7%, and dehydration in 7%.[44] Multicenter prospective complication data were reported by Teen-LABS investigators at 30 days and between 31 days and 3 years in 161 RYGB cases and 67 VSG cases (**Table 2**).[25,45] The most common operation was cholecystectomy, seen in 8% of the cohort. Most of the serious complications were observed in patients who underwent RYGB. Four VSG participants experienced reoperations including two with serious complications (a staple line leak requiring a stent, and one conversion to bypass for reflux). Timing of abdominal reoperations showed that 24%, 55%, and 21% occurred within the first, second, and third year, respectively.

The most significant long-term complications of adolescent bariatric surgery are nutritional deficiencies, which have been associated with all three procedures. Preoperative deficiencies place patients at increased risk for worsened postoperative deficiencies, which is why it is essential to identify and correct any vitamin and micronutrient deficiency during the preoperative period. Other contributors to postoperative deficiencies include reduced food intake, poor adherence with supplement regimens, and altered digestion and absorption. One adolescent study found mean adherence during the 6-month study to be 30%.[46] The most common vitamin deficiencies after RYGB are vitamin B$_{12}$, thiamine, and vitamin D.[47] Other deficiencies include vitamin A, folic acid, iron, copper, and zinc. Teen-LABS data showed 37% of patients were vitamin D deficient at baseline and 43% of RYGB and VSG patients remained deficient at 3 years. Vitamin B$_{12}$ deficiency had a statistically significant increase 3 years postsurgery, 1% at baseline versus 8% at 3 years ($P = .005$). Additionally, low ferritin levels were seen in 5% of patients at baseline compared with 57% at 3 years after surgery ($P<.001$). There was an 8% increase in vitamin A deficiency 3 years postsurgery (6% vs 13%).[25] Life-long nutritional monitoring and vitamin supplementation is recommended for all bariatric patients. Recommendations for supplementation are based on

Table 2
Early and late complications in patients undergoing Roux-en-y gastric bypass and sleeve gastrectomy

	Total (n = 228) N (%)	Bypass (n = 161) N (%)	Sleeve (n = 67) N (%)
Early (30 d)			
Reoperation for GI leak/sepsis	5 (2)	3 (2)	2 (3)
GI leak, not requiring reoperation	3 (1)	3 (2)	—
Gastrojejunal anastomotic stricture	6 (3)	6 (4)	—
Reoperation for bowel obstruction/bleeding	3 (1)	3 (2)	—
Reoperation for suspected sepsis	1 (<1)	1 (<1)	—
Wound infection	5 (2)	3 (2)	2 (3)
Unplanned splenectomy for injury	1 (<1)	1 (<1)	0
Solid organ injury not requiring intervention	3 (1)	1 (<1)	2 (3)
Bowel injury	1 (<1)	1 (<1)	—
Postoperative bleeding requiring transfusion	4 (2)	4 (2)	—
Postoperative bleeding not requiring transfusion	2 (<1)	2 (1)	—
Abdominal pain/dehydration/diarrhea/nausea	11 (5)	9 (6)	2 (3)
Late (31 d–3 y)			
Cholecystectomy	18 (8)	15 (9)	3 (4)
Gastrostomy	4 (2)	4 (2)	—
Lysis of adhesions	4 (2)	4 (2)	—
Exploratory laparotomy	3 (1)	3 (1)	—
Repair of internal hernia	3 (1)	3 (1)	—
Bowel resection or diversion	2 (1)	2 (1)	—
Wound drainage	2 (1)	1 (1)	1 (1)
Luminal stent for leak	1 (<1)	—	1 (1)
Ventral hernia repair	1 (<1)	—	1 (1)
Conversion to bypass	1 (1)	n/a	1 (1)

Abbreviations: GI, gastrointestinal; n/a, not applicable.

Data from Mechanick JI, Youdim A, Jones DB, et al. Clinical practice guidelines for the perioperative nutritional, metabolic, and nonsurgical support of the bariatric surgery patient—2013 update: cosponsored by American Association of Clinical Endocrinologists, the Obesity Society, and American Society for Metabolic & Bariatric Surgery. Endocr Pract 2013;19(2):337–72; and Inge TH, Courcoulas AP, Jenkins TM, et al. Weight loss and health status 3 years after bariatric surgery in adolescents. N Engl J Med 2015;374(2):113–23.

expert opinion and include two multivitamins, 1200 to 1500 mg of elemental calcium, 3000 IU of vitamin D, and 45 to 60 mg of elemental iron for menstruating women. Other supplements are based on results of monitoring.[24]

LIMITATIONS AND FUTURE DIRECTIONS

Longitudinal studies with sufficient sample sizes to have meaningful outcome data from important gender, racial, ethnic, and disease subpopulations are needed to truly assess the long-term benefit and risks of adolescent bariatric surgery. Aside from the Teen-LABS data, most of the studies thus far have been short-term retrospective analyses and have suffered from significant patient dropout and missing data. There is significant heterogeneity in definitions of comorbidities, resolution of comorbidities, and complications; standardized definitions would be beneficial. In addition qualitative data reporting patient perspectives are currently lacking.

SUMMARY

The three most commonly performed adolescent bariatric procedures are RYGB, AGB, and VSG. Considerable evidence now strongly suggests that clinically significant and durable weight loss is achieved for adolescents undergoing bariatric operations for treatment of severe obesity. In addition, improvement in key health conditions and weight-related quality of life are apparent. These benefits must be viewed in the context of risks of nutritional deficiencies and need for future reoperation, particularly following RYGB. Longer term data elucidating durability of weight loss, comorbidity improvements, and risk of relapse of prior comorbidities are needed. Although use of VSG is increasing, more studies are needed to determine the best operation for individual patients. In addition, long-term assessments of adverse events, including reoperations and nutritional deficiencies, bone health, substance use, and psychological outcomes, are needed to best understand the role of bariatric surgery in the treatment of adolescent severe obesity.

REFERENCES

1. Ogden CL, Carroll MD, Kit BK, et al. Prevalence of childhood and adult obesity in the United States, 2011-2012. JAMA 2014;311(8):806–14.
2. Ogden CL, Carroll MD, Kit BK, et al. Prevalence of obesity and trends in body mass index among US children and adolescents, 1999-2010. JAMA 2012; 307(5):483–90.
3. Kohler MJ, Thormaehlen S, Kennedy JD, et al. Differences in the association between obesity and obstructive sleep apnea among children and adolescents. J Clin Sleep Med 2009;5(6):506–11.
4. May AL, Kuklina EV, Yoon PW. Prevalence of cardiovascular disease risk factors among US adolescents, 1999-2008. Pediatrics 2012;129(6):1035–41.
5. Holterman A, Gurria J, Tanpure S, et al. Nonalcoholic fatty liver disease and bariatric surgery in adolescents. Semin Pediatr Surg 2014;23(1):49–57.
6. Juonala M, Magnussen CG, Berenson G, et al. Childhood adiposity, adult adiposity, and cardiovascular risk factors. N Engl J Med 2011;365(20):1876–85.
7. Baker S, Barlow S, Cochran W, et al. Overweight children and adolescents: a clinical report of the North American Society for Pediatric Gastroenterology, Hepatology and Nutrition. J Pediatr Gastroenterol Nutr 2005;40(5):533–43.
8. Gulati AK, Kaplan DW, Daniels SR. Clinical tracking of severely obese children: a new growth chart. Pediatrics 2012;130(6):1136–40.
9. Flegal KM, Wei R, Ogden CL, et al. Characterizing extreme values of body mass index-for-age by using the 2000 centers for disease control and prevention growth charts. Am J Clin Nutr 2009;90(5):1314–20.
10. Skinner AC, Skelton JA. Prevalence and trends in obesity and severe obesity among children in the United States, 1999-2012. JAMA Pediatr 2014;168(6): 561–6.
11. Freedman DS, Mei Z, Srinivasan SR, et al. Cardiovascular risk factors and excess adiposity among overweight children and adolescents: the Bogalusa Heart Study. J Pediatr 2007;150(1):12–7.e2.
12. The NS, North KE, Popkin BM, et al. Association of adolescent obesity with risk of severe obesity in adulthood. JAMA 2010;304(18):2042–7.

13. Spear BA, Barlow SE, Ervin C, et al. Recommendations for treatment of child and adolescent overweight and obesity. Pediatrics 2007;120(Suppl 4):S254–88.

14. Kelly AS, Barlow SE, Rao G, et al. Severe obesity in children and adolescents: identification, associated health risks, and treatment approaches: a scientific statement from the American Heart Association. Circulation 2013;128(15):1689–712.

15. Danielsson P, Kowalski J, Ekblom Ö, et al. Response of severely obese children and adolescents to behavioral treatment. Arch Pediatr Adolesc Med 2012; 166(12):1103–8.

16. Adams TD, Davidson LE, Litwin SE, et al. Health benefits of gastric bypass surgery after 6 years. JAMA 2013;308(11):1122–31.

17. Mason EE, Ito C. Gastric bypass in obesity. Surg Clin North Am 1967;47(6): 1345–51.

18. Greenstein R, Rabner J. Is adolescent gastric-restrictive antiobesity surgery warranted? Obes Surg 1995;5(2):138–44.

19. Tsai WS, Inge TH, Burd RS. Bariatric surgery in adolescents: recent national trends in use and in-hospital outcome. Arch Pediatr Adolesc Med 2007;161(3):217–21.

20. Zwintscher NP, Azarow KS, Horton JD, et al. The increasing incidence of adolescent bariatric surgery. J Pediatr Surg 2013;48(12):2401–7.

21. Woolford SJ, Clark SJ, Gebremariam A, et al. To cut or not to cut: physicians' perspectives on referring adolescents for bariatric surgery. Obes Surg 2010; 20(7):937–42.

22. Pratt JS, Lenders CM, Dionne EA, et al. Best practice updates for pediatric/adolescent weight loss surgery. Obesity (Silver Spring) 2009;17(5):901–10.

23. Michalsky M, Reichard K, Inge T, et al. ASMBS pediatric committee best practice guidelines. Surg Obes Relat Dis 2012;8(1):1–7.

24. Mechanick JI, Youdim A, Jones DB, et al. Clinical practice guidelines for the perioperative nutritional, metabolic, and nonsurgical support of the bariatric surgery patient-2013 update: cosponsored by American Association of Clinical Endocrinologists, the Obesity Society, and American Society for Metabolic & Bariatric Surgery. Endocr Pract 2013;19(2):337–72.

25. Inge TH, Courcoulas AP, Jenkins TM, et al. Weight loss and health status 3 years after bariatric surgery in adolescents. N Engl J Med 2015;374(2):113–23.

26. Elder KA, Wolfe BM. Bariatric surgery: a review of procedures and outcomes. Gastroenterology 2007;132(6):2253–71.

27. Buchwald H, Oien DM. Metabolic/bariatric surgery worldwide 2011. Obes Surg 2013;23(4):427–36.

28. ASMBS Clinical Issues Committee. Updated position statement on sleeve gastrectomy as a bariatric procedure. Surg Obes Relat Dis 2012;8(3):e21–6.

29. Black JA, White B, Viner RM, et al. Bariatric surgery for obese children and adolescents: a systematic review and meta-analysis. Obes Rev 2013;14(8): 634–44.

30. Inge TH, Jenkins TM, Zeller M, et al. Baseline BMI is a strong predictor of nadir BMI after adolescent gastric bypass. J Pediatr 2010;156(1):103–8.e1.

31. Alqahtani AR, Antonisamy B, Alamri H, et al. Laparoscopic sleeve gastrectomy in 108 obese children and adolescents aged 5 to 21 years. Ann Surg 2012;256(2): 266–73.

32. Odom J, Zalesin KC, Washington TL, et al. Behavioral predictors of weight regain after bariatric surgery. Obes Surg 2010;20(3):349–56.

33. Schauer PR, Kashyap SR, Wolski K, et al. Bariatric surgery versus intensive medical therapy in obese patients with diabetes. N Engl J Med 2012;366(17): 1567–76.

34. Buchwald H, Estok R, Fahrbach K, et al. Weight and type 2 diabetes after bariatric surgery: systematic review and meta-analysis. Am J Med 2009;122(3): 248–56.e5.
35. Alqahtani AR, Elahmedi MO, Al Qahtani A. Co-morbidity resolution in morbidly obese children and adolescents undergoing sleeve gastrectomy. Surg Obes Relat Dis 2014;10(5):842–50.
36. Boza C, Viscido G, Salinas J, et al. Laparoscopic sleeve gastrectomy in obese adolescents: results in 51 patients. Surg Obes Relat Dis 2012;8(2): 133–7 [discussion: 137–9].
37. Jen HC, Rickard DG, Shew SB, et al. Trends and outcomes of adolescent bariatric surgery in California, 2005-2007. Pediatrics 2010;126(4):e746–53.
38. Messiah SE, Lopez-Mitnik G, Winegar D, et al. Changes in weight and co-morbidities among adolescents undergoing bariatric surgery: 1-year results from the bariatric outcomes longitudinal database. Surg Obes Relat Dis 2013; 9(4):503–13.
39. Paulus GF, de Vaan LEG, Verdam FJ, et al. Bariatric surgery in morbidly obese adolescents: a systematic review and meta-analysis. Obes Surg 2015;25(5): 860–78.
40. Järvholm K, Olbers T, Marcus C, et al. Short-term psychological outcomes in severely obese adolescents after bariatric surgery. Obesity (Silver Spring) 2012;20(2):318–23.
41. Karlsson J, Taft C, Rydén A, et al. Ten-year trends in health-related quality of life after surgical and conventional treatment for severe obesity: the SOS intervention study. Int J Obes (Lond) 2007;31(8):1248–61.
42. Zeller MH, Reiter-Purtill J, Ratcliff MB, et al. Two-year trends in psychosocial functioning after adolescent Roux-en-Y gastric bypass. Surg Obes Relat Dis 2011; 7(6):727–32.
43. Varela JE, Hinojosa MW, Nguyen NT. Perioperative outcomes of bariatric surgery in adolescents compared with adults at academic medical centers. Surg Obes Relat Dis 2007;3(5):537–40.
44. Miyano G, Jenkins TM, Xanthakos SA, et al. Perioperative outcome of laparoscopic Roux-en-Y gastric bypass: a children's hospital experience. J Pediatr Surg 2013;48(10):2092–8.
45. Inge TH, Zeller MH, Jenkins TM, et al. Perioperative outcomes of adolescents undergoing bariatric surgery: the teen-longitudinal assessment of bariatric surgery (Teen-LABS) study. JAMA Pediatr 2014;168(1):47–53.
46. Modi AC, Zeller MH, Xanthakos SA, et al. Adherence to vitamin supplementation following adolescent bariatric surgery. Obesity (Silver Spring) 2013;21(3): E190–5.
47. Saltzman E, Karl JP. Nutrient deficiencies after gastric bypass surgery. Annu Rev Nutr 2013;33:183–203.

The Psychosocial Burden of Obesity

David B. Sarwer, PhD*, Heather M. Polonsky, BS

KEYWORDS

- Obesity • Bariatric surgery • Psychosocial functioning • Weight loss

KEY POINTS

- Numerous studies have demonstrated a positive association between obesity and various mental health issues, including depression, eating disorders, anxiety, and substance abuse.
- Obesity impacts individuals' quality of life, with many sufferers experiencing increased stigma and discrimination because of their weight.
- Patients frequently make unrealistic weight loss goals; conducting psychological evaluations before treatment allows clinicians to temper expectations and identify contraindications to success.
- Psychological implications of bariatric surgery are mixed. Although body image and depressive symptoms often improve, suicide ideation and substance abuse have been shown to increase.

Obesity is associated with several comorbidities, including cardiovascular disease, type 2 diabetes, sleep apnea, osteoarthritis, and several forms of cancer. Because of the staggering health care costs associated with these conditions, some authorities predict that these diseases pose a legitimate threat to the health of the American economy over the next several decades. Furthermore, the US Surgeon General has posited that obesity and its associated diseases could decrease the average life expectancy of Americans for the first time in history.

Obesity and its comorbidities also come with a significant psychosocial burden, impacting numerous areas of psychosocial functioning. Thus, the evaluation of psychosocial functioning is an important part of the assessment and treatment planning for the patient with obesity, particularly in the case of bariatric surgery. Although weight loss is associated with improvements in psychosocial functioning for most individuals, a small number of patients experience untoward psychological symptoms after weight reduction.

Disclosure Statement: Dr D.B. Sarwer has consulting relationships with BAROnova, Kythera, Medtronic, and Neothetics. Ms H.M. Polonsky has no relationships to disclose.
Center for Obesity Research and Education, Temple University College of Public Health, 3223 North Broad Street, Suite 175, Philadelphia, PA 19140, USA
* Corresponding author.
E-mail address: dsarwer@temple.edu

PSYCHOSOCIAL FUNCTIONING OF PERSONS WITH OBESITY

Several comprehensive reviews have suggested that between 20% and 60% of persons with obesity, and extreme obesity in particular, suffer from a psychiatric illness.[1-5] These percentages are typically greater than those seen in the general population.

Depression

Previous research suggests a relationship between excess body weight and depression.[6-9] Persons with extreme obesity, for example, are almost five times more likely to have experienced an episode of major depression in the past year as compared with those of average weight.[10] This relationship between obesity and depression seems to be stronger for women than men,[6] perhaps because of society's emphasis on thinness as a characteristic of female beauty.

Approximately one-third of candidates for bariatric surgery report clinically significant symptoms of depression at the time of surgery, whereas about 50% report a lifetime history of depression.[11,12] The reasons for this high prevalence are not well understood, but may include the experience of weight-related stigma and discrimination (discussed later), the presence of physical pain or other impairments in quality of life, or the occurrence of disordered eating.[13]

Eating Disorders

Disordered eating is common among persons with obesity. Many patients presenting for weight loss treatment report that they engage in eating for emotional reasons; others report having difficulty controlling the frequency of their eating, portion sizes, or eating behavior in response to the bombardment of food cues from modern society. Somewhat surprising to some, only a small minority have formally recognized eating disorders. The most common eating disorder among persons with obesity is binge-eating disorder. Binge-eating disorder is characterized by the consumption of a large amount of food in a brief period of time (less than 2 hours), during which the individual experiences a loss of control. As a result, the individual eats much faster than normal, until uncontrollably full, in the absence of hunger, and often eats alone. After eating, the individual often reports disgust.[14]

Early reports suggested that a large minority of persons with obesity who sought weight loss treatment, and up to half of patients who presented for bariatric surgery, had binge-eating disorder.[15-18] More recent studies have suggested that the disorder occurs in 5% to 15% of candidates for bariatric surgery.[19] Smaller percentages of patients with obesity have bulimia nervosa, where the binge eating is accompanied by self-induced vomiting or other compensatory behaviors, such as excessive exercise. Approximately 5% of persons with obesity suffer from the night eating syndrome, an eating, sleep, and mood disorder defined as a delay in the circadian pattern of food intake caused by awakenings in the night to eat.[20,21]

The presence of binge eating can negatively impact weight loss efforts. The presence of binge eating is associated with either suboptimal weight losses or premature weight regain following bariatric surgery. Binge eating is not considered a contraindication to bariatric surgery or other weight loss treatment.[22] It is, however, considered a potential poor prognostic indicator of weight loss treatment outcome, particularly in the absence of lifestyle modification strategies or pharmacotherapy specifically designed to address the behavior.

Anxiety

Anxiety disorders are common among patients who present for bariatric surgery; the occurrence among those presenting for nonsurgical treatment is less well established. The most common anxiety disorder in candidates for bariatric surgery is social anxiety disorder, found in 9% of patients.[2] In light of Western society's emphasis on thinness as a marker of physical beauty, it is not surprising that people with extreme obesity report increased anxiety in social situations.[23] Nevertheless, social anxiety, unless of crippling intensity, is not believed to contraindicate weight loss treatment. However, intuitive thought and clinical experience suggests that uncontrolled anxiety may negatively impact engagement in weight loss treatment in all its forms.

Substance Abuse

A small minority of individuals with obesity present for weight loss treatment actively abusing substances.[2] Active use or abuse is considered a contraindication to weight loss treatment. Approximately 10% of candidates for bariatric surgery report a history of illicit drug use or alcoholism, a percentage higher than seen in the general population. Surprisingly, two studies suggest that persons with extreme obesity and a lifetime history of substance abuse experience larger weight losses than those without a history of substance abuse.[24,25] It is believed that these individuals have likely developed impulse control and self-regulation strategies that helped them overcome their struggles with drugs and alcohol and that similarly serve them well in controlling their eating habits after bariatric surgery.

Mental Health Treatment

Many patients with obesity have turned to mental health treatment to modify their eating habits or address the emotional consequences of the disease. Approximately 50% of candidates for bariatric surgery report a history of mental health treatment and up to 40% report some form of treatment (either psychotherapy or pharmacotherapy) at the time of surgery.[24,26–29] The use of psychiatric medications, particularly antipsychotics and some classes of antidepressants, can contribute to weight gain and/or negatively impact weight loss efforts. Presently, little is known about how these medications interact with the different bariatric surgical procedures.[30,31] Changes in absorption of these medications may occur after surgery and rapid changes in body weight and fat mass may also affect the efficacy and tolerability of the medications.

Self-Esteem

Obesity can impact an individual's self-esteem. For some individuals, it may be difficult to recognize and appreciate talents and abilities because of their struggles with their weight. For others, obesity has relatively little impact. These individuals may be comfortable with their work and home life, but their weight has been the one area where they have not been successful.

Quality of Life and Body Image

Obesity also negatively impacts health-related quality of life.[32] Numerous studies have shown a relationship between excess body weight and decreases in quality of life.[33–36] Individuals often report significant difficulties with physical and occupational functioning. These impairments likely motivate many individuals to seek weight loss treatment.

Body image is an important aspect of quality of life for many individuals. Body image dissatisfaction is common for individuals who are overweight, as it is for women and girls of average weight. The degree of dissatisfaction seems to be directly related to the amount of excess weight a person has, although persons can report dissatisfaction with their entire bodies or with specific features.[33,36–38] Even in the presence of significant weight-related health problems, body image dissatisfaction is believed to play an influential role in the decision to seek weight loss treatment.[13]

Sexual Abuse, Physical Abuse, and Emotional Neglect

There seems to be a modest association between sexual abuse and obesity.[39] Studies have suggested that between 16% and 32% of bariatric surgery candidates reported a history of sexual abuse, which seems to be higher than seen in the general population.[39,40] Physical abuse is similarly common among persons with obesity. Approximately 50% of persons with extreme obesity report some form of emotional neglect during their childhood, ranging from verbal abuse, emotional neglect, or other family dysfunction associated with separation, divorce, substance abuse, or incarceration of a member of the nuclear family.

Stigma and Discrimination

Obesity, and extreme obesity in particular, can contribute to the experience of discrimination. Individuals with obesity are less likely to complete high school, are less likely to marry, and typically earn less money compared with persons of average body weight.[41,42] Persons who are obese are frequently subjected to discrimination in several settings, including educational, employment, and even health care settings. These experiences may be even more common among those suffering from severe obesity.

MOTIVATIONS FOR AND EXPECTATIONS OF WEIGHT LOSS TREATMENT

Improvement in health and longevity are likely a central motivation for weight loss treatment for many individuals with obesity. At the same time, concerns about physical appearance and body image likely influence the decision to engage in treatment.[13]

These issues may be particularly relevant with respect to bariatric surgery. Patients who present for surgery should be "internally" motivated to seek surgery for improvements in their health and well-being.[43] Patients who are "externally" motivated for surgery, such as those interested in surgery for some secondary gain, such as saving a troubled marriage, may not be psychologically appropriate for surgery. These individuals may have unrealistic beliefs about the impact of the weight loss on other areas of their lives and may become disappointed or despondent if those beliefs are not realized.

Although the weight losses associated with all of the bariatric surgical procedures are impressive when compared with those seen with lifestyle modification or pharmacotherapy, individuals who present for bariatric surgery often have unrealistic expectations regarding the amount of weight they will lose.[44] These unrealistic expectations were once thought to put individuals at risk for weight regain. However, studies have suggested that they are unrelated to postoperative weight losses.

Individuals interested in bariatric surgery may have expectations about the impact of surgery on other areas of their lives. Many people who present for surgery do so with the hope that it will improve not only their health, but also their physical appearance. Individuals who lose weight, regardless of the treatment approach, typically report improvements in their body image.[33,35,36,45,46] However, the massive weight loss typically seen with bariatric surgery may result in the development of loose and/or sagging skin of the abdomen, thighs, legs, and arms that may lead to body image dissatisfaction. This may lead some patients to present to a plastic surgeon for body contouring surgery (discussed later). Others may have expectations about the impact of weight loss on their interpersonal relationships. Many people may intuitively think that as they lose weight, and feel better about themselves, their social and/or romantic relationships will improve. This does occur for many individuals. However, for some, the experience of a major weight loss becomes an unsettling experience. Some individuals may experience unwanted attention related to their weight loss and physical appearance that may make them uncomfortable. Others may be upset or angry that people who treated them as if they were "invisible" before, now are friendly and sociable. Individuals seeking weight loss treatment should consider the potential impact of their weight loss on their marital and sexual relationships. Intuitively, most people would think that these relationships would improve with weight loss. However, body weight can play a much more complex role in some relationships.

EVALUATION OF PSYCHOSOCIAL FUNCTIONING BEFORE WEIGHT LOSS TREATMENT

Given the psychosocial burden of obesity, psychological status and functioning of the patient presenting for weight loss treatment should be evaluated before the onset of treatment.[43] Basic screening can be conducted by several professionals who may be part of a multidisciplinary treatment team. Many of these teams include mental health professional who often conduct more thorough evaluations before the onset of treatment. These professionals also are frequently involved in the delivery of treatment, either lifestyle modification counseling or supportive psychotherapy.

Most bariatric surgery programs in the United States request that candidates undergo a mental health evaluation before surgery.[47–51] These evaluations are often required by insurance companies, who do not provide reimbursement for surgery without mental health clearance. Most of these evaluations are performed by psychologists and social workers. Ideally, these professionals have an appropriate working knowledge of the psychosocial issues involved in obesity and bariatric surgery.

In general, the psychosocial evaluation serves two purposes.[51,52] First, it can identify potential contraindications to surgery, such as substance abuse, poorly controlled depression, or other major psychiatric illness. The evaluation can also help identify potential postoperative challenges and facilitate behavioral changes that can enhance long-term weight management.

In this regard, the evaluation takes on more of a psychoeducational component. Although there are published recommendations regarding the structure and content of these evaluations, consensus guidelines have yet to be established. Almost all evaluations rely on clinical interviews with patients; approximately two-thirds also include instrument or questionnaire measures of psychiatric symptoms and/or objective tests of personality or psychopathology.[28,51,53,54] More comprehensive evaluations assess the patient's knowledge of bariatric surgery, weight and dieting history, eating and activity habits, and potential obstacles and resources that may influence postoperative outcomes.

CHANGES IN PSYCHOSOCIAL FUNCTIONING FOLLOWING WEIGHT LOSS

Weight loss is associated with improvements in morbidity and mortality. Weight losses of 3% to 5% are considered to be clinically significant if associated with improvements in weight-related comorbidities.[49] Larger weight losses, particularly those seen with bariatric surgery, are often associated with dramatic improvements in many weight-related health conditions.[55]

Weight loss also is associated with significant improvements in psychosocial status. Most psychosocial characteristics (including symptoms of depression and anxiety, health- and weight-related quality of life, self-esteem, body image, and sexual functioning) improve with weight loss. These improvements are particularly profound in persons who undergo bariatric surgery. The substantial weight losses seen in the first 6 to 12 months after surgery are associated with dramatic changes in psychosocial status and often endure several years postoperatively.[56]

The impact of weight loss on formal psychopathology is less clear. Psychosocial distress that is secondary to obesity, such as significant body image dissatisfaction or distress about weight-related limitations on functioning, may facilitate weight loss following surgery.[57] In contrast, the presence of significant psychopathology that is independent from the degree of obesity, such as major depression, may inhibit patients' ability to make the necessary dietary and behavioral changes to have the most successful postoperative outcome possible.[2,58,59]

Nevertheless, significant psychopathology is believed to contraindicate weight loss treatment[56]; this issue is most salient when bariatric surgery is considered. In general, active substance abuse, active psychosis, bulimia nervosa, and severe uncontrolled depression are widely considered contraindications to bariatric surgery.[22] However, the presence of severe psychopathology must be balanced with the severity of the obesity and related health problems. Although individuals with severe psychopathology and/or other neurocognitive issues may have less-than-optimal outcomes compared with those persons without those conditions, they still may experience weight losses and improvements in physical and mental health more dramatic than those seen with lifestyle modification or pharmacotherapy.

PSYCHOLOGICAL COMPLICATIONS FOLLOWING WEIGHT LOSS

Although most studies suggest that the psychosocial impact of weight loss is largely positive, these experiences are not universal. Just as some patients experience medical complications, some experience poor behavioral or psychological outcomes. These issues have received the most attention among individuals who have undergone bariatric surgery.

Suboptimal Weight Loss

Approximately 25% of persons who undergo bariatric surgery fail to reach the typical postoperative weight loss or begin to regain large amounts of weight within the first few postoperative years.[13] Suboptimal results are typically attributed to psychosocial and/or behavioral issues, such as poor adherence to the postoperative diet or a return of maladaptive eating behaviors, rather than to surgical factors. Several studies have found that adherence to the postoperative diet is poor and caloric intake often increases significantly during the postoperative period.[13,60,61] Encouragingly, there are a growing number of studies that suggest that behavioral and psychosocial interventions can reverse weight gain after bariatric surgery.[43,62]

Depression and Suicide

Several studies have identified a relationship between depression, suicidality, and obesity.[6,10,63–65] For example, women with obesity are significantly more likely to experience suicidal ideation and to make suicide attempts than their normal-weight counterparts.[6] Persons with extreme obesity have been found to be more likely to attempt suicide than persons in the general population.[7,64]

In general, weight loss is associated with improvements in depressive symptoms. However, several studies have found a higher than expected rate of suicide among persons who have undergone bariatric surgery.[66–69] Given the typically positive relationship between weight loss and psychosocial functioning, these reports are counterintuitive and concerning. Unfortunately, little is known about the psychosocial factors and/or life events that may have contributed to these suicides. In the absence of this information, these findings underscore the importance of ensuring that patients who have psychiatric disorders receive appropriate mental health care before and after bariatric surgery.

Body Image Dissatisfaction

Weight loss is typically associated with improvements in body image.[32] Unfortunately some patients who lose large amounts of weight report, most typically after bariatric surgery, residual body image dissatisfaction associated with loose, sagging skin of the breasts, abdomen, thighs, and arms. Most postbariatric surgery patients consider the development of excess skin to be a negative consequence of surgery. This dissatisfaction likely motivates individuals to present to a plastic surgeon for body contouring procedures, something done by more than 50,000 individuals in 2014.[70]

Substance Abuse

There is concern that some individuals develop substance abuse problems after bariatric surgery. Several years ago, the mass media coined the term "addiction transfer." This term refers to the idea that patients who undergo bariatric surgery may develop addictions to substances, gambling, sex, and so forth to replace their preoperative "addiction" to food. "Addiction transfer" is not an accepted clinical or scientific term. The term and construct have several shortcomings, as detailed by Sogg.[71] Chief among these is that the view of food as an addictive substance, or eating as an addictive behavior, is by no means supported by scientific consensus. Additionally, there is little support for the notion that a treated symptom (eg, compulsive eating) will resurface in a different form (eg, compulsive drinking or shopping) unless the psychological basis for the original problem is resolved.

However, there is some evidence to suggest that individuals who undergo bariatric surgery are at increased risk of problematic substance use. In a seminal study on this issue, using data from approximately 2000 patients across 10 bariatric surgery programs in the United States, King and colleagues[72] found that although the prevalence of alcohol use disorder remained the same 1 year before and after surgery, prevalence increased during the second postoperative year. This increased odds of alcohol use disorder was particularly pronounced in Roux-en-Y gastric bypass procedure patients (as compared with laparoscopic adjustable banding patients); male patients; younger patients; patients who were smokers, regular alcohol consumers, or recreational drug users preoperatively; and patients with a low sense of belonging preoperatively. Furthermore, studies that have found an increased risk of death by suicide following bariatric surgery also have found an elevated risk of accidental death.[66] It is not known how many of those accidental deaths were substance related. Clearly, the effect of bariatric surgery on the risk of substance use disorders is an area in need of further research.

SUMMARY

This article provides an overview of the psychological aspects of obesity. The disease of obesity is associated with a significant psychosocial burden. Many individuals who have obesity also struggle with issues related to their mood, self-esteem, quality of life, and body image. This emotional distress likely plays a role in treatment seeking but also can impact successful treatment. For these reasons, most multidisciplinary obesity treatment teams include mental health professionals who can assess and treat these issues in patients as needed.

Encouragingly, weight loss is typically associated with improvements in psychosocial status and functioning. These positive changes are often most profound among those who have lost large percentages of their weight, as is often seen with bariatric surgery. Unfortunately, some individuals who lose weight experience a return of pre-existing psychopathology or the development of new psychosocial issues. Those who experience weight regain, regardless of the approach to weight loss, also remain at risk for the return of unwanted psychological symptoms. The unfortunate, ubiquitous nature of weight regain reminds all treatment providers of the need to assess psychosocial functioning at the onset of treatment, monitor changes during weight loss, and remain alert for worsening of symptoms with weight regain.

REFERENCES

1. Jones-Corneille LR, Wadden TA, Sarwer DB, et al. Axis I psychopathology in bariatric surgery candidates with and without binge eating disorder: results of structured clinical interviews. Obes Surg 2012;22(3):389–97.
2. Kalarchian MA, Marcus MD, Levine MD, et al. Psychiatric disorders among bariatric surgery candidates: relationship to obesity and functional health status. Am J Psychiatry 2007;164(2):328–34.
3. Legenbauer T, De Zwaan M, Benecke A, et al. Depression and anxiety: their predictive function for weight loss in obese individuals. Obes Facts 2009;2(4): 227–34.
4. Mitchell JE, Selzer F, Kalarchian MA, et al. Psychopathology before surgery in the Longitudinal Assessment of Bariatric Surgery-3 (LABS-3) psychosocial study. Surg Obes Relat Dis 2012;8(5):533–41 [Research Support, N.I.H., Extramural].
5. Rosenberger PH, Henderson KE, Grilo CM. Correlates of body image dissatisfaction in extremely obese female bariatric surgery candidates. Obes Surg 2006;16(10):1331–6 [Research Support, N.I.H., Extramural Research Support, Non-U.S. Gov't].
6. Carpenter KM, Hasin DS, Allison DB, et al. Relationships between obesity and DSM-IV major depressive disorder, suicide ideation, and suicide attempts: results from a general population study. Am J Public Health 2000;90(2):251–7 [Research Support, Non-U.S. Gov'tResearch Support, U.S. Gov't, P.H.S.].
7. Dong C, Li W, Li D, et al. Extreme obesity is associated with attempted suicides: results from a family study. Int J Obes 2006;30(2):388–90.
8. Faith MS, Matz PE, Jorge MA. Obesity–depression associations in the population. J Psychosom Res 2002;53(4):935–42.
9. Stunkard AJ, Faith MS, Allison KC. Depression and obesity. Biol Psychiatry 2003; 54(3):330–7.
10. Onyike CU, Crum RM, Lee HB, et al. Is obesity associated with major depression? Results from the Third National Health and Nutrition Examination Survey. Am J Epidemiol 2003;158(12):1139–47 [Research Support, U.S. Gov't, P.H.S.].
11. Pawlow LA, O'Neil PM, White MA, et al. Findings and outcomes of psychological evaluations of gastric bypass applicants. Surg Obes Relat Dis 2005;1(6):523–7 [discussion: 528–9].

12. Wadden TA, Butryn ML, Sarwer DB, et al. Comparison of psychosocial status in treatment-seeking women with class III vs. class I-II obesity. Surg Obes Relat Dis 2006;2(2):138–45 [Research Support, N.I.H., Extramural].

13. Sarwer DB, Dilks RJ, Ritter S. Bariatric surgery for weight loss. In: Cash TF, editor. Encyclopedia of body image and human appearance, vol. 1. Cambridge (MA): Academic Press; 2012. p. 36–42.

14. American Psychiatric Association. Diagnostic and statistical manual of mental disorders: DSM-5 Arlington. Washington, DC: American Psychiatric Publishing; 2013.

15. Adami GF, Gandolfo P, Bauer B, et al. Binge eating in massively obese patients undergoing bariatric surgery. Int J Eat Disord 1995;17(1):45–50.

16. Hsu LK, Sullivan SP, Benotti PN. Eating disturbances and outcome of gastric bypass surgery: a pilot study. Int J Eat Disord 1997;21(4):385–90.

17. Kalarchian MA, Wilson GT, Brolin RE, et al. Binge eating in bariatric surgery patients. Int J Eat Disord 1998;23(1):89–92.

18. Kalarchian MA, Wilson GT, Brolin RE, et al. Effects of bariatric surgery on binge eating and related psychopathology. Eat Weight Disord 1999;4(1):1–5.

19. Mitchell JE, King WC, Pories W, et al. Binge eating disorder and medical comorbidities in bariatric surgery candidates. Int J Eat Disord 2015;48(5):471–6.

20. Allison KC, Wadden TA, Sarwer DB, et al. Night eating syndrome and binge eating disorder among persons seeking bariatric surgery: prevalence and related features. Obesity (Silver Spring) 2006;14(S3):77S–82S.

21. Stunkard AJ, Allison KC. Two forms of disordered eating in obesity: binge eating and night eating. Int J Obes 2003;27(1):1–12.

22. Mechanick JI, Youdim A, Jones D, et al. AACE/TOS/ASMBS Bariatric Surgery Clinical Practice Guidelines. Endocr Pract 2013;19(2):1–36.

23. Sarwer DB, Moore RH, Spitzer JC, et al. A pilot study investigating the efficacy of postoperative dietary counseling to improve outcomes after bariatric surgery. Surg Obes Relat Dis 2012;8(5):561–8 [Randomized Controlled Trial Research Support, N.I.H., Extramural].

24. Clark MM, Balsiger BM, Sletten CD, et al. Psychosocial factors and 2-year outcome following bariatric surgery for weight loss. Obes Surg 2003;13(5): 739–45.

25. Heinberg LJ, Ashton K. History of substance abuse relates to improved postbariatric body mass index outcomes. Surg Obes Relat Dis 2010;6(4):417–21.

26. Glinski J, Wetzler S, Goodman E. The psychology of gastric bypass surgery. Obes Surg 2001;11(5):581–8.

27. Larsen JK, Geenen R, Van Ramshorst B, et al. Psychosocial functioning before and after laparoscopic adjustable gastric banding: a cross-sectional study. Obes Surg 2003;13(4):629–36.

28. Sarwer DB, Cohn NI, Gibbons LM, et al. Psychiatric diagnoses and psychiatric treatment among bariatric surgery candidates. Obes Surg 2004;14(9):1148–56 [Research Support, U.S. Gov't, P.H.S.].

29. Stout AL, Applegate KL, Friedman KE, et al. Psychological correlates of obese patients seeking surgical or residential behavioral weight loss treatment. Surg Obes Relat Dis 2007;3(3):369–75.

30. Sarwer DB, Faulconbridge LF, Steffen KJ, et al. Managing patients after surgery: changes in drug prescription, body weight can affect psychotropic prescribing. Curr Psychiatr 2010;10(1):3–9.

31. Steffen KJ, Sarwer DB, Thompson JK, et al. Predictors of satisfaction with excess skin and desire for body contouring after bariatric surgery. Surg Obes Relat Dis 2012;8(1):92–7.

32. Sarwer DB, Lavery M, Spitzer J. A review of the relationships between extreme obesity, quality of life, and sexual function. Obes Surg 2012;22(4):668–76.

33. Fabricatore AN, Wadden TA, Sarwer DB, et al. Health-related quality of life and symptoms of depression in extremely obese persons seeking bariatric surgery. Obes Surg 2005;15(3):304–9 [Research Support, N.I.H., Extramural Research Support, U.S. Gov't, P.H.S.].

34. Fontaine KR, Barofsky I. Obesity and health-related quality of life [review]. Obes Rev 2001;2(3):173–82.

35. Kolotkin RL, Head S, Hamilton M, et al. Assessing impact of weight on quality of life. Obes Res 1995;3(1):49–56 [Research Support, Non-U.S. Gov't].

36. Kolotkin RL, Meter K, Williams GR. Quality of life and obesity. Obes Rev 2001; 2(4):219–29.

37. Foster GD, Wadden TA, Vogt RA. Body image in obese women before, during, and after weight loss treatment. Health Psychol 1997;16(3):226–9 [Comparative Study Research Support, U.S. Gov't, P.H.S.].

38. Sarwer DB, Wadden TA, Foster GD. Assessment of body image dissatisfaction in obese women: specificity, severity, and clinical significance. J Consult Clin Psychol 1998;66(4):651–4 [Research Support, U.S. Gov't, P.H.S.].

39. Gustafson TB, Gibbons LM, Sarwer DB, et al. History of sexual abuse among bariatric surgery candidates. Surg Obes Relat Dis 2006;2(3):369–74.

40. Grilo CM, Masheb RM, Brody M, et al. Childhood maltreatment in extremely obese male and female bariatric surgery candidates. Obes Res 2005;13(1): 123–30.

41. Friedman KE, Ashmore JA, Applegate KL. Recent experiences of weight-based stigmatization in a weight loss surgery population: psychological and behavioral correlates. Obesity (Silver Spring) 2008;16(S2):S69–74.

42. Sarwer DB, Fabricatore AN, Eisenberg MH, et al. Self-reported stigmatization among candidates for bariatric surgery. Obesity (Silver Spring) 2008;16(Suppl 2):S75–9 [Research Support, N.I.H., Extramural].

43. Sarwer DB, Butryn ML, Forman EF, et al. Behavioral treatment/lifestyle modification. In: Still C, Sarwer DB, Blankenship J, editors. The ASMBS textbook of bariatric surgery, vol. 2. New York: Springer; 2014. p. 147–57.

44. Foster GD, Wadden TA, Vogt RA, et al. What is a reasonable weight loss? Patients' expectations and evaluations of obesity treatment outcomes. J Consult Clin Psychol 1997;65(1):79–85 [Research Support, U.S. Gov't, P.H.S.].

45. Boan J, Kolotkin RL, Westman EC, et al. Binge eating, quality of life and physical activity improve after Roux-en-Y gastric bypass for morbid obesity. Obes Surg 2004;14(3):341–8.

46. Sarwer DB, Wadden TA, Fabricatore AN. Psychosocial and behavioral aspects of bariatric surgery. Obes Res 2005;13(4):639–48 [Research Support, N.I.H., Extramural Research Support, U.S. Gov't, P.H.S. Review].

47. Buchwald H. Bariatric surgery for morbid obesity: health implications for patients, health professionals, and third-party payers. J Am Coll Surg 2005;200(4): 593–604.

48. Hubbard VS, Hall WH. Gastrointestinal surgery for severe obesity. Obes Surg 1991;1(3):257–65.

49. Jensen MD, Ryan DH, Apovian CM, et al. 2013 AHA/ACC/TOS guideline for the management of overweight and obesity in adults: a report of the American College of Cardiology/American Heart Association Task Force on Practice Guidelines and the Obesity Society. J Am Coll Cardiol 2014;63(25 Pt B):2985–3023.

50. LeMont D, Moorehead MK, Parish MS, et al. Suggestions for the pre-surgical psychological assessment of bariatric surgery candidates. Gainesville (FL): American Society for Bariatric Surgery; 2004. p. 129.

51. Wadden TA, Sarwer DB. Behavioral assessment of candidates for bariatric surgery: a patient-oriented approach. Obesity (Silver Spring) 2006;14:53S–62S.

52. Sarwer DB. Cosmetic surgery. In: Block AR, Sarwer DB, editors. Presurgical psychological screening: understanding patients, improving outcomes. Washington, DC: American Psychological Association; 2013. p. 253–71.

53. Bauchowitz AU, Gonder-Frederick LA, Olbrisch M, et al. Psychosocial evaluation of bariatric surgery candidates: a survey of present practices. Psychosom Med 2005;67(5):825–32.

54. Fabricatore AN, Crerand CE, Wadden TA, et al. How do mental health professionals evaluate candidates for bariatric surgery? Survey results. Obes Surg 2006;16(5):567–73.

55. Jensen MD, Ryan DH, Hu FB, et al. 2013 AHA/ACC/TOS guideline for the management of overweight and obesity in adults. Circulation 2013;129:S102–38.

56. Sarwer DB, Allison KC, Bailer BA. Psychosocial characteristics of bariatric surgery candidates: volume 2 integrated health. In: Still C, Sarwer DB, Blankenship J, editors. The ASMBS textbook of bariatric surgery, vol. 2. New York: Springer; 2014. p. 3–11.

57. Herpertz S, Kielmann R, Wolf A, et al. Do psychosocial variables predict weight loss or mental health after obesity surgery? A systematic review. Obes Res 2004; 12(10):1554–69.

58. de Zwaan M, Enderle J, Wagner S, et al. Anxiety and depression in bariatric surgery patients: a prospective, follow-up study using structured clinical interviews. J Affect Disord 2011;133(1–2):61–8 [Research Support, Non-U.S. Gov't].

59. Legenbauer T, Petrak F, de Zwaan M, et al. Influence of depressive and eating disorders on short- and long-term course of weight after surgical and nonsurgical weight loss treatment. Compr Psychiatry 2011;52(3):301–11 [Multicenter Study].

60. Sarwer DB, Wadden TA, Moore RH, et al. Preoperative eating behavior, postoperative dietary adherence, and weight loss after gastric bypass surgery. Surg Obes Relat Dis 2008;4(5):640–6 [Comparative Study Research Support, N.I.H., Extramural].

61. Sheets CS, Peat CM, Berg KC, et al. Post-operative psychosocial predictors of outcome in bariatric surgery [review]. Obes Surg 2015;25(2):330–45.

62. Livhits M, Mercado C, Yermilov I, et al. Preoperative predictors of weight loss following bariatric surgery: systematic review. Obes Surg 2012;22(1):70–89.

63. Bhatti JA, Nathens AB, Thiruchelvam D, et al. Self-harm emergencies after bariatric surgery: a population-based cohort study. JAMA Surg 2015;151(3):226–32.

64. Heneghan HM, Heinberg L, Windover A, et al. Weighing the evidence for an association between obesity and suicide risk [review]. Surg Obes Relat Dis 2012;8(1):98–107.

65. Mather AA, Cox BJ, Enns MW, et al. Associations of obesity with psychiatric disorders and suicidal behaviors in a nationally representative sample. J Psychosom Res 2009;66(4):277–85.

66. Adams TD, Gress RE, Smith SC, et al. Long-term mortality after gastric bypass surgery. N Engl J Med 2007;357(8):753–61.

67. Arterburn DE, Olsen MK, Smith VA, et al. Association between bariatric surgery and long-term survival. JAMA 2015;313(1):62–70 [Research Support, U.S. Gov't, Non-P.H.S.].

68. Mitchell JE, Crosby R, de Zwaan M, et al. Possible risk factors for increased suicide following bariatric surgery. Obesity (Silver Spring) 2013;21(4):665–72.

69. Tindle HA, Omalu B, Courcoulas A, et al. Risk of suicide after long-term follow-up from bariatric surgery. Am J Med 2010;123(11):1036–42 [Research Support, N.I.H., Extramural].

70. Plastic Surgery Statistics Report. ASPS National Clearinghouse of Plastic Surgery Procedural Statistics. Arlington Heights (IL): American Society of Plastic Surgeons; 2014.

71. Sogg S. Alcohol misuse after bariatric surgery: epiphenomenon or "Oprah" phenomenon? Surg Obes Relat Dis 2007;3(3):366–8.

72. King WC, Chen J, Mitchell JE, et al. Prevalence of alcohol use disorders before and after bariatric surgery. JAMA 2012;307(23):2516–25.

Energy and Nutrient Timing for Weight Control
Does Timing of Ingestion Matter?

Megan A. McCrory, PhD*, Ayla C. Shaw, MS, Joy A. Lee, MS, RD, LD

KEYWORDS

- Eating frequency • Meals • Snacks • Breakfast skipping • Irregular eating
- Meal pattern • Eating pattern • Reported energy intake plausibility

KEY POINTS

- Observational studies on eating patterns for weight control are inconclusive.
- Breakfast is poorly, or inconsistently, defined across studies.
- Experimental studies on the effects of changes in the frequency and timing of eating to weight control are inconclusive and longer-term studies are needed.
- Improved tracking of participant compliance with eating pattern interventions using objective methods is needed.

INTRODUCTION

In 2011 to 2014, the prevalence of adult obesity in the United States was 36.5% and, especially among those aged 20 to 59 years, was higher in women (38%) compared with men (34%).[1] Up by 7.7% since 1999 to 2000, the continued rise in adult obesity is a constant reminder that a solution to the obesity epidemic remains elusive. Increasingly, factors, such as sleep duration and quality[2,3] and the frequency and timing of energy and nutrient intakes,[4,5] are being studied as possible contributors to the epidemic and, therefore, as potential targets for interventions to prevent and treat obesity. The extent to which eating patterns, such as meal skipping, snacking, irregular eating, and the frequency or timing of eating, confer any disadvantage to weight control remains poorly understood. Both the Academy of Nutrition and Dietetics[6] and the 2015 Dietary Guidelines Advisory Committee[7] have recently called attention to these factors, stating that more research is needed on these issues.

The state of the existing research on eating patterns related to frequency and timing is reviewed. This articles focuses on studies in which self-selected diets are

The authors have nothing to disclose.
Department of Nutrition, Georgia State University, PO Box 3995, Atlanta, GA 30302-3995, USA
* Corresponding author.
E-mail address: mmccrory@gsu.edu

Endocrinol Metab Clin N Am 45 (2016) 689–718
http://dx.doi.org/10.1016/j.ecl.2016.04.017   **endo.theclinics.com**

consumed, with the exception of the eating pattern manipulated in experimental studies, and includes observational as well as intervention studies.

EPIDEMIOLOGY OF EATING PATTERNS

The US Department of Agriculture Economic Research Service estimates the per capita energy availability from the food supply (adjusted for spoilage and waste) in the United States increased from 2039 kcal/d in 1970 to 2544 kcal/d in 2010, an increase of 505 kcal/d, or 25%.[8] Other sources, based on US national survey data, show either similar[9,10] or smaller[11,12] increases in energy intake as well as a slight decrease since 2003 to 2004 of 65 kcal/d to 74 kcal/d.[12,13] The increase in energy intake from 1977 to 2006 may have been due to increases in portion size (65 g) and eating frequency (1.1 eating occasions/d).[9] Alternatively, other data[14] show that from 1971 to 2010 (**Fig. 1**), the mean eating frequency has remained at approximately 5 eating occasions per day. These differences in estimates may be attributed to differences in the baseline data set used. **Fig. 1** also shows the mean number of meals per day has stayed consistently at approximately 2.75 meals per day, indicating some individuals do not adhere to the traditional breakfast, lunch, and dinner meal pattern and skip meals, whereas the mean number of snacks has decreased from 2.5 to 2.25 snacks per day for men but increased from 2 to 2.3 snacks per day for women.[14] **Fig. 2** shows that the prevalence of skipping each of the 3 meal occasions increased from the early 1970s to the mid-1990s, then steadily decreased thereafter, although levels remain higher than baseline, with the most common meal skipped being lunch and the least common meal skipped being dinner for both men and women. Approximately two-thirds of Americans report eating breakfast, lunch, and dinner daily, representing a 10% decrease in the prevalence of eating all 3 meals in a day since 1971. The percentages of women consuming greater than or equal to 1 snack per day or greater than or equal to 2 snacks per day have increased, whereas the percentage of men snacking 1 or more times a day has not changed (see **Fig. 2**). Finally, concerning when people are eating, the data show that Americans are consuming breakfast, lunch, and snacks between breakfast and lunch and snacks between lunch and dinner later than previously and that dinner time has not changed, but a snack after dinner is consumed earlier than previously (**Fig. 3**). Overall, eating patterns have shifted toward more meal skipping and more snacking, especially among women, and all eating occasions before dinner are now consumed later, whereas an after-dinner snack is consumed earlier.

EATING FREQUENCY

Eating frequency, or the number of eating occasions per day, is commonly regarded as important for weight control. Specifically, it is said that a higher eating frequency assists with weight control by reducing appetite and/or increasing the metabolic rate or thermic effect of feeding. Studies in which energy intake is controlled, however, often have small sample sizes and are typically, although not always, of short duration.[15] Leidy and Campbell,[16] in reviewing controlled studies, concluded that eating more often than 3 times a day has minimal, if any, benefits to appetite control, and that eating less often than twice a day may have a negative impact on appetite control.

Many of the purported benefits of weight control come from cross-sectional studies in which a large number show an inverse association between eating frequency and adiposity.[17] Bellisle and colleagues[18] in the late 1990s, however, recognized that this association could be an artifact of implausible energy intake reporting, whereby individuals who reported eating less frequently had a higher body mass index (BMI) but also reported a lower total energy intake per day compared with those who

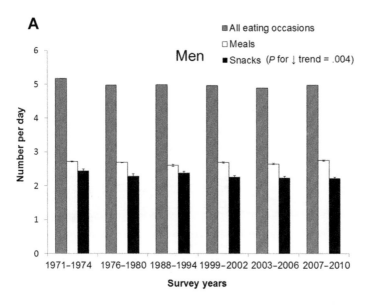

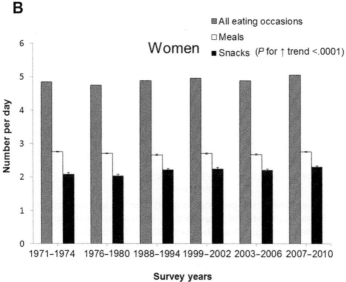

Fig. 1. Changes over time in the number of meals and snacks per day consumed by US men (A) and women (B). (*Data from* Kant AK, Graubard BI. 40-Year trends in meal and snack eating behaviors of American adults. J Acad Nutr Diet 2015;115(1):50–63.)

reported eating more frequently (**Fig. 4**). Such coexisting conditions are impossible because individuals with higher BMI have higher energy expenditure, and, therefore, a high BMI cannot be maintained on a low-energy intake.[19,20] **Tables 1** and **2** show summaries of cross-sectional studies on eating frequency in relation to self-selected energy intake and adiposity, grouped into 2 categories: studies in **Table 1** made no mention of or did not account for implausible energy intake reporting,[21–38] and studies in **Table 2** used a method[28,39] to identify and account for implausible

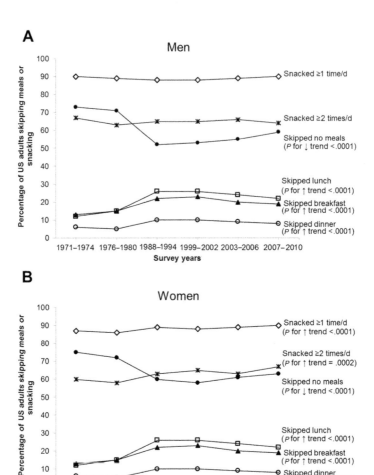

Fig. 2. Changes over time in the percentage of US men (*A*) and women (*B*) skipping meals and snacking. (*Data from* Kant AK, Graubard BI. 40-Year trends in meal and snack eating behaviors of American adults. J Acad Nutr Diet 2015;115(1):50–63.)

energy intake reporters in the analysis.[40–52] These methods rely on the first law of thermodynamics, which states that energy cannot be created or destroyed, so that reported energy intake (rEI) plus the energy cost of weight change equals energy expenditure. Thus, if no weight change ensues, rEI must equal energy expenditure. The data in **Tables 1** and **2** indicate that in the overwhelming majority of study groups (male [M], female [F], or M,F), in which the relationship between eating frequency and energy intake was reported, the relationship was positive.[23,28–31,37,42–48] There was a nonsignificant association in a few of the study groups,[25,26,38,42,51] whereas only 1 had an inverse relationship.[40] Concerning the relationship between eating frequency and adiposity, the findings were more mixed. In **Table 1**, a majority of study groups showed an inverse relationship between eating frequency and adiposity,[27,29,30,32–38] which is consistent with the common belief about this relationship. In **Table 2**, however, approximately half the study groups had nonsignificant relationships,[42–45,47,51,52]

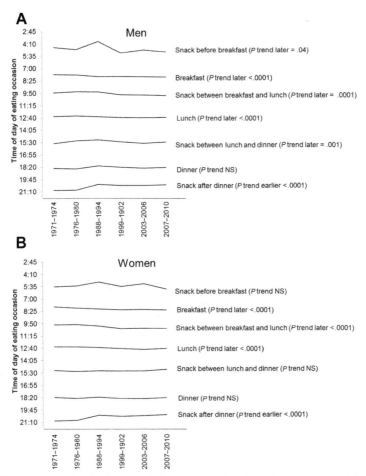

Fig. 3. Changes over time in the time of day that meals and snacks are consumed by US men (A) and women (B). NS, not significant. (*Data from* Kant AK, Graubard BI. 40-Year trends in meal and snack eating behaviors of American adults. J Acad Nutr Diet 2015;115(1):50–63.)

and the remainder were evenly split between positive[28,46,48,49] and inverse relationships.[40–42,45,50] Thus, in studies in which implausible energy intake reporting is taken into consideration during the analysis, the association between eating frequency and adiposity is inconclusive.

Given the findings by Bellisle and coworkers (see **Fig. 4**), the studies in **Tables 1** and **2** were grouped into those that reported inverse, positive, or nonsignificant associations and plotted against the mean rEI as a percentage of energy requirements (ER %). The mean rEI/ER% weighted for the number of subjects included in each analysis was also calculated. In these studies, if energy requirement or energy expenditure was not reported (NR), the energy requirement derived from the Dietary Reference Intake (DRI) equations was used to estimate total energy expenditure, called estimated energy requirement [EER].[53] Average EER of the participants was either provided by the study or estimated using several methods. If a study provided the gender, average age, height, and weight of participants, the appropriate equation for a combined

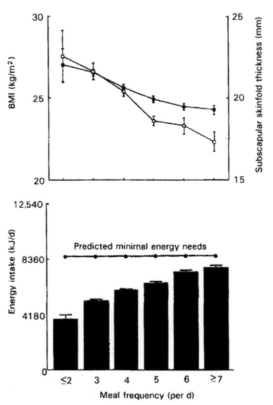

Fig. 4. Measures of adiposity and rEI in the NHANES I Epidemiologic Follow-up Study. Data for women only (*n* 4567). Values are means with their standard errors represented by vertical bars. Predicted minimal energy needs estimated as 1.4× predicted BMR. (●), BMI; (○), subscapular skinfold thickness. BMR, basal metabolic rate. (*From* Bellisle F, McDevitt R, Prentice AM. Meal frequency and energy balance. Br J Nutr 1997;77(Suppl 1):S57–70; with permission.)

nonobese and obese population was used. If any of these values was missing, EER was estimated using DRI tables for 30-year-old men or women with assumed population mean heights of 1.75 m for men and 1.625 m for women and a low active physical activity level, unless mean height was reported. An even distribution between BMI data points was assumed to extrapolate EER values. If enough information was not provided or too many assumptions had to be made, EER was designated as NR. Given a positive relationship between energy intake and eating frequency, a positive relationship would be expected between eating frequency and adiposity, all else being equal. **Fig. 5** shows that studies with negative associations between eating frequency and adiposity have a lower weighted mean rEI/ER% (82.0%) than studies with nonsignificant (85.8%) or positive associations (88.4%). Thus, these combined results suggest that the observed relationship between eating frequency and adiposity in community-dwelling studies may depend on the degree of reported plausibility of energy intake reported by the study sample. A study on secular trends offers support to this suggestion, showing that the inverse association of number of eating episodes with the likelihood of obesity in either men or women was not significant after statistical adjustment for implausible energy intake reporting.[54] Two longitudinal studies, however, have been conducted, both showing a higher number of eating occasions was associated with significantly greater risk of weight gain over 10 years.[29,55] In neither of these studies was energy intake reporting plausibility addressed.

Several randomized controlled trials of the effects of eating frequency on self-selected energy intake and body weight have been conducted (**Table 3**). The older studies tended to be of shorter duration, but, more recently, studies of medium and longer duration have been conducted. Additionally, later studies have included pre-scribed energy restriction, whereas those published before 2008 did not. Five of the 6 studies that reported the energy intake outcome showed no significant effect of eating frequency on energy intake,[56–60] whereas 1 showed a higher energy intake with higher eating frequency.[61] Concerning the effects of eating frequency on weight loss, 6 of the studies showed no significant effect,[56,58,59,62,63] and 4 showed a signif-icant effect.[57,60,64,65] Of the latter, 3 studies showed greater weight loss with higher eating frequency,[57,64,65] whereas 1 showed the opposite.[60] All these studies are prob-lematic in that most were short duration, and compliance with the prescribed eating frequency regimens was either self-reported[56–59,62,66] or NR in the articles.[60,61,63–65] Additionally, meal timing, meal size, dietary composition, and physical activity may have been confounding factors.

IRREGULAR EATING AND SKIPPING MEALS
Irregular Eating

Most intervention studies on eating frequency have eating episodes spaced relatively evenly throughout a day with regard to timing, with approximately the same amount of energy at each eating occasion. In support of this pattern, some evidence exists to suggest that not eating in a regular fashion could be detrimental for body weight and other outcomes, but little work has been done in this area. A cross-sectional study on 3170 adults 60 years old[67] showed that irregular eaters had a higher BMI than reg-ular eaters. Energy intake was NR, but irregular eaters had lower intakes of healthful foods, such as fruits, vegetables, and fish, as well as wine, with no differences in un-healthful foods, such as fatty meats and bacon, between the 2 types of eaters. Those data are consistent with a recent study,[68] which described 4 temporal patterns of intake consumed by 9326 adult National Health and Nutrition Examination Survey (NHANES) 1999 to 2004 participants aged 20 to 65 years. A more evenly spaced pattern of 3 meals per day with no snacks was more strongly associated with a lower prevalence of overweight and obesity and a nutritionally higher-quality diet, as indi-cated by the Healthy Eating Index (2005), than the 3 other temporal patterns, which demonstrated less regularity. More recently, both cross-sectional and longitudinal studies using data from the British Birth Cohort showed associations of eating irreg-ularity with energy intake, BMI, and metabolic syndrome risk, and those associations persisted even after implausible energy intakes were taken into account.[69,70] In 2 small and relatively short randomized controlled trials, unfavorable effects of irregular eating on metabolic and biochemical factors were demonstrated.[71–73] Nine lean[71,72] and 10 obese[73] women followed either a regular meal pattern (6 eating occasions/d) or an irregular meal pattern (3, 6, or 9 eating occasions/d) for 14 days, each using a random-ized crossover study design. The irregular eating pattern resulted in a lower thermic effect of feeding; higher fasting total cholesterol, low-density lipoprotein cholesterol, insulin peak, and insulin area under the curve after a test meal; and additionally, in obese women, a higher energy intake, compared with the regular pattern. Taken together, the results of these studies warrant further investigation of irregular eating patterns.

Table 1
Summary of associations of eating frequency with reported energy intake and adiposity in cross-sectional studies in healthy, nonpregnant, nonlactating adults in which implausible reported energy intakes were not taken into account

Reference, Year	Gender	N	Age, Mean or Range (y)[a]	Body Mass Index, Mean (kg/m²)[a]	Reported Energy Intake (% of Estimated Energy Requirement)[ab]	Eating Frequency Relation with Reported Energy Intake	Eating Frequency Relation with Adiposity
Fabry et al,[27] 1964	M	379	60-64	NR	NR	NR	–
Metzner et al,[33] 1977	M	948	46.4	NR	98[c]	NR	–
	F	1080	45.6	NR	83[c]	NR	–
Dreon et al,[25] 1988	M	155	44.3	29.8	87	NS	NS
Edelstein et al,[26] 1992	M,F	2034	70.4	25.1	84	NS	NS
Kant et al,[29] 1995	M	2580	44.5	25.9	86[c]	+	–
	F	4567	45.9	25.3	69[c]	+	–
Ortega et al,[34] 1998	M,F	150	73.5	26.3	NR	NR	NS[d] –[e]
Wahlqvist et al,[38] 1999	M,F	293	≥70	NR	NR	NS	–
Amosa et al,[21] 2001	F	80	18-27	29.9	NR	NR	NS
Titan et al,[37] 2001	M	6890	57.8	26.4	78[c]	+	–
	F	7776	56.4	25.9	86[c]	+	+

Berteus Forslund et al,[23] 2002	F	177	48.7	31.9	110	+	+
Ma et al,[32] 2003	M	251	48.0	28.6	77[c]	NR	—
	F	248	48.0	26.6	72[c]	NR	—
Berteus Forslund et al,[23] 2005	M	2396	46.6[a]	34.7[a]	98	+	+
	F	2955	44.5[a]	35.4[a]	103	+	+
Huang et al,[28] 2005	M,F	6499	46.5	25.9	83	NR	NS
Kerver et al,[31] 2006	M,F	10,893	≥20	NR	NR	+	NR
Berg et al,[22] 2009	M,F	3610	25–74	NR	NR	NR	NS
Smith et al,[36] 2012	M	1273	31.7	26.7	NR	NR	—
	F	1502	31.5	24.6	NR	NR	NS
Reicks et al,[35] 2014	M,F	2702	18–80	26.8	NR	NR	—
Karatzi et al,[30] 2015	M,F	164	46.8	27.0	84[c]	+	—[f]

Abbreviations: —, negative association; +, positive association; EF, eating frequency; NR, values or information not reported or unable to calculate values due to missing information; NS, not statistically significant.

[a] Values are shown separately for M and F if reported as such in the original publication.
[b] Values are calculated means weighted for N in study groups based on weight status.
[c] EER estimated from DRI equations or tables (see text for method).
[d] Men.
[e] Women.
[f] Study did not adjust for physical activity or age.

Table 2
Summary of associations of eating frequency with reported energy intake and adiposity in cross-sectional studies in healthy, nonpregnant, nonlactating adults in which implausible reported energy intakes were taken into account during analysis

Reference, Year	Gender	N	Age, Mean or Range (y)[a]	Body Mass Index, Mean (kg/m²)[a]	Reported Energy Intake (% of Estimated Energy Requirement or Total Energy Expenditure)[ab]	Eating Frequency Relation with Reported Energy Intake	Eating Frequency Relation with Adiposity
Summerbell et al,[51] 1996	M	71	13–91	22.2	80[c]	NS	NS
	F	149	13–91	23.7	81[c]	NS	NS
Drummond et al,[42] 1998	M	42	37.4	25.3	95	NS	−
	F	37	34.0	22.8	93	+	NS
Ruidavets et al,[50] 2002	M	330	45–64	26.5	84[c]	NR	−
Huang et al,[28] 2005 Howarth et al,[46] 2007	M,F	2685	49.3	25.3	96	+	+[d]
Yannakoulia et al,[52] 2007	F[e]	64	38.6	24.4	83[g]	+	NS (BMI) NS (%BF)
	F[f]	50	57.5	28.0	77[g]	+	NS (BMI) + (%BF)
Duval et al,[43] 2008	F	69	50.0	23.0	95[h]	+	−[d] NS
Hartline-Grafton et al,[44] 2010	F	329	47.3	29.1	88[c]	+	NS

Holmback et al,[45] 2010	M	1355	57.4	NR	97c	+	–
	F	1654	57.1	NR	94c	+	NS
Mills et al,[47] 2011	F	1099	49.6	27.7	93c	+	NS
Bachman et al,[41] 2011	M,F	257	48.4i	25.6i	89c	NR	–d
Murakami & Livingstone,[48] 2014	M	678	42.4	27.3	81c	+	+j
	F	809	42.4	26.8	73c	+	+j
Aljuraiban et al,[40] 2015	M,F	2385	48.9	28.3	99c	–	–
Murikami & Livingstone,[49] 2015	M	9397	≥20	28.6	89	NR	+j
	F	9568	≥20	28.6	82	NR	+j

Abbreviations: −, negative association; %BF, percentage body fat; +, positive association; EF, eating frequency; EI, energy intake; NR, values or information not reported or unable to calculate values due to missing information; NS, not statistically significant; PAEE, physical activity energy expenditure; REE, resting energy expenditure; TEE, total energy expenditure.

a Values are shown separately for M and F if reported as such in the original publication.

b Values are calculated means weighted for N in study groups based on weight status.

c EER estimated from DRI equations or tables (see text for method).

d Not adjusted for physical activity.

e Premenopausal.

f Postmenopausal.

g TEE estimated by Yannakoulia and colleagues from a questionnaire.[52]

h TEE used as reported in Duval and colleagues calculated as 1.11*(PAEE + REE).[43]

i Values are calculated means weighted for N in weight-reduced, normal weight, and overweight groups.

j Significant only after additionally adjusting for EI:TEE.

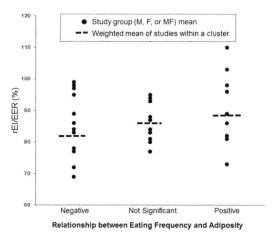

Fig. 5. Relationships between eating frequency and adiposity in cross-sectional studies in relation to the plausibility of self-reported intake. Data shown in **Tables 1** and **2**.

Skipping Meals/Breakfast

Studies on meal skipping associations with energy intake and/or BMI are equivocal.[46,74–76] Most studies on meal skipping have focused on isolating the breakfast meal. It is often cited that individuals who have successfully maintained a weight loss of greater than or equal to 13.6 kg for greater than or equal to 1 year report eating breakfast regularly among other lifestyle habits.[77] Yet, there has been much debate about the importance of breakfast consumption to weight control,[78–81] in particular, whether or not breakfast skipping plays a causal role in weight gain. Cross-sectional studies on breakfast skipping in relation to energy intake and BMI are summarized in **Table 4**. Only 12 of 25 studies reported on the association between breakfast skipping and energy intake.[23,82–93] A majority showed that skipping breakfast was associated with a lower energy intake relative to consuming any breakfast[82,83,85,86,89,91,92] or to specific types of breakfasts,[88,91] whereas 1 reported a higher energy intake with skipping breakfast,[87] and 3 reported a nonsignificant association.[23,90,93] Concerning the association between breakfast skipping and adiposity, findings are somewhat mixed. Fourteen studies showed skipping is associated with higher adiposity (1 in women but not men) relative to consuming any breakfast[75,84,87,89,94–101] or to specific types of breakfasts but not other types,[88,91] whereas 8 showed a nonsignificant association.[23,82,83,85,92,102–104] On the other hand, in 5 prospective studies with follow-ups ranging from 1 year to 10 years (see **Table 4**), all[32,55,84,90] but 1[105] showed that breakfast skipping was associated with greater weight gain. The association between skipping breakfast and energy intake was only reported in 1 of these studies and the association was not significant.[32] The prospective design of these studies, the fact that most controlled for confounding lifestyle factors, and their overall consistency in results lend some support to the possibility of a causal role of breakfast in weight control. Particularly important to the interpretation of the relationship between breakfast skipping and energy intake, however, unlike in at least some of the studies on eating frequency, is that none of these studies took into account the degree of plausibility of rEI. The authors previously reported importance of this issue[17,46] and demonstrated that when energy intake at breakfast, lunch, dinner, and snacks was related to weight status in the total sample, these relationships were positive for only lunch and dinner, but when only the plausible reporters were included, energy intake at all meals and snacks was positively associated with weight status. This analysis suggests that the energy intake may have largely been misreported at breakfast and snacks. The notion that energy intake maybe disproportionately under-reported at these eating occasions is consistent with the observation that fat and sugar are nutrients that tend to be underreported,[106] because breakfasts and snacks often consist of foods high in fat and sugar.

Experimental studies on breakfast skipping are limited. Seven studies in which the intervention period was greater than 1 day are summarized in **Table 5**. Of the 3 that reported energy intake 1 study showed energy intake was higher after the breakfast skipping treatment compared with the breakfast eating treatment,[107] and 2 showed the opposite.[108,109] Of the 6 studies that reported on body weight change,[107,108,110-113] a majority showed no impact of breakfast skipping. In 1 of these studies, in which energy restriction was not prescribed, weight gain was greater in the skipping treatment compared with the 2 eating treatments.[113] In the other study, in which energy restriction was prescribed, there was no main effect of breakfast skipping on weight loss, but there was a marginal interaction effect of the treatment with habitual breakfast habit such that participants whose breakfast treatment differed from their usual habit of skipping or eating breakfast lost more weight than participants whose breakfast treatment was consistent with their usual habit.[111] Usual breakfast habit did not, however, affect the outcome in 2 other intervention studies in which this variable was considered.[109,112]

Many of these studies suffer from methodological limitations besides implausible energy intake reporting. First, breakfast is either defined inconsistently across studies or is not defined by the investigators in most studies, as summarized in **Tables 4** and **5**. Two definitions have been proposed[114,115] but neither of them has been tested for their benefit to weight control or other outcomes. Another problem is that in a majority of observational studies, breakfast skipping was assessed by a questionnaire in which participants recalled how often they usually ate breakfast, and the answers were categorized crudely as well as inconsistently across studies. Additionally, in the intervention studies, compliance with the breakfast skipping or breakfast eating regimens was assessed only by self-report (except in 1 study[113]). The use of new technologies for tracking intake[116-118] should help circumvent this problem in the future.

In addition to the methodological issues, 1 reason why the role of breakfast skipping in energy balance has not been elucidated to date is that breakfast skipping may be a marker for other healthful eating practices that benefit weight control. Furthermore, breakfast skipping is associated with other eating patterns that may also be important for weight control.[89,90,119] For example, in a recent experimental study on the effects of breakfast skipping on eating patterns, it was observed that habitual breakfast skippers ate later in the evening than habitual breakfast eaters, regardless of whether they were undergoing the breakfast skipping or breakfast eating regimen.[109] In another study,[84] the percent of total daily energy intake (%TEI) consumed at breakfast was inversely correlated with %TEI consumed in the evening. Statistical adjustment for %TEI in the evening marginally attenuated the inverse association between %TEI at breakfast and weight change, showing that evening %TEI partly explained that association. As reviewed elsewhere, there is some evidence that a shifted pattern of eating later in the day, due to circadian disruption, may increase the risk for obesity,[120,121] although this may depend on the size of the meal.[122] Thus, breakfast skipping may combine with other eating patterns to affect energy balance. Consistent with this idea, data from a large observational study in Japan[100] showed that the combination of breakfast skipping and late night eating increased the risk for obesity to a greater extent than either of these behaviors alone (**Fig. 6**). Thus, the role of breakfast skipping in weight control is likely complex and requires further study.

Table 3
Summary of effects of eating frequency on changes in reported energy intake and body weight in adults given dietary counseling to follow low or high eating frequencies in randomized controlled trials

Reference, Year	Gender	Physio-Logic or Disease State	N	Age, Mean or Range (y)[a]	Body Mass Index, Mean at Baseline (kg/m²)[a]	Design	Duration of Intervention (wk)	Low Eating Frequency, Goal/Mean Reported (no/d)	High Eating Frequency, Goal/Mean Reported (no/d)	Effects of Eating Frequency on Reported Energy Intake?	Effects of Eating Frequency on Weight Loss?
Without energy restriction											
Arnold et al,[56] 1993	M,F	H	19	32.1	22.2	C	2	3[a]/3.2	9/8.3	N	N
Arnold et al,[57] 1994	M,F	HC	16	49.9	23.7	C	4	3[a]/3.2	9/8.2	N	High > low
McGrath & Gibney,[66] 1994	M	H	23	29.6	25.3	P	3	3/3.3	6/5.9	NR	NR
Arnold et al,[62] 1997	M,F	T2D or IGT	13	46–70	22.8	C	4	3/3.1	9/7.9	NR	N
Thomsen et al,[61] 1997	M,F	T2D	10	60	26.5	C	2	3/NR	8[b]/NR	High > low	N
With energy restriction											
Berteus Forslund et al,[59] 2008	M,F	NR	93	41.2	25.3	P	52	3/3.6	6/5.3	N	N

Study	Sex	Health	N	Age		Design	Weeks				Result
Cameron et al,[63] 2010	M,F	H	16	35.5	23.0	P	8	3/NR	6/NR	NR	N
Bachman & Raynor,[58] 2012	M,F	H	51	51.0	29.1	P	24	3/3	GR[c]/5.8	N	N
Kahleova et al,[60] 2014[d]	M,F	T2D	54	59.4	32.6	C	12	2/NR	6/NR	N	Low > high
Saheli et al,[65] 2014	M,F	T2D	84	35–65	NR	P	12	5[e]/NR	6[e]/NR	NR	High > low
Hatami Zargaran et al,[64] 2014	M,F	H	90	37	30.6	P	12	5[e]/NR	6[e]/NR	NR	High > low

Abbreviations: EF, eating frequency; GR, grazing; H, healthy; HC, hypercholesterolemic; IGT, impaired glucose tolerance; L, lactating; N, no; NR, values or information not reported or unable to calculate values due to missing information; RCT, randomized controlled trial; T2D, type 2 diabetic; Y, yes.
[a] One 36-kJ or two 18-kJ snacks were also allowed.
[b] Food provided for 5 of 8 eating occasions.
[c] Defined as consuming ≥100 kcal every 2 to 3 h.
[d] Food provided for half the participants.
[e] Three large meals and 2 small snacks versus 6 isocaloric eating occasions.

Table 4
Summary of associations of breakfast skipping with energy intake, adiposity, and weight change in cross-sectional and prospective studies in healthy, nonpregnant, nonlactating adults in which implausible reported energy intakes were not taken into account

Reference, Year	Gender	N	Age, Mean or Range (y)[a]	Breakfast Definition	Breakfast Skipping Definition	Method to Assess Breakfast	Energy Intake, Skippers Relative to Consumers	Adiposity, Skippers Relative to Consumers
Cross-sectional studies								
Berteus Forslund et al,[23] 2002	F	177	48.7	Meal eaten 6:00 AM–9:59 AM	No meal usually eaten 6:00 AM–9:59 AM	Meal Pattern grid	NS[a]	NS[a]
Keski-Rahkonen et al,[94] 2003	M,F	4660	32.2–69.8	Meal eaten before going to school or work	BF eaten ≤1×/wk or "a few" ×/wk	Q	NR	NS (OW) ↑ (OB)
Song et al,[82] 2005	M,F	4218	50.4	By participant	No BF	1× MP24hDR	↓	NS (OW + OB)
Williams,[83] 2005	M,F	10,851	≥19	By participant	BF eaten <5 d/wk	Q	↓[b]	NS[b]
Marin-Guerrero et al,[75] 2008	M,F	34,974	43.5	By participant	Not eaten BF regularly in past 6 mo	Q7d diary	NR	↑
Purslow et al,[84] 2008	M,F	6764	61.4	By participant	Q1 of EI at BF or before BF, 0%–11% of total EI	7d diary	↓[b]	↑[b]
Hingorjo et al,[95] 2009	M,F	192	18.9	By participant	NR	Q	NR	↑[b]

Study	Sex	N	Age	BF definition	BF comparison	Method	Outcome	Outcome
Nishiyama et al,[102] 2009	M,F	493	52.0	By participant	Not eating BF >3×/wk	Q	NR	NS[a]
Huang et al,[96] 2010	M,F	15,340	38.7	By participant	BF eaten ≤1×/wk	Q	NR	↑ (OB)
Min et al,[85] 2011	M,F	415	42.7	Meal eaten in the morning	BF eaten ≤1 of 3 d	1× MP24hDR + 2d diary	↓	NS[a]
Fugelstad et al,[103] 2012	M,F	419	47.0	By participant	BF eaten <7 d/wk	Q	NR	NS[a]
Mesas et al,[86] 2012	M,F	10,791	46.3	By participant	Never eat food at BF	Q	→	NR
Azadbakht et al,[87] 2013	F	411	20	Food or beverage (except water) before 10 AM	BF eaten <5 d/wk	Q	↑	↑[b]
Deshmukh-Taskar et al,[88] 2013	M,F	5316	NR	By participant	No intake besides water at BF or brunch	1× MP24hDR	↓ (vs RTEC) NS (other BF)	↑ (vs RTEC) NS (other BF)
Mekary et al,[89] 2013	M	29,206	58.1	Ey participant	BF not usually eaten in past 1 y	Q	→	↑
Odegaard et al,[90] 2013	M,F	3598	32.1	Ey participant	BF eaten 0–3 d/wk or 4–6 d/wk	Q	NS	NR
Smith et al,[98] 2013	M,F	15,747	≥17	Ey participant	BF eaten ≤5 d/wk	Q	NR	↑ (weight gain in past 1 y)

(continued on next page)

Table 4
(continued)

Reference, Year	Gender	N	Age, Mean or Range (y)[a]	Breakfast Definition	Breakfast Skipping Definition	Method to Assess Breakfast	Energy Intake, Skippers Relative to Consumers	Adiposity, Skippers Relative to Consumers
Bjornara et al,[97] 2014	M,F	6512	41	By participant	BF eaten <7 d/wk	Q	NR	NS (OW)[a] ↑ (OB)[a]
Goyal & Julka,[99] 2014	M,F	186	46.5	By participant	NR	Q	NR	↑[b]
Kutsuma et al,[100] 2014	M,F	60,800	43.8	By participant	BF eaten <4 d/wk	Q	NR	↑ (OB)
O'Neil et al,[91] 2014	M,F	18,988	NR	By participant	No intake besides water at BF	1× MP24hDR	↓ (vs 4 of 11 BF types)[c] NS (vs other BF)	↑ (vs 4 of 11 BF types)[d] NS (vs other BF)
Watanabe et al,[92] 2014	M,F	766	55	By participant	BF not usually eaten	Q	↓	NS[a]
Thomas et al,[93] 2015	F	18	29	By participant	BF <5 d/wk	Q	NS	NR[b]
Witbracht et al,[104] 2015	F	65	18–45	≥15% of est. total energy needs in solid food between 4:00 AM–10:00 AM ≥6×/wk	No intake of solid food 4–10 AM ≥4 d/wk	3× 24hDR	NR	NS[a]
Maksimovic et al,[101] 2016	M,F	12,461	≥20	By participant	NR	Q	NR	↑ (OW, OB F) NS (OW, OB M)

Prospective studies

Study	Sex	N	Age		Definition	Method		Outcome
Ma et al,[32] 2003	M,F	499	48	By participant	No BF on 75% of DR days	3 × 24hDR baseline and every 3 mo	NS	↑ (1 y weight gain)
Nooyens et al,[105] 2005	M	288	54.8	By participant	Number of d/wk BF not eaten	Q	NR	NS (5 y weight gain)
Van der Heijden et al,[55] 2007	M	20,064	57.3	By participant	BF not usually eaten in past 1 y	Q	NR	↑ (10 y weight gain)[a]
Purslow et al,[84] 2008	M,F	6764	61.4	By participant	Q1 of EI at BF or before BF, 0%–11% of total EI	7d diary	NR	↑ (3.7 y weight gain)
Odegaard et al,[90] 2013	M,F	3598	32.1	By participant	BF eaten 0–3 d/wk or 4–6 d/wk	Q	NR	↑ (vs daily) NS (vs 4–6 d/wk for 7 y weight gain)

Abbreviations: "by participant", no definition given by investigator or participant self-defined; BF, breakfast; DR, dietary recall; MP, multiple pass; NR, values or information not reported or unable to calculate values due to missing information; NS, not statistically significant; PA, physical activity; Q, question(s) or questionnaire; RTEC, ready-to-eat cereal.

[a] Not controlled for PA.

[b] Study did not control for any covariates.

[c] Grain/fruit juice; grain; presweetened RTEC with lower-fat milk; RTEC/lower-fat milk/whole fruit/fruit juice; coffee with cream anc sugar/sweets.

[d] Grain/fruit juice; grain; presweetened RTEC with lower-fat milk; RTEC/lower-fat milk/whole fruit/fruit juice; cooked cereal.

Table 5
Summary of effects of breakfast skipping on changes in reported energy intake and body weight in adults in randomized controlled trials lasting greater than 1 day

Reference, Year	Gender	N	Age, Mean or Range (y)[a]	Body Mass Index, Mean at Baseline (kg/m²)[a]	Design	Duration of Intervention (wk)	Breakfast Treatment	Breakfast Skipping Treatment	Effects of Breakfast Skipping on Reported Energy Intake?	Effects of Breakfast Skipping on Weight Loss?
With energy restriction										
Schlundt et al,[111] 1992	F	52	NR	30.5	P	12	BF cereal provided plus advice to eat 3 meals/d for a total of 1200 kcal/d	Bran muffins for eating occasions other than BF provided plus advice to eat lunch and dinner, for a total of 1200 kcal/d	NR	NS; marginally significant BF × habitual BF pattern (P = .10); those who changed pattern lost more weight[a]
Without energy restriction										
Tuttle et al,[110] 1950	M	11	22–28	NR	C	3	750 kcal BF provided at 7:00 AM–8:00 AM	No food 8:00 AM–12:00 PM	NR	NS
Farshchi et al,[107] 2005	F	10	25.5	23.2	C	2	Cereal + milk provided at 7:00 AM–8:00 AM; snack provided at 10:30 AM–11:00 AM	Snack provided at 10:30 AM–11:00 AM Cereal + milk provided at 12:00 PM–12:30 PM	BFS > BF	NS

Study	Sex	N			Design	Wk	BF	BFS		
Betts et al,[108] 2014	M,F	22	36	22.4	P	6	Instructions to consume ≥700 kcal before 11:00 AM, at least half consumed within 2 h of waking.	Instructions to fast until 12:00 PM	BF > BFS	NS
Dhurandhar et al,[112] 2014	M,F	283	41.6	32.4	P	16	Instructions to consume BF before 10:00 AM[ab]	Instructions not to consume any calories before 11:00 AM[ab]	NR	NS
Geliebter et al,[113] 2014	M,F	36	33.9	32.8	P	4	352 kcal cereal BF provided to 2 groups: coffee[c] + oat porridge or frosted flakes	11 kcal coffee[c]	NR	BFS > both BF groups
Reeves et al,[109] 2014	M,F	37	29.5 (NW) 36.2 (OW)	21.6 (NW) 26.9 (OW)	C	1	Instructions to consume BF daily within 1 h of waking[a]	Instructions not to eat until mid-day[a]	BF > BFS	NR

Abbreviations: BF, breakfast; BFS, breakfast skipping; C, crossover; EF, eating frequency; N, no; NR, values or information not reported or unable to calculate values due to missing information; NW, normal weight; OW, overweight; P, parallel; RCT, randomized controlled trial; Y, yes.

[a] BF and BFS groups were stratified so that half the participants in each group were habitual BF eaters and half were habitual BF skippers.

[b] Both groups and an additional control group were given a "Let's Eat for the Health of It" pamphlet.

[c] Plus 12 mL nondairy creamer and 1 artificial sweetener packet.

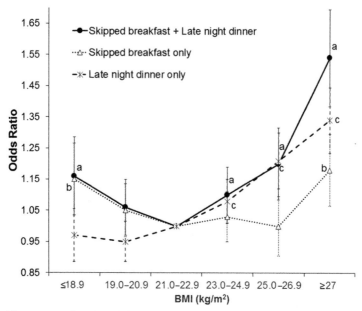

Fig. 6. Odds ratios predicting risk for obesity in individuals who skipped breakfast only, ate late at night only, or did both. a, skipped breakfast + late night dinner; b, skipped breakfast only; c, late night dinner. (*Data from* Kutsuma A, Nakajima K, Suwa K. Potential association between breakfast skipping and concomitant late-night-dinner eating with metabolic syndrome and proteinuria in the Japanese population. Scientifica (Cairo) 2014;2014:253581.)

FUTURE CONSIDERATIONS/SUMMARY

As the obesity prevalence has increased among the American population, eating patterns have also changed toward more frequent snacking and meal skipping, eating later, and larger portions. Observational studies of associations of self-selected eating patterns with energy intake and adiposity are largely inconclusive due to mixed findings and shortcomings, including a lack of standardized approaches toward defining and measuring eating occasions and implausible reporting of energy intake. Although implausible reporting can be accounted for by several approaches during analysis, most researchers have not taken advantage of the opportunity to do so. Experimental studies mostly show little impact of eating frequency and skipping breakfast on adiposity, but few studies have been done, most intervention periods were only a few weeks, and all suffered from inadequate monitoring of compliance with the intervention. In many studies, other eating patterns that covary with the one being examined have not been controlled. Improvement of methodology is necessary in future studies before firm conclusions can be made. An emerging body of research suggests that irregular eating patterns and the distribution of energy throughout the day may be important for weight control, and further study is required in these areas. Additionally, investigations should be performed to identify the extent to which personal and/or lifestyle factors, such as genetics,[123–125] chronotype,[126] and sleep habit,[127] influence the impact of energy and nutrient timing on weight control. Finally, limited experimental evidence in humans suggests that other qualities related to timing, including the relative size of meals in the morning versus evening[128–130] and the macronutrient distribution at selected eating occasions or times of day,[131–133] may also be important for weight control. These issues require further study.

REFERENCES

1. Ogden CL, Carroll MD, Fryar CD, et al. Prevalence of obesity among adults and youth: United States, 2011-2014. NCHS Data Brief 2015;(219):1–8.

2. Capers PL, Fobian AD, Kaiser KA, et al. A systematic review and meta-analysis of randomized controlled trials of the impact of sleep duration on adiposity and components of energy balance. Obes Rev 2015;16(9):771–82.

3. Chaput JP. Sleep patterns, diet quality and energy balance. Physiol Behav 2014;134:86–91.

4. Gletsu-Miller N, McCrory MA. Modifying eating behavior: novel approaches for reducing body weight, preventing weight regain, and reducing chronic disease risk. Adv Nutr 2014;5(6):789–91.

5. Schoenfeld BJ, Aragon AA, Krieger JW. Effects of meal frequency on weight loss and body composition: a meta-analysis. Nutr Rev 2015;73(2):69–82.

6. Raynor HA, Champagne CM. Position of the Academy of Nutrition and Dietetics: Interventions for the Treatment of Overweight and Obesity in Adults. J Acad Nutr Diet 2016;116(1):129–47.

7. Committee on Dietary Guidelines for Americans, 2005. Scientific report. Available at: http://health.gov/dietaryguidelines/2015-scientific. Accessed December 31, 2015.

8. ERS/USDA. Average daily per capita calories from the U.S. food availability, adjusted for spoilage and other waste. 2015. Available at: http://ers.usda.gov/data-products/food-availability-(per-capita)-data-system/.asp. Accessed December 31, 2015.

9. Duffey KJ, Popkin BM. Energy density, portion size, and eating occasions: contributions to increased energy intake in the United States, 1977-2006. PLoS Med 2011;8(6):e1001050.

10. Yancy WS Jr, Wang CC, Maciejewski ML. Trends in energy and macronutrient intakes by weight status over four decades. Public Health Nutr 2014;17(2):256–65.

11. Austin GL, Ogden LG, Hill JO. Trends in carbohydrate, fat, and protein intakes and association with energy intake in normal-weight, overweight, and obese individuals: 1971-2006. Am J Clin Nutr 2011;93(4):836–43.

12. Ford ES, Dietz WH. Trends in energy intake among adults in the United States: findings from NHANES. Am J Clin Nutr 2013;97(4):848–53.

13. Ng SW, Slining MM, Popkin BM. Turning point for US diets? Recessionary effects or behavioral shifts in foods purchased and consumed. Am J Clin Nutr 2014;99(3):609–16.

14. Kant AK, Graubard BI. 40-year trends in meal and snack eating behaviors of American adults. J Acad Nutr Diet 2015;115(1):50–63.

15. Mattson MP. The need for controlled studies of the effects of meal frequency on health. Lancet 2005;365:1978–80.

16. Leidy HJ, Campbell WW. The effect of eating frequency on appetite control and food intake: brief synopsis of controlled feeding studies. J Nutr 2011;141(1):154–7.

17. McCrory MA, Howarth NC, Roberts SB, et al. Eating frequency and energy regulation in free-living adults consuming self-selected diets. J Nutr 2011;141(1):148–53.

18. Bellisle F, McDevitt R, Prentice AM. Meal frequency and energy balance. Br J Nutr 1997;77(Suppl 1):S57–70.

19. Das SK, Saltzman E, McCrory MA, et al. Energy expenditure is very high in extremely obese women. J Nutr 2004;134(6):1412–6.

20. Lichtman SW, Pisarska K, Berman ER, et al. Discrepancy between self-reported and actual caloric intake and exercise in obese subjects. N Engl J Med 1992; 327:1893–9.

21. Amosa T, Rush E, Plank L. Frequency of eating occasions reported by young New Zealand Polynesian and European women. Pac Health Dialog 2001;8(1): 59–65.

22. Berg C, Lappas G, Wolk A, et al. Eating patterns and portion size associated with obesity in a Swedish population. Appetite 2009;52(1):21–6.

23. Berteus Forslund H, Lindroos AK, Sjostrom L, et al. Meal patterns and obesity in Swedish women-a simple instrument describing usual meal types, frequency and temporal distribution. Eur J Clin Nutr 2002;56(8):740–7.

24. Berteus Forslund H, Torgerson JS, Sjostrom L, et al. Snacking frequency in relation to energy intake and food choices in obese men and women compared to a reference population. Int J Obes 2005;29(6):711–9.

25. Dreon DM, Frey-Hewitt B, Ellsworth N, et al. Dietary fat: carbohydrate ratio and obesity in middle aged men. Am J Clin Nutr 1988;47:995–1000.

26. Edelstein SL, Barrett-Connor EL, Wingard DL, et al. Increased meal frequency associated with decreased cholesterol concentrations; Rancho Bernardo, CA 1984-1987. Am J Clin Nutr 1992;55:664–9.

27. Fabry P, Fodor J, Hejl Z, et al. The frequency of meals: its relation to overweight, hypercholesterolaemia, and decreased glucose-tolerance. Lancet 1964;2: 614–5.

28. Huang TT, Roberts SB, Howarth NC, et al. Effect of screening out implausible energy intake reports on relationships between diet and BMI. Obes Res 2005; 13(7):1205–17.

29. Kant AK, Schatzkin A, Graubard BI, et al. Frequency of eating occasions and weight change in the NHANES I Epidemiologic Follow-Up Study. Int J Obes 1995;19:468–74.

30. Karatzi K, Yannakoulia M, Psaltopoulou T, et al. Meal patterns in healthy adults: Inverse association of eating frequency with subclinical atherosclerosis indexes. Clin Nutr 2015;34(2):302–8.

31. Kerver JM, Yang EJ, Obayashi S, et al. Meal and snack patterns are associated with dietary intake of energy and nutrients in US adults. J Amer Diet Assoc 2006; 106:46–53.

32. Ma Y, Bertone ER, Stanek EJI, et al. Association between eating patterns and obesity in a free-living US adult population. Am J Epidemiol 2003;158:85–92.

33. Metzner HL, Lamphiear DE, Wheeler NC, et al. The relationship between frequency of eating and adiposity in adult men and women in the Tecumseh Community Health Study. Am J Clin Nutr 1977;30:712–5.

34. Ortega RM, Redondo MR, Zamora MJ, et al. Relationship between the number of daily meals and the energy and nutrient intake in the elderly. Effect on various cardiovascular risk factors. Nutr Hosp 1998;13(4):186–92 [in Spanish].

35. Reicks M, Degeneffe D, Rendahl A, et al. Associations between eating occasion characteristics and age, gender, presence of children and BMI among U.S. adults. J Am Coll Nutr 2014;33(4):315–27.

36. Smith KJ, Blizzard L, McNaughton SA, et al. Daily eating frequency and cardiometabolic risk factors in young Australian adults: cross-sectional analyses. Br J Nutr 2012;108(6):1086–94.

37. Titan SMO, Bingham S, Welch A, et al. Frequency of eating and concentrations of serum cholesterol in the norfolk population of the European prospective investigation into cancer (EPIC-Norfolk): cross-sectional study. BMJ 2001;323:1–5.

38. Wahlqvist ML, Kouris-blazos A, Wattanapenpaiboon N. The significance of eating patterns: an elderly Greek case study. Appetite 1999;32(1):23–32.

39. Black AE. Critical evaluation of energy intake using the Goldberg cut-off for energy intake:basal metabolic rate. A practical guide to its calculation, use and limitations. Int J Obes 2000;24:1119–30.

40. Aljuraiban GS, Chan Q, Oude Griep LM, et al. The impact of eating frequency and time of intake on nutrient quality and body mass index: the INTERMAP Study, a Population-Based Study. J Acad Nutr Diet 2015;115(4):528–36.e1.

41. Bachman JL, Phelan S, Wing RR, et al. Eating frequency is higher in weight loss maintainers and normal-weight individuals than in overweight individuals. J Am Diet Assoc 2011;111(11):1730–4.

42. Drummond SE, Crombie NE, Cursiter MC, et al. Evidence that eating frequency is inversely related to body weight status in male, but not female, non-obese adults reporting valid dietary intakes. Int J Obes 1998;22:105–12.

43. Duval K, Strychar I, Cyr MJ, et al. Physical activity is a confounding factor of the relation between eating frequency and body composition. Am J Clin Nutr 2008; 88(5):1200–5.

44. Hartline-Grafton HL, Rose D, Johnson CC, et al. The influence of weekday eating patterns on energy intake and BMI among female elementary school personnel. Obesity 2010;18(4):736–42.

45. Holmback I, Ericson U, Gullberg B, et al. A high eating frequency is associated with an overall healthy lifestyle in middle-aged men and women and reduced likelihood of general and central obesity in men. Br J Nutr 2010;104(7):1065–73.

46. Howarth NC, Huang TTK, Roberts SB, et al. Eating patterns and dietary composition in relation to BMI in younger and older adults. Int J Obes 2007;31:675–84.

47. Mills JP, Perry CD, Reicks M. Eating frequency is associated with energy intake but not obesity in midlife women. Obesity 2011;19(3):552–9.

48. Murakami K, Livingstone MB. Eating frequency in relation to body mass index and waist circumference in British adults. Int J Obes 2014;38(9):1200–6.

49. Murakami K, Livingstone MB. Eating frequency is positively associated with overweight and central obesity in US adults. J Nutr 2015;145(12):2715–24.

50. Ruidavets JB, Bongard V, Bataille V, et al. Eating frequency and body fatness in middle-aged men. Int J Obes 2002;26:1476–83.

51. Summerbell CD, Moody RC, Shanks J, et al. Relationship between feeding pattern and body mass index in 220 free-living people in four age groups. Eur J Clin Nutr 1996;50:513–9.

52. Yannakoulia M, Melistas L, Solomou E, et al. Association of eating frequency with body fatness in pre- and postmenopausal women. Obesity 2007;15(1): 100–6.

53. Institute of Medicine. Dietary reference intakes for energy, carbohydrate, fiber, fat, fatty acids, cholesterol, protein, and amino acids, Part I. Washington, DC: National Academy of Sciences; 2005.

54. Kant AK, Graubard BI. Secular trends in patterns of self-reported food consumption of adult americans: NHANES 1971-1975 to NHANES 1999-2002. Am J Clin Nutr 2006;84:1215–23.

55. van der Heijden AA, Hu FB, Rimm EB, et al. A prospective study of breakfast consumption and weight gain among U.S. men. Obesity 2007;15(10):2463–9.

56. Arnold LA, Bell MJ, Duncan AW, et al. Effect of isoenergetic intake of three or nine meals on plasma lipoproteins and glucose metabolism. Am J Clin Nutr 1993;57:446–51.

57. Arnold L, Ball M, Mann J. Metabolic effects of alterations in meal frequency in hypercholesterolaemic individuals. Atherosclerosis 1994;108(2):167–74.

58. Bachman JL, Raynor HA. Effects of manipulating eating frequency during a behavioral weight loss intervention: a pilot randomized controlled trial. Obesity 2012;20(5):985–92.

59. Berteus Forslund H, Klingstrom S, Hagberg H, et al. Should snacks be recommended in obesity treatment? A 1-year randomized clinical trial. Eur J Clin Nutr 2008;62(11):1308–17.

60. Kahleova H, Belinova L, Malinska H, et al. Eating two larger meals a day (breakfast and lunch) is more effective than six smaller meals in a reduced-energy regimen for patients with type 2 diabetes: a randomised crossover study. Diabetologia 2014;57(8):1552–60.

61. Thomsen C, Christiansen C, Rasmussen OW, et al. Comparison of the effects of two weeks' intervention with different meal frequencies on glucose metabolism, insulin sensitivity and lipid levels in non-insulin-dependent diabetic patients. Ann Nutr Metab 1997;41:173–80.

62. Arnold L, Mann JI, Ball MJ. Metabolic effects of alterations in meal frequency in type 2 diabetes. Diabetes Care 1997;20(11):1651–4.

63. Cameron JD, Cyr MJ, Doucet E. Increased meal frequency does not promote greater weight loss in subjects who were prescribed an 8-week equi-energetic energy-restricted diet. Br J Nutr 2010;103(8):1098–101.

64. Hatami Zargaran Z, Salehi M, Heydari ST, et al. The effects of 6 isocaloric meals on body weight, lipid profiles, leptin, and adiponectin in overweight Subjects (BMI > 25). Int Cardiovasc Res J 2014;8(2):52–6.

65. Salehi M, Kazemi A, Hasan Zadeh J. The effects of 6 isocaloric meals pattern on blood lipid profile, glucose, hemoglobin a1c, insulin and malondialdehyde in type 2 diabetic patients: a randomized clinical trial. Iran J Med Sci 2014; 39(5):433–9.

66. McGrath SA, Gibney MJ. The effects of altered frequency of eating on plasma lipids in free-living healthy males on normal self-selected diets. Eur J Clin Nutr 1994;48:402–7.

67. Sierra-Johnson J, Unden AL, Linestrand M, et al. Eating meals irregularly: a novel environmental risk factor for the metabolic syndrome. Obesity 2008; 16(6):1302–7.

68. Eicher-Miller HA, Khanna N, Boushey CJ, et al. Temporal dietary patterns derived among the adult participants of the national health and nutrition examination survey 1999-2004 are associated with diet quality. J Acad Nutr Diet 2016; 116(2):283–91.

69. Pot GK, Hardy R, Stephen AM. Irregular consumption of energy intake in meals is associated with a higher cardiometabolic risk in adults of a British birth cohort. Int J Obes 2014;38(12):1518–24.

70. Pot GK, Hardy R, Stephen AM. Irregularity of energy intake at meals: prospective associations with the metabolic syndrome in adults of the 1946 British birth cohort. Br J Nutr 2016;115(2):315–23.

71. Farshchi HR, Taylor MA, Macdonald IA. Regular meal frequency creates more appropriate insulin sensitivity and lipid profiles compared with irregular meal frequency in healthy lean women. Eur J Clin Nutr 2004;58:1071–7.

72. Farshchi HR, Taylor MA, Macdonald IA. Decreased thermic effect of food after an irregular compared with a regular meal pattern in healthy lean women. Int J Obes 2004;28:653–60.

73. Farshchi HR, Taylor MA, Macdonald IA. Beneficial metabolic effects of regular meal frequency on dietary thermogenesis, insulin sensitivity, and fasting lipid profiles in healthy obese women. Am J Clin Nutr 2005;81(1):16–24.

74. Carels RA, Young KM, Coit C, et al. Skipping meals and alcohol consumption. The regulation of energy intake and expenditure among weight loss participants. Appetite 2008;51(3):538–45.

75. Marin-Guerrero AC, Gutierrez-Fisac JL, Guallar-Castillon P, et al. Eating behaviours and obesity in the adult population of Spain. Br J Nutr 2008;100(5):1142–8.

76. Kuroda T, Onoe Y, Yoshikata R, et al. Relationship between skipping breakfast and bone mineral density in young Japanese women. Asia Pac J Clin Nutr 2013;22(4):583–9.

77. Wing RR, Phelan S. Long-term weight loss maintenance. Am J Clin Nutr 2005; 82(Suppl):222S–5S.

78. Brown AW, Bohan Brown MM, Allison DB. Belief beyond the evidence: using the proposed effect of breakfast on obesity to show 2 practices that distort scientific evidence. Am J Clin Nutr 2013;98(5):1298–308.

79. Zilberter T, Zilberter EY. Breakfast: to skip or not to skip? Front Public Health 2014;2:59.

80. Casazza K, Brown A, Astrup A, et al. Weighing the evidence of common beliefs in obesity research. Crit Rev Food Sci Nutr 2015;55(14):2014–53.

81. Levitsky DA. Breaking the feast. Am J Clin Nutr 2015;102(3):531–2.

82. Song WO, Chun OK, Obayashi S, et al. Is consumption of breakfast associated with body mass index in US adults? J Am Diet Assoc 2005;105:1373–82.

83. Williams P. Breakfast and the diets of Australian adults: an analysis of data from the 1995 National Nutrition Survey. Int J Food Sci Nutr 2005;56(1):65–79.

84. Purslow LR, Sandhu MS, Forouhi N, et al. Energy intake at breakfast and weight change: prospective study of 6,764 middle-aged men and women. Am J Epidemiol 2008;167(2):188–92.

85. Min C, Noh H, Kang YS, et al. Skipping breakfast is associated with diet quality and metabolic syndrome risk factors of adults. Nutr Res Pract 2011;5(5):455–63.

86. Mesas AE, Guallar-Castillon P, Leon-Munoz LM, et al. Obesity-related eating behaviors are associated with low physical activity and poor diet quality in Spain. J Nutr 2012;142(7):1321–8.

87. Azadbakht L, Haghighatdoost F, Feizi A, et al. Breakfast eating pattern and its association with dietary quality indices and anthropometric measurements in young women in Isfahan. Nutrition 2013;29(2):420–5.

88. Deshmukh-Taskar P, Nicklas TA, Radcliffe JD, et al. The relationship of breakfast skipping and type of breakfast consumed with overweight/obesity, abdominal obesity, other cardiometabolic risk factors and the metabolic syndrome in young adults. The National Health and Nutrition Examination Survey (NHANES): 1999-2006. Public Health Nutr 2013;16(11):2073–82.

89. Mekary RA, Giovannucci E, Cahill L, et al. Eating patterns and type 2 diabetes risk in older women: breakfast consumption and eating frequency. Am J Clin Nutr 2013;98(2):436–43.

90. Odegaard AO, Jacobs DR Jr, Steffen LM, et al. Breakfast frequency and development of metabolic risk. Diabetes Care 2013;36(10):3100–6.

91. O'Neil CE, Nicklas TA, Fulgoni VL 3rd. Nutrient intake, diet quality, and weight/adiposity parameters in breakfast patterns compared with no breakfast in adults: National Health and Nutrition Examination Survey 2001-2008. J Acad Nutr Diet 2014;114(12 Suppl):S27–43.

92. Watanabe Y, Saito I, Henmi I, et al. Skipping breakfast is correlated with obesity. J Rural Med 2014;9(2):51–8.

93. Thomas EA, Higgins J, Bessesen DH, et al. Usual breakfast eating habits affect response to breakfast skipping in overweight women. Obesity 2015;23(4): 750–9.

94. Keski-Rahkonen A, Kaprio J, Rissanen A, et al. Breakfast skipping and health-comprimising behaviors in adolescents and adults. Eur J Clin Nutr 2003;57: 842–53.

95. Hingorjo MR, Syed S, Qureshi MA. Overweight and obesity in students of a dental college of Karachi: lifestyle influence and measurement by an appropriate anthropometric index. J Pak Med Assoc 2009;59(8):528–32.

96. Huang CJ, Hu HT, Fan YC, et al. Associations of breakfast skipping with obesity and health-related quality of life: evidence from a national survey in Taiwan. Int J Obes 2010;34(4):720–5.

97. Bjornara HB, Vik FN, Brug J, et al. The association of breakfast skipping and television viewing at breakfast with weight status among parents of 10-12-year-olds in eight European countries; the ENERGY (EuropeaN Energy balance Research to prevent excessive weight Gain among Youth) cross-sectional study. Public Health Nutr 2014;17(4):906–14.

98. Smith TJ, Dotson LE, Young AJ, et al. Eating patterns and leisure-time exercise among active duty military personnel: comparison to the Healthy People objectives. J Acad Nutr Diet 2013;113(7):907–19.

99. Goyal R, Julka S. Impact of breakfast skipping on the health status of the population. Indian J Endocrinol Metab 2014;18(5):683–7.

100. Kutsuma A, Nakajima K, Suwa K. Potential association between breakfast skipping and concomitant late-night-dinner eating with metabolic syndrome and proteinuria in the Japanese Population. Scientifica (Cairo) 2014;2014:253581.

101. Maksimovic MZ, Gudelj Rakic JM, Vlajinac HD, et al. Relationship between health behaviour and body mass index in the Serbian adult population: data from National Health Survey 2013. Int J Public Health 2016;61(1):57–68.

102. Nishiyama M, Muto T, Minakawa T, et al. The combined unhealthy behaviors of breakfast skipping and smoking are associated with the prevalence of diabetes mellitus. Tohoku J Exp Med 2009;218(4):259–64.

103. Fuglestad PT, Jeffery RW, Sherwood NE. Lifestyle patterns associated with diet, physical activity, body mass index and amount of recent weight loss in a sample of successful weight losers. Int J Behav Nutr Phys Act 2012;9:79.

104. Witbracht M, Keim NL, Forester S, et al. Female breakfast skippers display a disrupted cortisol rhythm and elevated blood pressure. Physiol Behav 2015; 140:215–21.

105. Nooyens AC, Visscher TL, Schuit AJ, et al. Effects of retirement on lifestyle in relation to changes in weight and waist circumference in Dutch men: a prospective study. Public Health Nutr 2005;8(8):1266–74.

106. Poppitt SD, Swann D, Black AE, et al. Assessment of selective under-reporting of food intake by both obese and non-obese women in a metabolic facility. Int J Obes 1998;22:303–11.

107. Farshchi HR, Taylor MA, Macdonald IA. Deleterious effects of omitting breakfast on insulin sensitivity and fasting lipid profiles in healthy lean women. Am J Clin Nutr 2005;81(2):388–96.

108. Betts JA, Richardson JD, Chowdhury EA, et al. The causal role of breakfast in energy balance and health: a randomized controlled trial in lean adults. Am J Clin Nutr 2014;100(2):539–47.

109. Reeves S, Huber JW, Halsey LG, et al. Experimental manipulation of breakfast in normal and overweight/obese participants is associated with changes to nutrient and energy intake consumption patterns. Physiol Behav 2014;133: 130–5.

110. Tuttle WW, Daum K, Myers L, et al. Effect of omitting breakfast on the physiologic response of men. J Am Diet Assoc 1950;26:332–5.

111. Schlundt DG, Hill JO, Sbrocco T, et al. The role of breakfast in the treatment of obesity: a randomized clinical trial. Am J Clin Nutr 1992;55(3):645–51.

112. Dhurandhar EJ, Dawson J, Alcorn A, et al. The effectiveness of breakfast recommendations on weight loss: a randomized controlled trial. Am J Clin Nutr 2014; 100(2):507–13.

113. Geliebter A, Astbury NM, Aviram-Friedman R, et al. Skipping breakfast leads to weight loss but also elevated cholesterol compared with consuming daily breakfasts of oat porridge or frosted cornflakes in overweight individuals: a randomised controlled trial. J Nutr Sci 2014;3:e56.

114. Timlin MT, Pereira MA. Breakfast frequency and quality in the etiology of adult obesity and chronic diseases. Nutr Rev 2007;65(6 Pt 1):268–81.

115. O'Neil CE, Byrd-Bredbenner C, Hayes D, et al. The role of breakfast in health: definition and criteria for a quality breakfast. J Acad Nutr Diet 2014;114(12 Suppl):S8–26.

116. Dong Y, Hoover A, Scisco J, et al. A new method for measuring meal intake in humans via automated wrist motion tracking. Appl Psychophysiol Biofeedback 2012;37(3):205–15.

117. Fontana JM, Farooq M, Sazonov E. Automatic ingestion monitor: a novel wearable device for monitoring of ingestive behavior. IEEE Trans Biomed Eng 2014; 61(6):1772–9.

118. Gemming L, Utter J, Ni Mhurchu C. Image-assisted dietary assessment: a systematic review of the evidence. J Acad Nutr Diet 2015;115(1):64–77.

119. Cahill LE, Chiuve SE, Mekary RA, et al. Prospective study of breakfast eating and incident coronary heart disease in a cohort of male US health professionals. Circulation 2013;128(4):337–43.

120. Garaulet M, Gomez-Abellan P. Timing of food intake and obesity: a novel association. Physiol Behav 2014;134:44–50.

121. Mattson MP, Allison DB, Fontana L, et al. Meal frequency and timing in health and disease. Proc Natl Acad Sci U S A 2014;111(47):16647–53.

122. Kinsey AW, Ormsbee MJ. The health impact of nighttime eating: old and new perspectives. Nutrients 2015;7(4):2648–62.

123. Boraska V, Davis OS, Cherkas LF, et al. Genome-wide association analysis of eating disorder-related symptoms, behaviors, and personality traits. Am J Med Genet B Neuropsychiatr Genet 2012;159B(7):803–11.

124. Jaaskelainen A, Schwab U, Kolehmainen M, et al. Meal frequencies modify the effect of common genetic variants on body mass index in adolescents of the northern Finland birth cohort 1986. PLoS One 2013;8(9):e73802.

125. Garaulet M, Corbalan-Tutau MD, Madrid JA, et al. PERIOD2 variants are associated with abdominal obesity, psycho-behavioral factors, and attrition in the dietary treatment of obesity. J Am Diet Assoc 2010;110(6):917–21.

126. Corbalan-Tutau MD, Gomez-Abellan P, Madrid JA, et al. Toward a chronobiological characterization of obesity and metabolic syndrome in clinical practice. Clin Nutr 2015;34(3):477–83.

127. Kim NH, Shin DH, Kim HT, et al. Associations between metabolic syndrome and inadequate sleep duration and skipping breakfast. Korean J Fam Med 2015; 36(6):273–7.
128. Keim NL, Van Loan MD, Horn WF, et al. Weight loss is greater with consumption of large morning meals and fat-free mass is preserved with large evening meals in women on a controlled weight reduction regimen. J Nutr 1997;127(1):75–82.
129. Jakubowicz D, Froy O, Wainstein J, et al. Meal timing and composition influence ghrelin levels, appetite scores and weight loss maintenance in overweight and obese adults. Steroids 2012;77(4):323–31.
130. Jakubowicz D, Barnea M, Wainstein J, et al. High caloric intake at breakfast vs. dinner differentially influences weight loss of overweight and obese women. Obesity 2013;21(12):2504–12.
131. Leidy HJ, Bossingham MJ, Mattes RD, et al. Increased dietary protein consumed at breakfast leads to an initial and sustained feeling of fullness during energy restriction compared to other meal times. Br J Nutr 2009;101(6): 798–803.
132. Leidy HJ, Armstrong CL, Tang M, et al. The influence of higher protein intake and greater eating frequency on appetite control in overweight and obese men. Obesity 2010;18(9):1725–32.
133. Sofer S, Eliraz A, Kaplan S, et al. Greater weight loss and hormonal changes after 6 months diet with carbohydrates eaten mostly at dinner. Obesity 2011; 19(10):2006–14.

Index

Note: Page numbers of article titles are in **boldface** type.

A

AACE. See *American Association of Clinical Endocrinologists (AACE)*.
Abdominal reoperations, in adolescents, after bariatric surgery, 672–673
Abuse, obesity and, of substances. See *Substance abuse*.
    sexual, physical, and emotional, 680
Adaptive thermogenesis, 612
Addiction transfer, after bariatric surgery, 683
Adenosine monophosphate–activaed protein kinase, leptin-leptin receptor activation of, 634
Adenosine triphosphate (ATP), energy stored as, 608
Adipocytes, exercise impact on, 609–610
    leptin secretion by, 634
    thermogenic, in BAT, metabolic phenotype of, 606–608
Adipose tissues. See also *Fat mass*.
    in obesity, **605–621**. See also *Beige adipose tissue; Brown adipose tissue (BAT)*.
    leptin action in, 635
    white. See *White adipose tissue (WAT)*.
Adiposity, eating frequency and, 694–695, 700
    rEI and measures of, 693–694, 700
        summary of study associations, 696–699
    skipping breakfast associations with, 700, 704–707
        greater than one day, 701, 708–709
Adjustable gastric banding (AGB), for obesity, description of, 651–652
    eating behavior changes following, 546
    historical perspectives of, 540
    in adolescents, 668
        complications of, 672–673
        limitations of, 673–674
        outcomes of, 670–671
Adolescent bariatric surgery, for obesity, **667–676**
    background on, 667–668
    BMI and, 667–668
    definitions for, 667–668
    eligibility criteria for, 669
    future directions for, 673–674
    key points of, 667
    limitations of, 673–674
    outcomes of, 670–673
    preoperative evaluation for, 669
    prevalence of, 668
    role of, 668
    weight loss procedures in, 669–670

Endocrinol Metab Clin N Am 45 (2016) 719–749
http://dx.doi.org/10.1016/S0889-8529(16)30079-2
0889-8529/16/$ – see front matter

X

Z

Moving?

Make sure your subscription moves with you!

To notify us of your new address, find your **Clinics Account Number** (located on your mailing label above your name), and contact customer service at:

Email: **journalscustomerservice-usa@elsevier.com**

800-654-2452 (subscribers in the U.S. & Canada)
314-447-8871 (subscribers outside of the U.S. & Canada)

Fax number: 314-447-8029

Elsevier Health Sciences Division
Subscription Customer Service
3251 Riverport Lane
Maryland Heights, MO 63043

*To ensure uninterrupted delivery of your subscription, please notify us at least 4 weeks in advance of move.

Printed and bound by CPI Group (UK) Ltd, Croydon, CR0 4YY

08/05/2025

01864686-0002